Strategies to Protect the Health of DEPLOYED U.S. FORCES

Assessing Health Risks to Deployed U.S. Forces

Workshop Proceedings

Board on Environmental Studies and Toxicology
Commission on Life Sciences
National Research Council

NATIONAL ACADEMY PRESS
Washington, D.C.

NATIONAL ACADEMY PRESS • 2101 Constitution Ave., N.W. • Washington, D.C. 20418

NOTICE: The project that is the subject of this report was approved by the Governing Board of the National Research Council, whose members are drawn from the councils of the National Academy of Sciences, the National Academy of Engineering, and the Institute of Medicine. The members of the committee responsible for the report were chosen for their special competences and with regard for appropriate balance.

This project was supported by Contract No. DASW01-97-C-0078 between the National Academy of Sciences and the Department of Defense. Any opinions, findings, conclusions, or recommendations expressed in this publication are those of the author(s) and do not necessarily reflect the view of the organizations or agencies that provided support for this project.

International Standard Book Number 0-309-06876-2

Additional copies of this report are available from:

National Academy Press
2101 Constitution Ave., NW
Box 285
Washington, DC 20055

800-624-6242
202-334-3313 (in the Washington metropolitan area)
http://www.nap.edu

Copyright 2000 by the National Academy of Sciences. All rights reserved.

Printed in the United States of America

THE NATIONAL ACADEMIES

National Academy of Sciences
National Academy of Engineering
Institute of Medicine
National Research Council

The **National Academy of Sciences** is a private, nonprofit, self-perpetuating society of distinguished scholars engaged in scientific and engineering research, dedicated to the furtherance of science and technology and to their use for the general welfare. Upon the authority of the charter granted to it by the Congress in 1863, the Academy has a mandate that requires it to advise the federal government on scientific and technical matters. Dr. Bruce M. Alberts is president of the National Academy of Sciences.

The **National Academy of Engineering** was established in 1964, under the charter of the National Academy of Sciences, as a parallel organization of outstanding engineers. It is autonomous in its administration and in the selection of its members, sharing with the National Academy of Sciences the responsibility for advising the federal government. The National Academy of Engineering also sponsors engineering programs aimed at meeting national needs, encourages education and research, and recognizes the superior achievements of engineers. Dr. William A. Wulf is president of the National Academy of Engineering.

The **Institute of Medicine** was established in 1970 by the National Academy of Sciences to secure the services of eminent members of appropriate professions in the examination of policy matters pertaining to the health of the public. The Institute acts under the responsibility given to the National Academy of Sciences by its congressional charter to be an adviser to the federal government and, upon its own initiative, to identify issues of medical care, research, and education. Dr. Kenneth I. Shine is president of the Institute of Medicine.

The **National Research Council** was organized by the National Academy of Sciences in 1916 to associate the broad community of science and technology with the Academy's purposes of furthering knowledge and advising the federal government. Functioning in accordance with general policies determined by the Academy, the Council has become the principal operating agency of both the National Academy of Sciences and the National Academy of Engineering in providing services to the government, the public, and the scientific and engineering communities. The Council is administered jointly by both Academies and the Institute of Medicine. Dr. Bruce M. Alberts and Dr. William A. Wulf are chairman and vice chairman, respectively, of the National Research Council.

PRINCIPAL INVESTIGATOR

Lorenz Rhomberg, Gradient Corporation, Cambridge, Massachusetts (formerly of the Harvard School of Public Health, Boston, Massachusetts)

ADVISORY GROUP FOR STRATEGIES TO PROTECT THE HEALTH OF U.S. FORCES

Arthur J. Barsky, Brigham and Women's Hospital, Boston, Massachusetts
Germaine M. Buck, State University of New York at Buffalo, Buffalo, New York
William S. Cain, University of California, San Diego, California
John Doull, The University of Kansas Medical Center, Kansas City, Kansas
Ernest Hodgson, North Carolina State University, Raleigh, North Carolina
David H. Moore, Battelle Memorial Institute, Bel Air, Maryland
Roy Reuter, Life Systems, Inc., Cleveland, Ohio
Ken W. Sexton, University of Minnesota, Minneapolis, Minnesota
Robert E. Shope, University of Texas, Medical Branch, Galveston, Texas
Ainsley Weston, National Institute of Occupational Safety and Health, Morgantown, West Virginia

Staff

Carol A. Maczka, Project Director
Raymond A. Wassel, Program Director
Susan N.J. Pang, Staff Officer
Robert Crossgrove, Technical Editor
Catherine M. Kubik, Senior Project Assistant
Leah L. Probst, Project Assistant
Mirsada Karalic-Loncarevic, Information Specialist

Sponsor

U.S. Department of Defense

BOARD ON ENVIRONMENTAL STUDIES AND TOXICOLOGY

Gordon Orians (Chair), University of Washington, Seattle, Washington
Donald Mattison (Vice Chair), March of Dimes, White Plains, New York
David Allen, University of Texas, Austin, Texas
Ingrid C. Burke, Colorado State University, Fort Collins, Colorado
William L. Chameides, Georgia Institute of Technology, Atlanta, Georgia
John Doull, The University of Kansas Medical Center, Kansas City, Kansas
Christopher B. Field, Carnegie Institute of Washington, Stanford, California
John Gerhart, University of California, Berkeley, California
J. Paul Gilman, Celera Genomics, Rockville, Maryland
Bruce D. Hammock, University of California, Davis, California
Mark Harwell, University of Miami, Miami, Florida
Rogene Henderson, Lovelace Respiratory Research Institute, Albuquerque, New Mexico
Carol Henry, Chemical Manufacturers Association, Arlington, Virginia
Barbara Hulka, University of North Carolina, Chapel Hill, North Carolina
James F. Kitchell, University of Wisconsin, Madison, Wisconsin
Daniel Krewski, University of Ottawa, Ottawa, Ontario
James A. MacMahon, Utah State University, Logan, Utah
Mario J. Molina, Massachusetts Institute of Technology, Cambridge, Massachusetts
Charles O'Melia, Johns Hopkins University, Baltimore, Maryland
Willem F. Passchier, Health Council of the Netherlands
Kirk Smith, University of California, Berkeley, California
Margaret Strand, Oppenheimer Wolff Donnelly & Bayh, LLP, Washington, D.C.
Terry F. Yosie, Chemical Manufacturers Association, Arlington, Virginia

Senior Staff

James J. Reisa, Director
David J. Policansky, Associate Director and Senior Program Director for Applied Ecology
Carol A. Maczka, Senior Program Director for Toxicology and Risk Assessment
Raymond A. Wassel, Senior Program Director for Environmental Sciences and Engineering
Kulbir S. Bakshi, Program Director for the Committee on Toxicology
Lee R. Paulson, Program Director for Resource Management

COMMISSION ON LIFE SCIENCES

Michael T. Clegg (Chair), University of California, Riverside, California
Paul Berg (Vice Chair), Stanford University, Stanford, California
Frederick R. Anderson, Cadwalader, Wickersham & Taft, Washington, D.C.
Joanna Burger, Rutgers University, Piscataway, New Jersey
James E. Cleaver, University of California, San Francisco, California
David Eisenberg, University of California, Los Angeles, California
John Emmerson, Fishers, Indiana
Neal First, University of Wisconsin, Madison, Wisconsin
David J. Galas, Keck Graduate Institute of Applied Life Science, Claremont, California
David V. Goeddel, Tularik, Inc., South San Francisco, California
Arturo Gomez-Pompa, University of California, Riverside, California
Corey S. Goodman, University of California, Berkeley, California
Jon W. Gordon, Mount Sinai School of Medicine, New York, New York
David G. Hoel, Medical University of South Carolina, Charleston, South Carolina
Barbara S. Hulka, University of North Carolina, Chapel Hill, North Carolina
Cynthia Kenyon, University of California, San Francisco, California
Bruce R. Levin, Emory University, Atlanta, Georgia
David Livingston, Dana-Farber Cancer Institute, Boston, Massachusetts
Donald R. Mattison, March of Dimes, White Plains, New York
Elliot M. Meyerowitz, California Institute of Technology, Pasadena, California
Robert T. Paine, University of Washington, Seattle, Washington
Ronald R. Sederoff, North Carolina State University, Raleigh, North Carolina
Robert R. Sokal, State University of New York, Stony Brook, New York
Charles F. Stevens, The Salk Institute, La Jolla, California
Shirley M. Tilghman, Princeton University, Princeton, New Jersey
Raymond L. White, University of Utah, Salt Lake City, Utah

Staff

Warren R. Muir, Executive Director
Jacqueline K. Prince, Financial Officer
Barbara B. Smith, Administrative Associate
Kit W. Lee, Administrative Assistant

OTHER REPORTS OF THE BOARD ON
ENVIRONMENTAL STUDIES AND TOXICOLOGY

Waste Incineration and Public Health (1999)
Hormonally Active Agents in the Environment (1999)
Research Priorities for Airborne Particulate Matter: II. Evaluating Research Progress and Updating the Portfolio (1999)
Ozone-Forming Potential of Reformulated Gasoline (1999)
Risk-Based Waste Classification in California (1999)
Arsenic in Drinking Water (1999)
Research Priorities for Airborne Particulate Matter: I. Immediate Priorities and a Long-Range Research Portfolio (1998)
Brucellosis in the Greater Yellowstone Area (1998)
The National Research Council's Committee on Toxicology: The First 50 Years (1997)
Toxicologic Assessment of the Army's Zinc Cadmium Sulfide Dispersion Tests (1997)
Carcinogens and Anticarcinogens in the Human Diet (1996)
Upstream: Salmon and Society in the Pacific Northwest (1996)
Science and the Endangered Species Act (1995)
Wetlands: Characteristics and Boundaries (1995)
Biologic Markers (5 reports, 1989-1995)
Review of EPA's Environmental Monitoring and Assessment Program (3 reports, 1994-1995)
Science and Judgment in Risk Assessment (1994)
Ranking Hazardous Waste Sites for Remedial Action (1994)
Pesticides in the Diets of Infants and Children (1993)
Issues in Risk Assessment (1993)
Setting Priorities for Land Conservation (1993)
Protecting Visibility in National Parks and Wilderness Areas (1993)
Dolphins and the Tuna Industry (1992)
Hazardous Materials on the Public Lands (1992)
Science and the National Parks (1992)
Animals as Sentinels of Environmental Health Hazards (1991)
Assessment of the U.S. Outer Continental Shelf Environmental Studies Program, Volumes I-IV (1991-1993)
Human Exposure Assessment for Airborne Pollutants (1991)
Monitoring Human Tissues for Toxic Substances (1991)
Rethinking the Ozone Problem in Urban and Regional Air Pollution (1991)
Decline of the Sea Turtles (1990)

Copies of these reports may be ordered from
the National Academy Press
(800) 624-6242
(202) 334-3313
www.nap.edu

Contents

Background — 1

Collection and Use of Personal Exposure and Human Biological-Marker Information for Assessing Risks to Deployed U.S. Forces in Hostile Environments — 2
Morton Lippmann

Characteristics of the Future Battlefield and Deployment — 24
Edward D. Martin

The Nature of Risk Assessment and Its Application to Deployed U.S. Forces — 35
Joseph V. Rodricks

Future Health Assessment and Risk-Management Integration for Infectious Diseases and Biological Weapons for Deployed U.S. Forces — 59
Joan B. Rose

Approaches for Using Toxicokinetic Information in Assessing Risk to Deployed U.S. Forces — 113
Karl K. Rozman

Health Risks and Preventive Research Strategy for Deployed U.S. Forces from Toxicological Interactions Among Potentially Harmful Agents — 150
Raymond S.H. Yang

Appendix: Biographical Information on Commissioned Authors — 183

Background

The National Academy of Sciences (NAS) was asked to advise the Department of Defense (DOD) on a long-term strategy for protecting the health of the nation's military personnel when deployed to unfamiliar environments. As part of the academy's response to this request, the National Research Council's (NRC's) Board on Environmental Studies and Toxicology was asked to develop an analytical framework for assessing health risks to deployed forces.

Dr. Lorenz Rhomberg of Gradient Corporation (formerly of the Harvard University School of Public Health) served as the project's principal investigator. He was assisted by 10 advisers representing a variety of relevant disciplines.

To assist Dr. Rhomberg and the advisers, six papers were commissioned on topics identified as key issues: (1) possible scenarios of future deployments and battle considerations, (2) existing risk-assessment methods and their possible application to deployment situations, (3) approaches for collecting and using personal exposure and biological-marker information, (4) health assessment and risk management integration for biological agents, (5) toxicologic interactions among agents, and (6) possible paradigms for incorporating toxicokinetic information in risk assessment. The six papers were presented at a workshop on January 28-29, 1999 in Washington, DC. Over 60 participants from the military and scientific communities were present. The sessions were moderated by members of the advisory group, and the commissioned authors were asked to consider the comments and suggestions that arose during the workshop in revising their papers. The final papers were also reviewed by two members of the Commission on Life Sciences: Donald Mattison, March of Dimes and John Emmerson, Fishers, Indiana.

The commissioned papers were used as background for the NRC report *A Risk Assessment Framework for Protecting the Health of Deployed Forces*, which is being published concurrently with these proceedings. The findings, conclusions, and recommendations that appear in the workshop papers are solely those of the authors and should not be interpreted as those of the NRC.

Collection and Use of Personal Exposure and Human Biological-Marker Information for Assessing Risks to Deployed U.S. Forces in Hostile Environments

by Morton Lippmann[1]

ABSTRACT

Risk management is especially important for military forces deployed in hostile and/or chemically contaminated environments, and on-line or rapid turn-around capabilities for assessing exposures can create viable options for preventing or minimizing incapacitating exposures or latent disease or disability in the years after the deployment. With military support for the development, testing, and validation of state-of-the-art personal and area sensors, telecommunications, and data management resources, the DOD can (1) enhance its capabilities for meeting its novel and challenging tasks; and (2) create technologies that will find widespread civilian uses.

This review assesses currently available options and technologies for productive pre-deployment environmental surveillance, exposure surveillance during deployments, and retrospective exposure surveillance post-deployment, and introduces some opportunities for technological and operational advancements in technology for more effective exposure surveillance and effects management options for force deployments in future years. The issues discussed are (1) information needs for assessing personal exposures and risks for deployed forces; (2) options for pre-deployment baseline determinations, for collection of personal exposure related data during field deployment, and for post-deployment personal exposure assessments; (3) maximizing effective personal exposure data resources during and post-deployment; (4) technical capabilities for personal exposure assessment; and (5) assessing risks.

Advances in information technology have made it possible to envision the collection, maintenance, and utilization of a deployment data resource that would enable theater commanders and medical staff to recognize and evaluate environmental health hazards and to manage deployments so as to avoid or

---

[1]Human Exposure and Health Effects Program, New York University School of Medicine, 57 Old Forge Road, Tuxedo, NY 10987

minimize those hazards. Such data, together with a deployment sample archive, would also facilitate future epidemiological studies that could identify additional causal relationships between environmental factors and health outcomes.

Applications can include (1) on-line access to remote sensing and continuous monitoring data for tactical planning; (2) data review by medical staff personnel in order to arrange for monitoring military personnel for possible effects of toxicant exposures, provide countermeasures during deployments, and prioritize medical examinations and biomarker sample collections and analyses in the early post-deployment period; (3) additional sampling and/or monitoring, or analysis of archived samples, in order to be able to resolve ambiguities or conflicts concerning levels of exposure or environmental contamination; and (4) review of medical and environmental data by epidemiologists post-deployment in investigations of possible causal factors for delayed illness reports associated with service in a specific deployment.

Each of these applications could consume large amounts of resources, and the allocations should be decided according to pre-established priorities by an appropriate panel of peers, including military users and state-of-the-art research investigators with expertise in the emerging technologies.

INTRODUCTION

Exposure assessment is a key element in risk assessment and risk management, and is especially important for military forces deployed in hostile or uncharacterized environments. Furthermore, on-line or rapid turn-around capabilities for assessing exposures can provide military commanders with viable options for preventing or minimizing exposures that can incapacitate or degrade the on-site capabilities of deployed forces, or that can result in latent disease or disability in the months and years after the deployment. Delayed or latent adverse effects resulting from deployment exposures can degrade force readiness for future deployments as well as cause pain and suffering to force members and/or create compensatory costs needed to care for the force members and their families. Exposure assessments can therefore be valuable and cost-effective tools of primary disease and disability protection. The military could support and mobilize the high-technological resources that will be needed for the development, testing, and validation of state-of-the-art personal and area sensors, telecommunications devices, and data management resources. Such investments would not only help the Department of Defense (DOD) enhance its capabilities for meeting the novel and challenging tasks in deploying forces in the post-cold-war period, but also create technologies that will find productive new uses in other aspects of occupational and environmental health protection in the United States and around the world.

The military services have already established a core unit, the U.S. Army Center for Health Promotion and Preventive Medicine (USACHPPM). It fulfills many of the functions that are outlined in this paper through its Deployment Environmental Exposure Surveillance Program (DESP), which was established in July 1996. The scope of this program could be expanded to include a greater emphasis on personal exposure surveillance and the collection and archiving of environmental and biological samples for later laboratory analyses needed to resolve emerging questions about exposures and their health effects among deployed personnel. The sample archive envisioned here could be viewed as an expansion of the Armed Forces Serum Repository established in August 1997 under DOD Directive 6490.2 for the purpose of joint medical surveillance. The expanded repository would include blood cells for biological-marker (biomarker) analyses, as well as air-sampling filters and cartridges and soil and water samples.

Although this paper focuses on disease and non-battle injuries (DNBI), many of the high-technological capabilities developed for the nuclear, biological, and chemical (NBC) defense programs' spiral system developments can be envisioned as being applicable to force protection from unintentional exposures to environmental toxicants. This is especially the case for the fully integrated and digitized joint warning, reporting, and analysis architecture that the NBC program expects to implement in the next 3 to 5 years. Plans to acquire very light-weight hazard sensors under the NBC program will also advance measurement technologies that might have eventual applicability to on-site and personal detectors capable of measuring much lower concentrations of agents of concern with respect to DNBI.

This paper introduces and spells out, in a conceptual sense, currently available options and technologies for productive pre-deployment environmental surveillance, exposure surveillance during deployments, and retrospective post-deployment exposure surveillance. It also introduces some opportunities for technological and operational advancements in technology for more effective exposure surveillance and proposes some risk management options for force deployments in future years. The discussions that follow cover

- information needs for assessing personal exposures and risks for deployed forces,
- options for pre-deployment baseline determinations,
- options for collection of personal exposure data during field deployment,
- options for post-deployment personal exposure assessments,
- maximizing effective personal exposure data resource during deployment and post-deployment,
- current technical capabilities for personal exposure assessment, and
- assessing risks.

INFORMATION NEEDS FOR ASSESSING PERSONAL EXPOSURES AND RISKS FOR DEPLOYED FORCES

Environmental Quality Factors at Deployment Sites

The military is obligated to determine identifiable on-site risks whenever possible prior to the deployment of forces. Contaminated sites, such as abandoned gas works, chemical manufacturing sites and waste dumps, with the actual and potential risks of personnel contacting hazardous chemical residues should be avoided whenever mission options permit and less contaminated or noncontaminated alternate sites compatible with operational necessities are available.

Prescreening of potential deployment sites should be done at the candidate sites by appropriately trained environmental specialists or industrial hygienists whenever possible. When on-site surveys are not possible, remote sensors or scanners should be employed to the extent that they are technologically and operationally feasible. (See NRC 1999.)

Survey personnel should prepare guidance and background data on the extent or potential of site contamination to the military (or civilian) engineers assigned to site preparation for large-scale deployments. In turn, the military engineers should take care to prepare the site, to the extent feasible, in ways that prevent or minimize the potential for exposure to preexisting on-site contamination. Both the site survey and site preparation teams should create a record trail on on-site contamination that is accessible to hygienists, medical personnel, and epidemiologists in case subsequent actions or investigations are needed during on-site deployment or for post-deployment follow-up investigations.

During force deployments, the emphasis should shift to the collection of data on personal exposures to on-site contaminants, using personal samplers and monitors, as well as the collection of exposure biomarkers whenever appropriate equipment, sampling opportunities, analytical methods, and procedures are available. Because it will seldom, if ever, be feasible to collect personal exposure data on all members of a deployed force, a sampling strategy will be needed to identify suitable and willing individuals within the force who can serve effectively as representatives of their group for determinating exposure. There will also need to be plans and procedures to investigate and ameliorate the sources and extent of detected excessive exposure, as well as procedures for feasible countermeasures for documented excessive exposures.

Exposure-Reponse Relationships and Exposure Limits for Toxicants

For chemical agents of known toxicity, it is important to have or be able to develop exposure limits or guidelines to serve as benchmarks of excessive exposure for either short or long-term exposures. The recently prepared TG230A Short-Term Chemical Exposure Guidelines for Deployed Military Personnel (USACHPPM 1999a) and the RD230A Reference Document (USACHPPM 1999b) provide guidance for 1-h inhalation exposures for 43 chemicals, for 1-to 14-day exposures for 91 chemicals, and drinking-water concentration limits for 170 chemicals. Guidance for 1-h inhalation exposure limits for other chemicals is available from the American Industrial Hygiene Association (AIHA) in their Emergency Response Planning Guidelines (ERPGs). Currently, the U.S. Environmental Protection Agency (EPA) is supporting a National Research Council (NRC) Committee on Toxicology program to prepare Guidelines for Community Emergency Exposure Levels that will gradually be substituted for ERPGs where appropriate. Based upon the AIHA criteria of protection of "nearly all individuals" against "experiencing or developing irreversible or other serious health effects or symptoms that could impair. . . abilities to take protective action," the 1-h TG230A criteria are all conservative by factors ranging from 2 to 80. The American Conference of Governmental Industrial Hygenists (ACGIH) threshold limit values and biological exposure indices provide guidance for 15-min exposures and longer-term (8-h) exposures.

Descriptors of Deployed Forces

Deployed forces can be expected to vary greatly in age, ethnicity, genetic susceptibilities, and prior histories of exposures to toxicants and disease, as well as in possible allergic or stress reactions to exposures or countermeasures. The information resource that will be used to document known exposures and possible responses to these exposures should contain as much descriptive information on each person in the force as possible to facilitate primary medical management of individuals who develop health problems during deployment or post-deployment. It should also serve as a resource for epidemiologists who might be able to utilize population distributions of exposures and responses to establish criteria and standards that advance the military's capabilities for optimal force protection. In setting up a computerized data resource to serve such functions, consideration must be given to limiting access of sensitive personal information to those with an approved right-to-know.

The activity patterns of members of the force can be critically important determinants of the extent of the internal doses received as a result of toxicant exposures by dermal contact and inhalation. Dermal exposures can be significant during field exercises and combat situations, and inhalation doses can be greatly affected by the amounts of air inhaled, the frequency of respiration, and the depth of penetration of the air inhaled into the lungs. The selection of force members to serve as exposure sentinels, as noted previously, should be influenced by their known or expected activities and by the exposures they have encountered or are expected to encounter.

Descriptors, Locations, and Access to Data Resources

The emerging technological capabilities of the Information Age create opportunities for the effective collection, storage, and utilization of relevant information on personal exposures, activities, and constitutional risk factors of kinds and magnitudes that are unprecedented. As a result, relationships between exposures and health outcomes that had been impossible to establish for individuals might become apparent when the data from large numbers of exposed individuals are combined. Thus, it might be possible to derive secondary benefits from the results of deployment sampling and dose commitments in terms of new knowledge or insights on latent or chronic effects that can be detected only on a population basis. Consolidation of the diverse data elements needed for such powerful analyses will require a data-management strategy, that includes a system for reporting essential data elements in a uniform and consistent manner across the various commands and services in a given theater of operation.

The full potential of the database envisioned above will require coordination and discipline at all levels. Its ultimate potential will become manifest when theater commanders can readily access on-line area and personal monitor measurements for field-deployment decisions, and medical officers can make timely decisions on the administration of countermeasures to ameliorate the effects of recent exposures to contaminants. Epidemiologists will be able to optimally construct cohorts in appropriate exposure groupings for studies of the overall impacts of the deployments on the health status of active and retired veterans of deployment. Arrangements will need to be made to control access to all of this information to those with a need-to-know to protect the privacy of medical records and the information on deployments for military security reasons.

Framework for Data Analyses

To achieve all of the ambitious potential applications outlined above, there will need to be uniform frameworks for data management. The overall integration of some of the deployment risk-assessment elements is well illustrated in Figure 1, which appeared in the Deployment Toxicology Research and Development Master Plan in September 1997 (GEO CENTERS, Inc.). An approach to combining data resources for developing an overall exposure (and risk) assessment, developed by an ACGIH-AIHA task group (Lippmann et al. 1996) for occupational exposure applications, is illustrated in Figure 2.

OPTIONS FOR PRE-DEPLOYMENT BASELINE DETERMINATIONS

Health Baseline Data

If subtle changes in symptom frequency or physiological functions result from toxicant exposures during deployments, they will be almost impossible to detect without data on pre-deployment baseline levels in the same individuals. This is because of the enormous range of baseline values for such variables, even in the generally healthy young adults in the military services. If conventional batteries of function tests are performed, along with the collection of questionnaire data on signs and symptoms prior to deployment, comparisons of comparable data during deployment and post-deployment on a relatively small cohort of individuals might be sufficient to determine either the short-term effects or the long-term effects, or both.

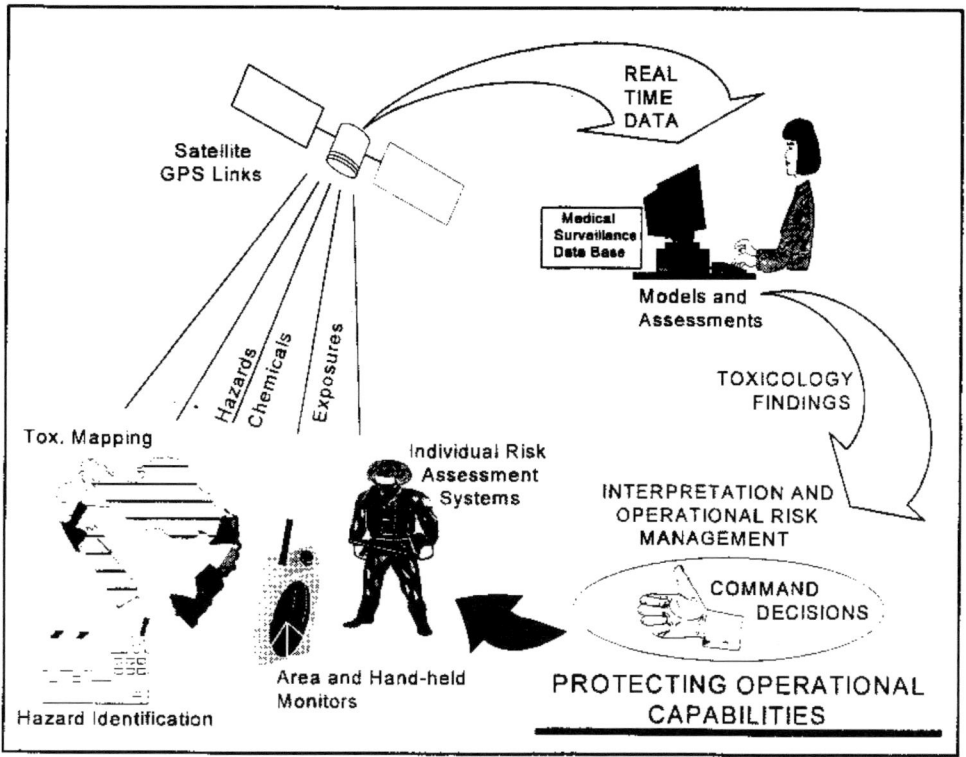

FIGURE 1 Deployment toxicology research and development master plan. (Source: GEO-CENTERS, Inc. 1997)

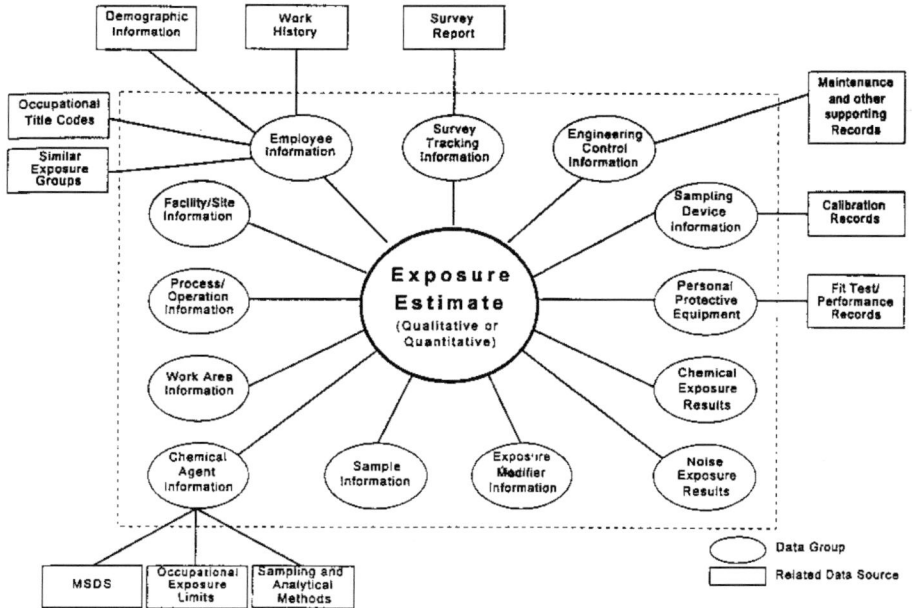

FIGURE 2 Data flowchart. This model illustrates the focus and scope of the recommended data elements for the occupational exposure database. (Source: Lippmann et al. 1996)

Collection of Biological Specimens for Archive and Future Analyses

For exposures to certain gases and aerosols producing acute responses, personal badges and monitors can provide sufficient exposure information. However, for agents that can penetrate the skin after dermal exposure, or for agents that are cumulative toxicants producing delayed effects, valuable information can best be derived from biological monitoring using samples of blood, urine, or hair. The analyses of these biological openings for a specific agent, its metabolites, enzymes induced, or adducts formed in endogenous proteins or DNA can indicate the presence of the agent or its metabolites in the body. For most, if not all of these analytes, there are likely to be broad variations in baseline levels, and the analyses can be quite expensive (Zhitkovich and Costa 1998).

Although analyses might be quite expensive, the collection and storage of the specimens is not, and a prudent precautionary sample collection procedure will permit sensitive determinations of the results of exposures that occurred during deployments. The process begins with the collection, identification, and archiving of samples of the biological materials during the pre-deployment clinical examinations. Comparable samples can be collected and archived during deployment or post-deployment to permit sensitive intercomparisons of assay results for evidence of changes in biomarkers that might have occurred as a result of exposures during the deployment, thus documenting the extent of the exposures or the effects that they produced.

For most purposes, the biomarker analyses will be performed on components of blood or urine. For other analyses, other biological materials that might be easier to collect in the field can also be useful; these include hair, fingernails, and sputum. Under some circumstances, other samples, such as exhaled air, nasal epithelium, and buccal cells might also be useful.

Exposure biomarkers are indicative of delivered toxicant doses and are focused on the early stages of the continuum illustrated in Figure 3, and tend to have higher degrees of agent-specificity (Table 1). An important factor in the practical use of biomarkers is a low and consistent background level of the biomarker response in nonexposed populations. Tight variance in biomarker measurements among unexposed subjects indicates that the biomarker is not strongly affected by unknown factors associated with, for example, diet or lifestyle. Sensitivity and low interindividual variability are the most important parameters influencing the statistical power of a biomarker. Taioli et al. (1994) provide a general strategy and useful examples as to how variability of biomarkers can be estimated, and offer an equation to calculate the minimal sample size. For example, DNA adduct-based assays require relatively small sample sizes, whereas gene expression biomarkers, with very large variability among unexposed individuals, require much larger populations.

Blood biomarkers are a heterogeneous group of biological measurements, including unmodified original chemicals, chemical-specific metabolites, stress hormones, modifications of proteins and DNA, and serum and intracellular components, with half-lives of up to about 10 days. Blood contains large quantities of hemoglobin and albumin, proteins that can be readily isolated in pure form. Carboxyl, amino, and sulfhydryl groups are typical sites of adduction by electrophilic compounds. Many protein adducts are stable under physiological conditions, providing an opportunity to assess cumulative exposure, because the life span of human hemoglobin is approximately 120 days. The biological half-lives of albumin adducts are shorter, due to a faster metabolic turnover of albumin (DeBord et al. 1992). Protein adducts, although not mechanistically involved in the pathway leading to disease, can be useful as long as the relationship between surrogate and mechanistic biomarkers is known.

Peripheral blood lymphocytes are the most frequently used cells to assess biomarkers related to potential genotoxic exposures. Lymphocytes contain DNA and circulate throughout the human body, and therefore they are exposed to any circulating genotoxic agent or its metabolites. These cells can integrate exposure over extended time intervals because they are long-lived (Braselmann et al. 1994)

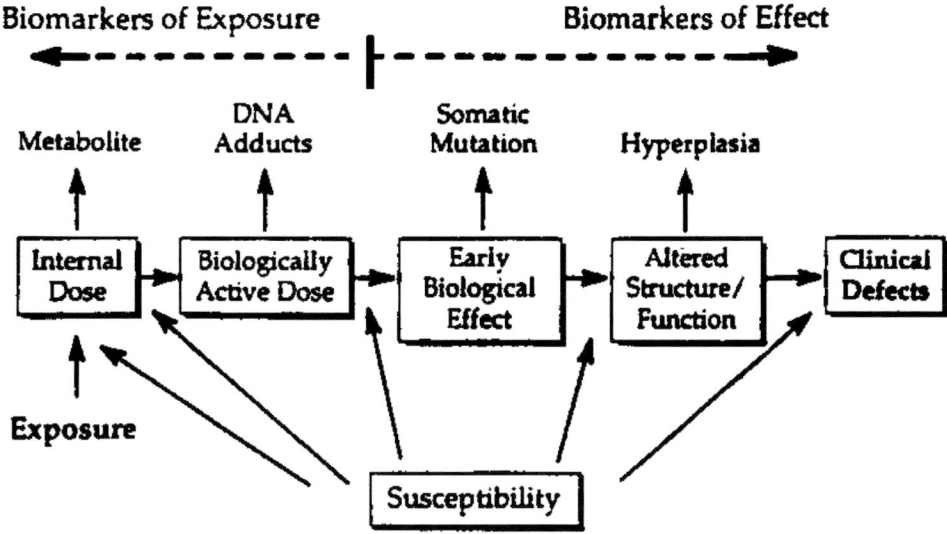

FIGURE 3 Relationship between exposure and disease. (Source: Zhitkovich and Costa 1998)

TABLE 1 Examples of Biomarkers With Different Agent-Specificity

Specificity	Biomarkers	Exposure
Low	Sister chromatid exchanges and chromosomal abberations in peripheral lymphocytes	Clastogens
	Micronuclei in buccal cells	Clastogens
	β-oxo dG in urine or lymphocytic DNA	Radiation and many chemicals
	N-acetyl-β-D-glucosaminidase in urine	Nephrotoxic agents
	Mutagenesis at HPRT locus in lymphocytes or glycophoryn A in erythrocytes	Mutagens
	Urinary malonialdehyde	Agents causing lipid peroxidation
Intermediate	Serum or urinary chromium	Toxic and dietary forms of chromium
	Urinary nitrosoproline	Nitrosamines
	Immunoassay for PAH-DNA adducts 1-hydroxypyrene in urine	PAH compounds
	Cholinergic muscarinic receptors or acetylcholinesterase activity	Organophosphorus insecticides
High	Original substance in biologic specimens	For example, cadmium
	Substance-specific metabolite	For example, S-phenylmercapturic acid for benzene
	Chemical-specific DNA or protein adducts	For example, styrene-hemoglobin for styrene exposure
	Biologic response characteristic of specific exposure	δ-Aminolevulinic acid in urine (lead exposure) Urinary porphyrins profiles (mercury exposure)

Source: Zhitkovich and Costa 1998

and do not divide in vivo. Many in vitro studies found that unstimulated lymphocytes have inefficient DNA repair capabilities (Barret et al. 1995; Freeman and Ryan 1988), permitting these cells to accumulate detectable DNA damage from very low exposures. Lymphocytes are also capable of metabolizing many important xenobiotics such as ρ-aminohipparic acids (PAHs) to DNA-reactive species (Gupta et al. 1988).

Measurements of biomarkers in urine samples generally reflect recent exposures, and can be useful for assessing accidental overexposures and psychological or physiological stresses. Analyses of spot urinary samples can be used to estimate exposures in populations, whereas individual exposures are best assessed using 24-h collections. Urinary biomarker measurements are corrected for a dilution factor by normalizing all determinations for a creatinine content. Most analyses of urine samples are based on detection of chemical exposure, and involve measurement of an original substance or its metabolite. A smaller group of urinary bioassays can also estimate a biologically effective dose. Exposure to a majority of carcinogens results in the formation of DNA adducts that later can be excised by cell-repair systems. For some chemicals, excised adducts are then excreted in urine, and determinations of these adducts can provide a measure of biologically effective doses.

Hair samples can provide a temporal history of peak exposures to toxic or trace metals and some organic species or DNA that are incorporated into the growing hair shaft. For personnel who do not get frequent military-style haircuts, hair samples can provide good evidence of previous exposure over periods of many months. In practice, this might apply primarily to female members of the force.

In selecting any biological marker, one should consider the predictive value, specificity, sensitivity, and occurrence of false positives and false negatives. The factors to consider are:

- Does the test measure or evaluate exposure to an agent?
- Does the test provide reproducible results?
- Is analytical error and biological variability small?
- Is the test quantitatively relatable to the relevant range of exposure?
- Have the convenience and risk factors (associated with administering the test) been considered?
- Are the concentrations of the agent measured quantitatively relatable to an adverse health effect or stress that could impair performance of critical tasks?

Actual analyses of samples from the archive would be done on a limited number of individuals' samples when evidence of effects points to the need for such analyses, and would initially be focused on the specific kinds of biomarkers that are likely to be most informative. Depending on the findings of such exploratory analyses, and their potential significance to the future health of the force members, a further expansion of the analysis program might be warranted, looking for other biomarkers and at samples from other individuals in the cohort. Some analyses might be indicated in the near term following deployment, and others might be needed far into the future for evidence of delayed chronic health effects that became apparent from epidemiological follow-ups, or when appropriate and more sensitive assays become available to answer questions that could not be resolved on the basis of the original assay analyses.

Environmental Quality

It might be possible to collect samples of air, soil, and surface waters, and to measure levels of background radiation prior to deployment to determine whether the deployment of forces at a given location would be unsafe or unwise. If such analyses do not indicate risks of contamination, and deployment is subsequently initiated, it would be prudent to store pre-deployment environmental samples in the deployed forces archive, and to collect and store additional samples during deployment and post-deployment to be able to determine if contamination occurred during deployment, either as a result of hostile actions or as a result of the deployment activities themselves. If evidence of such contamination is found, a determination will need to be made about whether it is sufficient to warrant decontamination or investigations of exposures to deployed forces or indigenous populations.

OPTIONS FOR COLLECTION OF DATA DURING FIELD DEPLOYMENTS

Remote Sensing

Remote sensing of air-contaminant levels and abnormal patterns of ground and vegetation surfaces associated with the presence of soil or water pollution can occur at various levels of spatial resolution using current military intelligence techniques and equipment. Civilian-sector technologies for measuring air concentrations in point- source plumes by LIDAR and by long-path infrared (IR) and ultraviolet (UV) spectroscopy can also be harnessed for air monitoring at deployment sites.

Personal Sampling and Monitoring by Field-Line or Duty Corpsmen

When one wants to know the exposure of an individual to chemical contaminants inhaled in the air, there is no good substitute for sampling or monitoring the air in the breathing zone of that individual. The breathing zone is typically defined as the space within about 1 foot (30 cm) of the nose or mouth, and small sampling heads or passive sampling badges are typically mounted on the lapel to monitor the breathing zone. When comparisons are made between the concentrations in the breathing zone and concentrations in the general area of the individual being monitored, personal exposure is often considerably higher than the concentration in the area, especially when the individual is engaged in activities that release or resuspend the chemicals from soil in the area or from accumulated contamination on the clothing of the individual. For collecting such samples from field personnel there will need to be well-trained field-line corpsmen responsible for issuing, collecting, labeling the sample, storing in short and long-term archives and assuring appropriate means of their delivery to appropriate laboratories for analysis.

Collection of Biological Specimens by Medical Personnel

Biological specimens collected in the field will also need to be collected by well-trained corpsmen, nurses, or other medical corps personnel. It is imperative that the samples are not contaminated by soil on the hands, that low-background sealable containers are used to contain the specimens, and that all samples are carefully and appropriately identified, for example, by unique bar code. For blood and urine samples, it is quite important to record the time of day that the collection took place in relation to recent activities and exposures, and to take appropriate precautions in sample handling and storage to preserve the integrity of the samples for both transit to a laboratory or preservation in a sample archive.

Collection of Samples of Environmental Media

If pre-deployment samples or direct measurements of air, soil, water, and background radiation were collected, and their subsequent analyses indicated potentially serious toxicant exposures, then comparable samples should be collected at one or more times during force deployment. These should then be analyzed for the toxicants of concern to assess the effect of deployment activities on the nature and extent of toxicant exposures to the troops, and the extent of the dispersion of the on-site toxicants from their initial reservoirs into the environmental media.

If pre-deployment samples did not indicate a serious concern for toxicant exposures during deployment, it still might be prudent to collect comparable samples for an archive to be able to determine whether deployment activities either uncovered previously undetected contamination, or created or released to the environment toxicants that should be cleaned up prior to departure. The samples might also be needed to document the results of intentional releases of toxicants by hostile forces during the deployment.

Performance Measures

Neurobehavioral performance measures can be used as biomarkers of exposure and biomarkers of operationally important responses to exposures. In either case, they can only be properly interpreted as changes in measures from baseline levels, as discussed previously. Exposures to some solvents, pesticides, and metals might alone, or together, or in combination with vaccines and prophylactic drugs, produce altered cognitive functions in the absence of clinical signs or symptoms, and signal the need for confirmatory evidence of exposure through assays of environmental media, air samples, or biological fluids. The effects produced by exposures to neurotoxicants among military personnel might be especially important to the performance of their assigned missions and to their ability to effectively and responsibly manage the weapons at their disposal.

The performance measures that can be quickly self-administered might be the only feasible means for many individuals in the deployed forces. Hand-held computers can be programmed to (1) administer appropriate tests of mental capacity, reaction times, or agility; (2) calculate performance indices; and (3) telemeter the results to a central medical evaluation unit. For further information on the state-of-the-art for assays of neurobehavioral performance in humans, see Anger et al. (1998).

It should also be noted that the U.S. Geological Survey is engaged in the development of physiological and behavioral measures of acute chemical neurotoxicity in aquatic organisms as part of the deployment toxicology research program, and that the indicators that they have developed could be used to assess environmental contamination and associated risks at deployment sites.

Use of Protective Measures

The military has carefully developed specifications for the purchase, supply, distribution, and maintenance of personal protective devices, such as respirators, faceshields and goggles, and protective clothing, which are issued to deployed forces in anticipation of expected exposures. Records of their actual use by individuals in the field should be part of their personnel records to facilitate such retrospective exposure assessments that might be needed in the post-deployment period. On days when there are indications that potentially damaging exposures might have occurred, it should be possible to arrange for the collection and archiving of respirator canisters or samples of protective gear for later laboratory analyses, with appropriate notation of the user's identification, times and locations where the protective device was worn or used, and remarks concerning known contaminant sources or releases relevant to the potential exposure. Analyses of these samples and associated information could prove invaluable to the military for determining (1) actual exposures of deployed individuals to specific agents; (2) indications of likely exposure to other individuals in the same general operational area who are not being monitored; and (3) the efficacy of the personal protective gear being provided to the forces for reducing or eliminating the uptake of toxicants from the working environment.

Records of Activity Profiles

Environmental exposure is an essential determinant of the amount of the contaminant taken up by an individual in that environment. However, uptake is also dependent on the individual's activities and the effect of any barriers to mass transfer from the environment to systemic uptake by the individual. Uptake of air contaminants is strongly dependent on the volumes inhaled and the lung depths to which it is drawn, which, in turn, is dependent on the activity level of the individual. It is also dependent on the use and effectiveness of any respiratory protective device that is supplied to the individual. It should be recognized that it might not be possible to attain the ultimate protective capacity of a demand-type respirator under the stress and exertion levels encountered by military personnel in the field.

Similarly, dermal exposure represents a potential for uptake that can be strongly modified by contact area, contact times, and the integrity of the skin barrier. Ingestion exposure is governed largely by the amounts consumed, and uptake from any contaminated food and drink that might be consumed by deployed forces is also affected by the amounts and nature of other elements of the diet. Thus, to the extent that it is feasible to collect and retain data on daily activities and meals for the deployed forces, such data might prove to be very useful in determining exposure profiles and estimating toxicant uptake for retrospective health risk evaluations.

OPTIONS FOR POST-DEPLOYMENT EXPOSURE ASSESSMENTS

The late deployment and early post-deployment period can be critically important for the collection of samples and data that can help the military draw the most important lessons about toxicant exposures that might have taken place during the deployment. This period is usually a time when the military emergency or urgent situation justifying a deployment is past and there might be time and resources available during the phase-down for filling data and knowledge gaps that could not be addressed when there were more urgent priorities and when access to deployed personnel for the collection of biological samples and activity logs was infeasible.

Collection of Biological Samples

Evidence for toxicant exposures during deployment will often be possible in the weeks and months after the exposure has taken place for those toxicants that (1) have cumulative effects; (2) accumulate in the body; or (3) produce metabolites or effects that persist in cells that remain in the blood stream, are excreted in the urine, or are fixed in growing hair. The results of post-deployment analyses can be of special significance and value when comparable samples are collected and analyzed or archived before and during the active phases of the deployment, because baseline values might vary greatly from person to person.

In any case, post-deployment biological samples that are collected soon after the deployment is completed could be very useful, even in the absence of pre-deployment reference samples, for analysis of the population distribution of exposures. A special opportunity to collect large numbers of samples can arise when the force is relocated on transport ships. Samples could be collected by unit corpsmen using the support available from the ship's facility for sample collection, processing, and storage. For troops being relocated by air, there might be opportunities for sample collection at intermediate sites with clinical facilities, or upon arrival at new duty sites.

Collection of Environmental Media Post-Deployment

The collection of samples of environmental media post-deployment can fill several potentially important needs. By comparison of the analyses of comparable samples collected pre-deployment, during deployment, and post-deployment, it might be possible to document the extent of unavoidable or avoidable exposures, due to the presence of background levels of toxicants in the environment. They may also make it possible to document the extent of environmental toxicant burdens created during the deployment, and thereby the need for or extent of remediation of deployment sites or following their return to local control.

Analyses and Comparisons of Pre-Deployment and Post-Deployment Samples

Sensitive and specific analyses of the contents of all of the biological and environmental samples that are archived during the pre-deployment, deployment, and post-deployment periods would be uneconomical and unwarranted. A strategic plan that sets priorities in the selection of samples for analysis will be needed. The priorities will be determined by the information needed to protect the health, welfare, and readiness of the forces that are deployed.

Samples that might warrant a high priority for early analysis include:

• Pre-deployment environmental media samples needed to determine whether there are likely to be exposures that could compromise the health of the forces and could be avoided or minimized.

• Biological and environmental samples collected during and immediately following deployment needed to determine if serious toxicant exposures have taken place, based on evidence such as unusual illness patterns, alarms sounded by areawide chemical or biological agent sensors, and suspicious activities by hostile forces.

• Biological samples collected during deployment and the early post-deployment period needed to investigate any unexplainable health problems that turn up among previously deployed forces, as happened with Gulf War Syndrome.

Depending upon the results obtained in such screening assays, analyses of additional samples from the archive, or analyses of additional analytes in the samples, might be warranted to obtain a fuller picture of the nature, extent, and significance of the exposures that might have occurred during deployment.

In developing a strategic plan for the maintenance and management of a sample archive, consideration must be given to the criteria for the disposal of unneeded samples at appropriate times after the deployment to be able to accommodate the needs for archiving samples in future deployments.

Analyses of Cumulative Exposures

Acute toxicant exposures and their consequences are expected to be obvious to area commanders and their medical support staffs. However, the effects of more slowly acting toxicants might not become evident during the deployment, and the exposure index might be more closely related to cumulative exposure than to peak exposure. Estimates of cumulative exposure can be derived from biomarker analyses. For inhalation exposures, estimates can also be derived or established from cumulative concentration-time products, with allowance for variable uptake due to activity level and deposition rates. Because continuous records of ambient air-concentrations are not likely to be available at any location, let alone for all individuals in the force, exposure models will need to be employed in making useful estimates of cumulative exposure using air concentration data.

Case-Control Studies

Case-control studies can be powerful forensic tools for elucidating causal relations between outcomes and exposures when reasonable and plausible exposure groupings can be identified. Unfortunately, this proved not to be possible in the investigations of the Gulf War Syndrome because of the lack of any useful data on the agents that might have been responsible or the means of retrospectively determining the exposures to those agents. Should such a mysterious pattern of post-deployment illness occur in the future, and if archived biological and environmental samples are available as outlined above, it should be possible to compare indices of exposure in those with illness with those in matched control populations, without illness, thereby identifying the exposure characteristics most closely associated with the pattern of illness.

MAXIMIZING EFFECTIVE USE OF SAMPLE AND DATA RESOURCES

Information technology developed in both the military and civilian sectors in recent years has made it possible to envision the construction, maintenance, and utilization of a deployment data resource that would enable theater commanders and medical staff to recognize and evaluate environmental health hazards and to manage deployments to avoid or minimize those hazards. Together with a deployment sample archive, it would also facilitate future epidemiological studies that could identify additional causal relationships between environmental factors and health outcomes, and thereby stimulate the development of means of recognizing additional risk factors warranting exposure controls in future deployments.

To take maximal advantage of these new technological capabilities, it is imperative that the biological and environmental samples and data elements that are needed for such applications are collected and maintained in uniform and readily interpretable forms, and that they are accessible to all authorized users. Applications will include:

• on-line access of deployment decision-makers to remote sensing and continuous monitoring data that they could consider in tactical planning;

• data review by medical staff personnel to arrange for monitoring military personnel for possible effects of toxicant exposure; provide countermeasures during deployments; and set priorities for medical examinations and biomarker sample collections and analyses in the early post-deployment period;

• on-line access and data review by industrial hygienists and environmental assessment specialists to arrange for additional sampling and monitoring, or analysis of archived samples, to resolve ambiguities or conflicts concerning levels of exposure or environmental contamination; and

• review of medical and environmental data by epidemiologists in post-deployment investigations of possible causal factors for delayed-illness reports associated with service in a specific deployment.

However, to accommodate all of these needs in a timely and efficient manner, it will be necessary to have a flexible system for sample and data management that can be adopted and applied uniformly by all of the military services. It could be an extension of the Defense Occupational Health Readiness System.

Constructing a Sample Archive

As noted earlier, USACHPPM's DESP is a logical repository for an expanded sample archive, as proposed here. It could incorporate an expanded version of the existing Armed Forces Serum Repository, as well as samples of blood cells, urine, hair, air sampling filters and vapor-collection canisters, soil, and locally available drinking water. Blood cells and urine and hair samples can provide DNA for future molecular-level biological assays, which might be critical in forensic toxicology investigations of possible delayed health effects that might occur among deployed force personnel. The strategic aspects of the design, maintenance, accessibility for sample analyses, minimal analytical efforts justifying use of the archived samples, and reporting data from the analyses should be established by USACHPPM staff with appropriate input from an external scientific advisory committee with expertise in exposure assessment, toxicology, epidemiology, analytical chemistry, molecular biology, and clinical medicine.

Constructing a Data Resource

There are a number of essential features for a data resource that can effectively serve a variety of primary and secondary users. The primary users must first be satisfied with data format, data reduction paradigms, and data access because they will be providing the financial and logistical support for data collection and entry. When the different branches of the military services are engaged in joint deployments, it is also essential that a harmonized array of data elements are adopted, so that the data sets can be merged and the results of data analyses can be uniformly interpreted.

In setting up a data-management system and defining a commonly agreed upon set of well-defined data elements, it is important to also consider the analytical needs of secondary users of the data resource. They might need more descriptive background information on the geography, topography, meterology, and history of the deployment sites than do the military command or medical units. Some of the considerations involved in setting up comprehensive and harmonized databases for personal exposures that could facilitate primary and secondary data users were described in detail by an ACGIH-AIHA task group (Lippmann et al. 1996) and by a European Community task group (Rajan et al. 1997) for occupational exposure data. In the environmental arena, the EPA (1998) has recently described a major initiative to facilitate increased use of its environmental data resources by secondary users.

In defining its essential data elements and constructing a format and procedure for entering, maintaining, and accessing its own data on exposure and health outcome related factors, the designers of the military databases should consider opportunities for commonalities with the database developments currently under way in the civilian arenas in the occupational health and environmental fields. This examination of recent ongoing activities should, of course, include the efforts already undertaken within each of the military services to broaden, expand, and utilize their own data resources on occupational exposures, and should bring in the perspectives of the services' own professionals who will be secondary users of the data resource.

Engaging Industrial Hygiene Expertise for Cumulative Exposure Assessments

There might need to be a component of the data resource devoted to the assessment of the cumulative exposure of each member of the deployed force to each of the toxicants encountered during the deployment that might account for excess illness observed among the cohort in the post-deployment period. Such assessments will involve the combination of measurement data, exposure models, and expert judgments. It might also involve the selection of air, biological, or environmental samples from the archive for follow-up analyses to fill in data gaps that limit such assessments. Thus, the creation of files on cumulative exposure assessment might be an iterative process that involves collaboration among hygienists, toxicologists, and epidemiologists.

Engaging Toxicological Expertise for Interpreting Biomarker Data

Currently, there are relatively few biomarkers that are specifically identified with toxic agents or stresses likely to be encountered during military deployments, and therefore few environmental or biological samples collected prior to, or during, a deployment are likely to be analyzed routinely. Most samples will be retained in the archive, to be analyzed when it is necessary to confirm or quantify exposures that are suspected of causing adverse effects. In deciding which samples to analyze and what analyses are appropriate and feasible, there will need to be input by toxicological experts, who will also be needed to interpret the analytical results obtained. They will need access to other parts of the database in forming their judgments about the extent and significance of the exposures indicated from the biomarker analyses, and the lessons they learn from each analysis might be useful in iterative upgrades of the data elements in the overall database and in its management.

Engaging Epidemiological Expertise for Data Analyses

Because the envisioned database is expected to be an unprecedently bountiful resource for military epidemiologists, it should be provided with significant input into the selection and format for certain of its data elements by them. This will be especially important for the construction of appropriate summaries of exposures for use in the exploration and definition of exposure-response relationships.

CURRENT TECHNOLOGICAL CAPABILITIES FOR PERSONAL EXPOSURE ASSESSMENT

Personal exposures can be measured continuously on-line for a limited number of gases and vapors, determined from time-integrated samples that are subsequently analyzed for a much broader array of agents in both gaseous and particulate forms, and inferred, albeit with greater uncertainty, from measured exposures to others in the same general area or from exposure models utilizing measured environmental levels and activity patterns within the monitored area. Estimates of personal exposure can also be developed from biomarker measurements when consideration is given to systemic uptake from the environment, knowledge of metabolic fate in relation to times of exposure and sample collection, and other knowledge about retention sites and half-lives in internal organs.

Personal Air Sample Collection

The technology for collecting personal air samples over periods ranging from hours to days is relatively well developed, and reliable devices for such sampling are widely available and relatively inexpensive. The easiest to use and most unobtrusive devices are the passive samplers for gases and vapors that collect the agent penetrating a diffusion barrier onto an adsorption surface at a rate dependent only on concentration and diffusion coefficient. The devices are small and easily worn on a lapel. Recordkeeping requirements for sample collection are limited to the person wearing the device, the times when the cover of the sampler is opened and closed, and the activities of the wearer during the time it was open for sample collection. In many cases, the samples can be analyzed subsequently in a field laboratory. In others, more sophisticated central laboratory analyses might be required. When the rate of sample collection is too low to determine the concentrations of the agent interest, active samplers that collect samples at higher rates might be needed.

An active sampler requires a battery-powered air mover and a flow meter as well as a sampling substrate, all of which increase the cost and complexity of the sampler and the burden on the wearer by at least a few pounds. However, active samplers sample air at much higher rates (up to ~ 5 L/min), permitting more sensitive assays with a broader range of analytes. Gases and vapors can be collected on adsorptive granules packed within presealed tubes or on chemically pretreated filters, and particles can be collected on a filter disc compatible with the analyses to be performed. Membrane filters are used to collect samples on their surfaces and are scanned by microscopy, x-ray fluorescence, or radioactivity, for viable organisms after incubation in an appropriate growth media. Aerosol samplers can also have an inertial precollector to collect samples restricted to specific aerodynamic particle sizes based on deposition probabilities in functionally distinct regions of the human respiratory tract. In any case, industrial hygiene or other field personnel will be needed to dispense and collect personal samplers and to check out the validity of sample start and end times, flow metering (if active sampling), the temporal and spatial coordinates of the sampling intervals, and the notation of relevant conditions and activities.

Personal Monitors With Electrical Signal Outputs

Opportunities to use personal sensors and transducers to identify gaseous chemical exposures of deployed forces will be increasing in the near future as the inherent capabilities of miniature sensors, circuits, and telecommunications devices mature and are developed in the form of conveniently usable hardware. Recent symposia have highlighted applications of miniaturized electrochemical sensors and interferometers to make sensitive and specific concentration measurements that can be telemetered, along with spatial location coordinates, to central sites, such as military command posts and medical commands, for their surveillance and appropriate responses. Position transducers are already available commercially, whereas the chemical sensors will need further refinement and validation before they are ready for widespread use by military forces.

Biological Sample Collection

The collection of biological samples, such as blood, urine, and hair, is best done under controlled conditions in which scrupulous sanitary and contamination-free control conditions can be exercised. For regularly scheduled collections in noncombatant environments, this might be possible for troops who are accessible to medical personnel. For those in more remote locations, it might be necessary to equip a military ambulance to go to the vicinity of the troops for sample collections and to have the facilities within them for sample identification, processing, and storage. The personnel collecting the samples must also be sensitive to the need to carefully collect the coordinate data on the recent activities and experiences of the individual providing the samples to help interpret the results of any analyses that are performed on the sample.

Temporal Considerations of Analytical Laboratory Capabilities

For each deployment, there will need to be at least one laboratory that collects and processes samples of air, soil, water, and biological fluids for either on-site analyses or transferral to theater-area labs in mobile army hospitals, modular field medical units, or hospital ships offshore, or to more remote central laboratories. For samples that can be adequately processed in the theater-area, the results can be fed back, within days, to field personnel for guiding further sampling, relocation of personnel or activities, or therapeutic interventions.

For analyses that require more sensitive or sophisticated laboratory facilities or specialized analyses, the turn-around time will be longer, and there will be fewer opportunities for prompt feedback to deployed forces for additional timely sample collection or reduction of ongoing exposures. There will be, however, significant advantages in terms of documenting the full nature and extent of agents that were present at very low concentrations.

Detection Limits of Analytical Laboratory Capabilities

The practical detection limits for a given sample depends on a number of factors whose influences will vary greatly from agent to agent and from one analysis to another. These factors relate to analytical sensitivity and specificity, the interferences produced by co-contaminants in the samples and components of the sampling substrates, the level and constancy of background readings of the sensing elements, the frequency and reliability of periodic recalibrations for span and zero readings, and the care taken to avoid sample and equipment contamination by the analysts. Thus, it is essential that the quality-assurance and quality-control procedures of the laboratory meet the highest standards of good laboratory practice.

Interpretation of Biomarker Changes

Exposure of biomarkers offer so many potential advantages over direct measures of exposure that they must eventually become more routinely used and more readily interpretable. However, it is essential that those relying on biomarker-based exposure estimates are fully aware of their inherent strengths and their fundamental limitations.

One major strength of biomarkers, especially for military deployment applications, is that they are influenced by past exposures, as opposed to direct measures of exposure over a given sampling interval. Thus, biomarker samples that are collected shortly after a suspected exposure has taken place can be used to "look back in time" to establish whether, in fact, the exposure actually occurred for the individual providing the sample and, by implication, for other individuals in the same group or area.

Another, sometimes realized, potential strength of biomarker analyses is the high degree of sensitivity that is possible. This is especially true for biomarkers based on characteristic responses to the exposure rather than the exposure agent itself. Highly sensitive tests for immunological responses and changes in DNA or protein structure are often much more sensitive than chemical analyses, and are longer lasting indicators of past exposures. A further potential advantage of exposure biomarkers is the relative absence of concern about stray contamination of the sample by the original exposure agent during the sample collection in the field. When reaction products are being measured, it is less likely that they will be produced during the sample processing or laboratory analysis. However, they might not be compound-specific.

The major limitations of biomarkers as indices of exposure involve the issues of the interpretability of the measurements that are made. One major potential limitation can be the absence of a benchmark or background level of the index being measured. This need not be a major problem for personnel in military deployments when pre-deployment background biomarker samples are collected, properly stored, and accessible for comparative evaluations.

In the absence of pre-deployment biomarker samples, the utility of biomarker samples collected during post-deployment will depend on the kinds of information that might be needed. If background levels of the biomarker of interest are very low, or if exposures are very high, the absence of a pre-deployment sample will not be important. For the more typical situation in which relatively low levels of exposure to an agent that can produce long-term chronic disease are known or suspected, there are several possibilities. One is to confine the analysis of the exposure to those individuals who have provided pre-deployment samples, and use their biomarker changes as indicative of others believed to be similarly exposed. Another possibility is to compare the distribution of biomarker levels in a large number of members of the deployed force with the distribution of levels in a matched population that has not been engaged in the same deployment. In this case, the level measured in a given member of the deployed force might not provide a personal index of disease risk, but the analyses might still provide valuable information on the average exposure of the deployed population and some indication on its distribution. The population approach might only be feasible, however, for assays that are reasonably inexpensive.

One unavoidable limitation of biomarker samples, however, is the fact that they are inherently "grab" samples collected at specific points in time. This is a relatively manageable problem for interpreting a brief peak exposure that occurred over a known time interval and in which the metabolic and translocation times are known, but it can be a major problem when the temporal pattern and extent of the relevant exposure is unknown. This is because the measured parameter can be highly variable over time and there is only one measurement made of a sample collected at an unknown time after the exposure. Thus, the analysis might be adequate to establish that an exposure took place, but unable to characterize the level of exposure. The problem is most severe for intermittant peak exposures whose timing is otherwise unknown, and least severe for steady-state exposures on which internal biomarker levels reach relatively stable levels.

ASSESSING RISKS FROM PERSONAL EXPOSURES

Within the broad spectrum of risks encountered by deployed U.S. forces on foreign soil, this paper has focused on the risks related to exposures to chemical compounds in environmental media at deployment sites. It has not dealt with chemical warfare agents for which the military services have long had plans for force protection and countermeasures. As a result of this distinction, the risks are generally more likely to be less obvious to the forces on the ground and more likely to produce delayed health effects than promptly observable effects. When delayed effects are seen, they are likely to be nonspecific in origin or causation and the search for causality might require careful sifting through records relating troop activities to areas having environmental contamination and personal exposures and relating those exposures to nonexposed or less-exposed matched control populations. The nature of the risks, and their often unanticipated relationships to exposures on foreign terrains, accounts for the emphasis in this paper on sample and record collection and retention for follow-up investigations to establish causal, dose-related relationships.

Combining Exposure Data with Exposure-Response Relationships

When sample analyses or environmental monitoring data indicate exposures to agents of known toxicity having established exposure limits, the risk analysis is relatively straightforward. If exposures exceed established standards or guidelines for such agents, the medical management of overexposed individuals should also be relatively routine. However, for exposure to agents that produce effects that have not previously been well characterized and whose long-term prognosis is uncertain, then prudent concern for the future health of the deployed force members warrants careful study and follow-up by military and Veteran's Department medical personnel and epidemiologists. Depending on the nature of the effects and their progression over time, this might require regularly scheduled clinical examination, biomarker sample collections, questionnaire responses, checks on vital status and, for the deceased, cause of death.

Research Needs

This paper envisions a long-term iterative process of exposure and health-status monitoring to identify and characterize health risks to military personnel during noncombat deployments on sites where characteristics of chemical agent exposures are unknown or poorly known. Initially the technological means for pre-deployment environmental or on-line personal exposure assessments are expected to be limited to the detection and characterization of a limited number of chemical toxicants, and quantitative exposure assessments will be delayed by the time it takes for sample collection and laboratory analyses, and by the sensitivity and specificity of the analyses that can be performed.

Table 2, from the Deployment Toxicology Research and Development Master Plan of September 1997 (GEO CENTERS, Inc. 1997), provides a thorough inventory of the technical challenges of exposure assessment for deployed forces and the kinds of advances that could be made through investments in research. Investments in further technological developments in miniature chemical sensors, microprocessors, and telecommunications devices could lead, within a relatively few years, to much greater technological capabilities for long-path area measurements and personal monitoring of a broad range of toxic gases and vapors, which would provide military commanders with options for force deployment that prevent or at least reduce times of exposures to toxic agents.

Investments in biomarker research, development, and validation could provide extraordinarily sensitive means of documenting exposures to toxicants as well as aspects of the biological responses to such exposures. To the extent that measured biomarker responses lie along a pathway leading directly to long-term changes and chronic disease, then it might be possible to prescribe therapeutic interventions that prevent, forestall, or ameliorate such late effects of the exposures.

Investments in the creation, management, and utilization of accessible sample and data archives related to exposures and their health consequences are also needed for various analytical and research purposes. These include (1) use of on-line exposure information for deployment decision-making; (2) use of on-line and sample analyses data for early actions on further sample collection needs and medical interventions for overexposed personnel; (3) identification of military personnel acccording to exposure category for future clinical or epidemiological follow-up; (4) identification of agents for which new sampling or analytical techniques are most urgently needed for risk-assessment purposes; and (5) identification of archived samples and sample analyses that can resolve issues that might arise from delayed reports of unusual illness patterns following deployments.

Each of these categories of research could consume large amounts of resources, and the allocations should be decided according to preestablished priorities by an appropriate panel of peers, including military users and state-of-the-art research investigators with expertise in the emerging technologies.

TABLE 2 Exposure Assessment Issues and Near- and Far-Term Capabilities

Technical Issues and Challenges	Capabilities (Near-Term)	Long-Term Vision

Personal Samplers and Monitors
  Instantaneous
  Grab
  Periodic
  Real-time/Continuous
  Passive
Area Samplers and Monitors
  Real-time results
  Remote vs. Local
  Media Sampled (air, water, soil)
  Statistical considerations
  Data Transfers
  Relevance to human uptake
  Hand-held
Biomarkers of Exposure
  Simple vs. Complex
  Recent vs. Past vs. Continuous
  Validation—biological relevance
  Sample: breath, urine, blood, dermal, transcutaneous, hair, etc.
Contaminant
  Form: gas, vapor, particulate, aerosol, fume, dissolved, suspended
  Mixtures
  Stability/Transformation
  Relevance of form to toxicity
Sources of exposure
  Rates and Distance
  Changing compositions
Exposure vs. Dose
  Exposure route contributions
  Absorption factors and rates
  Differential uptake or deposition
  Individual characteristics
  Respiratory rates/Activity
Exposure elimination
  Countermeasures vs. performance decrements
Military-unique exposure standards
Predeployment screening
Retrospective exposure tracking
	Sensor Technologies
	  Miniaturization
	  Weight reduction
	  Biosensors
	  Artificial nose
	  Passive dosimeters
	  Ultrasonic Flexural Plate Wave Devices
	  ELFFS
	  Computer Tomography/FTIR
	  Mini GC/MS
	
	Computer Hardware
	  Greater capacity and speed
	  Miniaturization
	  Portability
	
	Computer Software
	  Modeling and Simulations
	  Artificial intelligence
	  Available catalogs/databases
	
	Networks & Communications
	  Linking for data collection, transfer, and analysis
	  Remote/stand off capability
	  Ready access to experts and databases
	  On call/on demand data
	
	Molecular Biology
	  More and better biomarkers of exposure
	
	Exposure models to extrapolate from limited exposure measurements to large study populations and incorporate short-duration, high intensity exposures.
	
	Improved field methods for characterizing simultaneous exposures.
		Personal monitoring online
		
		Personal to population extrapolation
		
		Combined risk information systems
		  Warning
		  Summary statements
		  Risk avoidance
		
		Relationships of exposures to indicators of health effects database (extensive)
		
		Single biomonitoring device integrating measures of exposure and dose
		
		Exposure-Dose models that can anticipate associated problems with introduction of new chemical and bio toxins
		
		Personal Status Monitor (PSM): physiological stress indicators
		
		Genetic engineering for sensitive populations
		
		Universal micro-environmental suits
		
		Validated methods for measuring relevant exposure and total dose data directly from biological samples taken by non-invasive techniques
		
		Replacement breathing systems
		
		Biologically-based exposure assessment systems
		
		Technological advances that measure low concentration of chemicals and biomarkers in biological specimens linked to internal dose concentrations at target origins

Source: GEO-CENTERS, Inc. 1997.

REFERENCES

Anger, W.K., D. Storzbach, R.W. Amler, and O.J. Sizemore. 1998. Human behavioral neurotoxicity: Workplace and community assessments. Pp. 709-732. In: Environmental and Occupational Medicine, 3rd Ed., W.N. Rom, ed. Philadelphia: Lippincott-Raven.

Barret, J.M., P. Calsou and B. Salles. 1995. Deficient nucleotide excision repair activity in protein extracts from normal human lymphocytes. Carcinogenesis 16:1611-1616.

Braselmann, H., E. Schmid, and M. Bauchinger. 1994. Chromosome aberrations in nuclear power plant workers: The influence of dose accumulation and lymphocyte life-time. Mutat. Res. 306:197-202.

DeBord, D.G., T.F. Swearengin, K.L. Cheever, A.D. Booth-Jones, and L.A. Wissinger. 1992. Binding characteristics of ortho-toluidine to rat hemoglobin and albumin. Arch. Toxicol. 66:231-236.

EPA (U.S. Environmental Protection Agency). 1998. Data Suitability Assessment, Center for Environmental Information and Statistics. OPPE, EPA. Washington, DC. (Nov. 20)

Freeman, S.E. and S.L. Ryan. 1988. Excision repair of pyrimidine dimers in human peripheral blood lymphocytes: Comparison between mitogen stimulated and unstimulated cells. Mutat. Res. 194:143-150.

GEO-CENTERS, Inc. 1997. Deployment Toxicology Research and Development Master Plan. Prepared for U.S. Army Center for Environmental Health Research (Provisional). Contract No. DAMD 17-93-C-3006 and Subcontact No. GC-2533-93-001. (September).

Gupta, R.C., K. Earley and S. Sharma. 1988. Use of human lymphocytes to measure DNA binding capacity of chemical carcinogens. Proc. Natl. Acad. Sci. U.S.A. 85:3513-3517.

Lippmann, M., M.R. Gomez and G. Rawls. 1996. Data elements for occupational exposure databases: Guidelines and recommendations for airborne hazards and noise. Appl. Occup. Environ. Hyg. 11(11)1294-1311.

NRC (National Research Council) 1999. Strategies to Protect the Health of Deployed U.S. Forces: Technology and Methods for Detection and Tracking of Exposures to a Subset of Harmful Agents. Washington, DC: National Academy Press.

Rajan, B., R. Alesbury, B. Carton, M. Gerin, H. Litske, H. Marquart, E. Olsen, T. Scheffers, R. Stamm, and T. Woldback. 1997. European proposal for core information for the storage and exchange of workplace exposure measurements on chemical agents. Appl. Occup. Environ. Hyg. 12:31-39.

Taioli, E., P. Kinney, A. Zhitkovich, H.Fulton, V. Voitkun, G. Cosma, K. Frenkel, P. Toniolo, S. Garte and M. Costa. 1994. Application of reliability models to studies of biomarker validation. Environ. Health Perspect. 102:306-309.

USACHPPM (United States Army Center for Health Promotion and Preventive Medicine). 1999a. TG230A Short-term chemical exposure guidelines for deployed military personnel. Draft. USACHPPM, Aberdeen Proving Ground, Maryland. (March).

USACHPPM. (United States Army Center for Health Promotion and Preventive Medicine) 1999b. Reference document 230A: technical basis for USACHPPM technical guide 230A—Short term chemical exposure guidelines for deployed military personnel. Draft. USACHPPM, Aberdeen Proving Ground, Maryland. (March).

Zhitkovich, A. and M. Costa. 1998. Biologic markers. Pp. 177-186. In: Environmental and Occupational Medicine, 3rd Ed., W.N. Rom, ed., Philadelphia: Lippincott-Raven Publishers.

Characteristics of the Future Battlefield and Deployment

by Edward D. Martin[1]

ABSTRACT

In an era of unprecedented change, the military planner of today must prepare for contingencies involving operations by forces of a very large size to forces for special operations and operations other than war which may involve just a few soldiers, sailors, or airmen. The entire spectrum of geographic features and weather conditions must be accounted for in the plan. The typical linear battlefield will be replaced by a combat situation with a 360-degree threat, the potential for new high tech weapons, the use of chemicals and biologicals, and the use of non-traditional forces and terrorism.

With the gradual urbanization of the world's population, future battles will inevitably be fought within city limits geometrically compounding the planner's problem and the force commander's options. In addition to the threat from the opposing force, the field commander will face structural damage, local industrial hazards, and loss of mobility and degradation of communication links.

Combined, the future battle field and force deployment scenarios will, in spite of extensive training, provide for extremely high levels of stress. The threats from emerging bacteria and viruses, chemical weapons and industrial compounds and the urban battlefield will additionally inhibit and stress combat forces. Changes in force structure, national demographics, and the greater reliance on women in combat roles, will require minimal changes in force protection.

Natural or weaponized disease, non-battle injury, to include industrial hazard exposure, and stress will continue as the major threat to deployed forces in the future. Military and industrial intelligence of contested areas, modern equipment and extensive training, pre and post deployment health studies will provide the most successful means of force protection.

INTRODUCTION

The purpose of this paper is to briefly discuss the probable characteristics of future battlefields and deployment. In an era of unprecedented change in global economics and politics, military doctrine, and

---

[1]Edward Martin & Associates, Inc., 5309 North First Place, Arlington, VA 22203.

the rapid deployment of new and different technologies for use by combat forces and their support personnel, one could easily assume there would be great change in the nature of threats to combat forces when deployed. However, in spite of changes to military roles, missions, and technical capabilities, there will be more threats to deployed forces that will be the same as those threats experienced in the past.

TYPES OF WARFARE

Military planners will be required to continue to plan for the entire spectrum of warfare from two simultaneous major theater wars (MTWs) to the insertion and extraction of a very small tactical unit assigned to do a specific task in support of our National Command Authority. The former is possibly the easiest situation, in general terms, in which to protect deploying forces, due to the extensive planning and substantial deployment of assets involved.

In addition to the objectives and goals of each deployment, there will be specific risks to the deployed forces depending upon the geography and environment of the area in which the deployment is to be accomplished and the relative hostility and capability of the opposite force. Numerous contingency plans exist to cover operating in the varied environmental conditions experienced in most of the world's political hot spots and areas of potential conflict. These environmental conditions include arctic conditions, oppressive desert heat, flatlands and rolling hills, impassable mountain terrain, arid and dusty landscapes, and tropical rain forest and jungles. Due to the varied environmental and climatic conditions, a wide spectrum of military capabilities will be required, ranging from a large standing and well-trained force to special operations units trained to handle terrorist units. Whether any of the current plans will continue to be valid or even useful in 10 to 15 years is certainly debatable. What can be said for sure for the foreseeable future is that contingency planning will require constant updating in response to political, environmental, technical, and fiscal considerations. In general terms, the following will be the most likely major considerations:

A. Weaponry for U.S. Forces will become more accurate, mobile and lethal through the use of technology. The use of these weapons will require very specific and intensive technical and operational training and will require U.S. Force commanders to rely on seamless interoperability of multidisciplinary and multiservice forces.

B. Whenever possible, and particularly in an MTW, the deployment or insertion of ground forces into hostile areas will be preceded by an air campaign. The air campaign composed of United States and Allied Air and Naval Forces will initiate hostilities with appropriate standoff weaponry such as air and sea launched cruise missiles. If and when air superiority or air supremacy are established, and at the appropriate time in the battle plan, there will be maximum use of stealth and conventional aircraft for precision bombing of specific targets. Fighter aircraft and those carrying anti-radiation missiles like the HARM missile used in today's scenarios will provide cover for these attacks, followed by aerial and satellite reconnaissance to assess bomb damage. The risks for environmental contamination and disease for these airmen, seamen, and their support personnel will be, with very few exceptions, precisely the same as those found when flying from their normal garrisons. In fact, it is likely that many of the initial missions will be flown from the continental United States or from air bases that are frequently used by U.S. or Allied Air Forces. In most cases, existing and standard environmental health programs, in compliance with military, U.S. Occupational Safety and Health Administration (OSHA), and U.S. Environmental Protection Agency (EPA) standards, coupled with contingency training and command discipline, should provide the airman and sailor with the necessary environmental or disease protection.

One major exception to the rule would be the risk to the airman if his plane is damaged or shot down and he is forced to eject or land at an alternate field.

A successful air campaign will, by definition, result in the destruction in some or all of the enemy's

- command, control, and communications capabilities;
- industrial base for the production of weapons, power, fuels, and war-fighting materials; and
- infrastructure for the production of power, distribution of water, handling of waste material, and transportation capabilities such as roads, bridges, railheads, and docks.

This will not only put the enemy at risk for industrial hazards, but will also put any future occupying force on the ground at that same risk.

C. In most scenarios, however, ground forces will still be required to occupy specific territories at some time in the deployment. To fully utilize the mobility and technical advantage of weaponry, forces will be deployed in smaller functional units with highly reliable and secure communications and positioning equipment. Although there will be some individual battles directly facing an enemy in a linear fashion, the overall battlefield, or theater of operations, is likely not to be present in a linear fashion. Deployed forces, as such, must be aware of their location relative to friend and foe and must be prepared to move and fight in any direction.

D. Although it is unlikely, due to fiscal constraints, that large forces will be issued highly technical individual equipment by the year 2010, there will be some units issued the equipment available in today's development laboratories because of their special missions or their likelihood to be the first deployed in a variety of scenarios. In the Army's Land Warrior Program, for example, the individual soldier will be provided with lightweight protective material and a myriad of highly sophisticated equipment for physiological sensing, threat presentation, weapons control, and communications. Although each individual piece of equipment will be as light as possible, the amount of equipment that the individual might be required to carry, in addition to his or her weapon, is likely to increase. The resulting weight will require superb physical conditioning to prevent the most common musculoskeletal injuries and strains.

Additionally, through the use of this improved and new personal equipment, the individual soldier will be presented with data akin to that of an air traffic controller at O'Hare International Airport and will be required to assimilate and react to that data. The soldier will also be required to have the situational awareness to protect the lives of unknown airline passengers or airline flight paths, as well as their own lives, the lives of other members of their unit, and their mission objectives. New types of intensive individual training in simulators and in field combat conditions will therefore be an absolute necessity prior to the deployment of forces with this type of equipment, not only for technical purposes, but to minimize the possible stresses inherent in data overload.

E. The nonlinear battlefield, for a variety of sound and proven military reasons, will force commanders into ordering a greater dispersion of forces rather than concentrating their available forces near a specific point for the purposes of supply or support, including medical care. Additionally, again for a variety of reasons, some of which will be political and economic, the use of overwhelming force against an enemy in a linear fashion will often be replaced by the use of expeditionary forces tailored to the specific needs of the force commander and his tactical and strategic objectives. These forces will generally be smaller and more specialized than forces used in the overwhelming-force scenario and might well be less resilient relative to support forces, lines of supply, battlefield reserves, and medical units. In a 360-degree battlefield, a commander might not be able or willing to concentrate forces at a single point of attack. He might use the dispersion of his forces as a means to get greater utilization of modern weaponry and to disallow the enemy a simple targeting solution. This fact alone will be a source of increased anxiety for the individual soldier. Also, while in the dispersed location, data will be presented to the individual relative to his position on the battlefield, the positions of other elements of the friendly forces, the enemy's location and weapon array, and his order of battle. Because of the constant chatter or rapidly changing data presentations on communications links and his or her reliance on buddy care for injury rather than on an immediately available medical unit, the individual might experience further anxiety, a sense of isolation, and information overload degrading his ability to process the information presented to him.

F. For centuries, military planners have been careful not to bring the battle into the confines of cities when other means of movement, occupation of the area, or defeats of the enemy are possible. History is replete with great campaigns that ended with laying siege to or isolating the enemy's capital or major cities. Although most of these actions brought the final destruction of the enemy's force or government, some did not (Stalingrad). All did have in common great destruction, considerable causalities, and much loss of life. Today 50% of the world's population lives in urban areas. Demographers predict that by the year 2020 about 70% of the world's population will live in cities and at least 70% of these cities will be located within 300 miles of the world's coastlines. Thus, it is highly likely that specific operational capabilities and operations in urban areas will unfortunately be a requirement of ground forces. The U.S. Marine Corps has already begun specific training for that eventuality.

There are many good reasons as to why a military planner would wish to avoid fighting in a city, not the least of which is that urban warfare quickly equalizes the relative abilities of a small defending force opposing a large attacking force. This assumes, of course, that the attacking force does not wish to completely destroy the city with an air campaign or artillery. The ability for the defending force to use the cover of a city for sniper fire and similar operations can quickly demoralize an attacking force. Normal field operations for the attacking force, such as the use of rapid tactical mobility, the use of armored vehicles, logistic resupply, messing, and medical care, are restricted, whereas the defending force is presented with excellent fields of fire. A few of the obstacles, all of which can be experienced in exposures in buildings, streets, and alleyways, include structural damage, falling debris, building fires, the resulting smoke and poor visibility, booby traps, mines, use of nonlethal incapacitants, and civilian refugees. Such conditions will certainly limit the attacking force's progress and might be the cause of considerable injury and stress. Most important, with the attacking force highly dependent upon immediate and effective communications links and technologies, the city, in the best of circumstances, will degrade those communications links and, in some cases, make them ineffective and unusable. Tall structures, although providing the defending force with tactical advantage, will severely hamper locating the enemy force, limit the routes of attack for the occupying force, and severely restrict the location and evacuation of injured and wounded for both combatants. One can imagine trying to find a casualty in a modern tall building and, if found, carrying that casualty down 30 or 40 flights of stairs on a standard litter, all the time under the threat of constant attack from a hidden enemy. In addition to the difficulty of vertical evacuation down from a skyscraper, the tactical evacuation will encounter difficulty in moving over rubble-strewn streets using current vehicular technology.

Because none of these facts will be lost on the individual soldier, once again he or she will have the sense of isolation and separation from his or her combat unit in spite of specific training for this type of warfare. The city will present the attacking force with the additional potential for disease and industrial contamination from the destruction of the city's infrastructure. Fortunately, however, large urban areas more likely have been mapped in detail and surveyed for industrial production, and that information will have been provided to the attacking commander at some point prior to the attack.

OPERATIONS OTHER THAN WAR

It has become increasingly obvious from recent history that U.S. forces will continue to be deployed and used for operations other than war (OOTW), such as peacekeeping, natural disaster recovery, and other humanitarian support. In these roles, very small, and often very technical or specific capabilities, such as medical or engineering units, will be deployed with varying degrees of logistic support and will most likely represent the major role of U.S. forces in the foreseeable future. The lack of major logistic support for this type of deployment might result in the use of local resources for food, water, and supplies. Because of the unpredictability of such deployments relative to their timing and location, OOTW might also represent the most dangerous scenario for deployed forces relative to disease, non-battle-injury, environmental hazards, and even hostile action. Forces might be required to face situations ranging from very hostile and lethal nonuniformed guerrilla forces to exposure to unusual diseases, and often will face massive natural destruction and environmental conditions that will task their ability to perform the mission. Because this type of deployment is "on call" and will most likely be to areas not usually considered likely future deployment areas, there might be little time for commanders to obtain accurate intelligence on disease prevalence and the industrial base or to evaluate the host nation's infrastructure, such as water supplies, sanitation, and insect control. These deployments might well be to parts of the world considered "third world" and to areas of the globe where the emergence of new strains of bacteria or viruses is common. As such, it is imperative that global medical and industrial intelligence continue to be collected and shared by agencies such as the Central Intelligence Agency, the Defense Intelligence Agency, the World Health Organization, and the Centers for Disease Control and Prevention (CDC). These collections must be categorized, analyzed, and packaged for use by deploying force commanders and their medical personnel by the Armed Forces Medical Intelligence Center (AFMIC).

NON-TRADITIONAL WEAPONS

Although research on technologies such as lasers, microwaves, sonics, and microbiological and gene therapies (e.g., the development and use of antisense oligonucleotides) is generally intended to improve the human condition, it can be used to do just the opposite. In general, however, these are not the types of technologies that can be exploited in other than sophisticated laboratories. Additionally, the exploitation of these technologies requires resources, such as special equipment or unusually high amounts of electrical power, all of which will assist intelligence agencies in their discovery and identification. This is not to say that with determination and unlimited fiscal resources countries or political groups could not purchase one or all of these technologies in some type of operative or usable form. That said, the transfer of these advanced technologies into weapons to be used against a large deploying force, other than as a single-use terrorist weapon, will require an industrial base and infrastructure that today is limited to just a handful of potential enemies.

Although U.S. forces, by policy, will not bring nontraditional weapons to the battlefield, the use of nuclear weapons and chemical and biological agents, delivered as weapons or by acts of individual guerrilla or terrorist elements, cannot be ruled out. With the exception of nuclear weapons, the production of this type of threat is not limited to countries or organizations with extremely sophisticated technologies or infrastructures; their delivery to an area as a combat or terrorist weapon depends only upon the determination and will of the offending organization. U.S. forces have been trained to operate in the nuclear, chemical, and biological environment, but they can handle the situation best when the chemical or biological agent has been identified and its source is known. Operating continually in chemical-biological protective gear, even with fielded and forthcoming improvements, moderately to severely degrades the effectiveness of the deploying force, and this will be especially true in the urban or climatically severe environment. Today, the rapid identification of the presence of an agent of a biological or chemical nature, from a weapon or an industrial source, or in a field of combat, a city, or a specific building, is, at best, modestly successful. To prevent deploying forces in the future from the requirement for passive protection, continued commitment and emphasis on research on detection systems is an absolute requirement to provide that type of information immediately to the force commander.

For the foreseeable future, U.S. forces and their allies will continue to use obscurants to hide tactical movements, smoke to signal locations of friendly forces, and chemicals for pest control and sanitation. All of these, when properly applied, should not pose a major immediate health threat to ground forces, but will inhibit visibility, cause minor eye or respiratory irritation, and might cause long-term effects yet unknown.

Although appalling to most of the world's cultures, the use of nuclear devices as a tactical or political weapon is still possible and, in the view of some planners, even likely. The outcome of the use of this type of weapon is well known and, depending upon the location and timing of the detonation, might well cause massive casualties that would instantly overwhelm existing medical services and be an extremely effective psychological weapon for the remaining fighting or recovery force. Additionally, there will be a political response of some type, either in the United States or the United Nations, that could result in the additional use of nuclear weapons and additional support to deployed forces.

Although the debate continues as to the long-term effects of the military vaccination program in the face of an increasing number of potential new agents, there is little doubt that future deployed U.S. forces will be vaccinated against biological agents known to be endemic to the area of deployment. Vaccination would also be used against those agents known to be available for use as weapons if and when that threat is identified and a safe vaccine exists. However, vaccinating troops against all known and emerging types of biological and viral threats will be practically impossible. Therefore, data, particularly on emerging disease agents, obtained from various intelligence sources and compiled by AFMIC and CDC, must therefore be immediately shared with industry and the academic community to provide for the basic research necessary in epidemiology, vaccine development, and treatment options. Because OOTW are "on call," starting the process of study when the deployment is eminent will be of little value.

Forces deployed and prepared to fight in high-threat chemical environments will require accurate and reliable intelligence of opposing forces and their ability and willingness to use chemicals as a battlefield weapon. Additionally, an in-depth knowledge of the industrial base of the areas to which U.S. forces will be deployed will be an absolute requirement prior to deployment for protection against inadvertent chemical exposure at toxic or subtoxic levels. This will be particularly true for forces deployed in OOTW and for forces required for operating in the urban environment. Force commanders must have the information necessary to select and destroy targets of military importance without putting their own forces at risk for chemical or industrial contamination and, if the risk is unavoidable, to prospectively protect their forces during and after the attack.

PHYSICAL EFFECTS

The physical conditioning of U.S. forces prior to deployment has generally never been better. Active-duty forces are maintained in excellent physical and dental health and this state will be absolutely required, as previously mentioned, as new technologies are brought to the battlespace. The trend in downsizing the standing forces and relying more on National Guard and Reserve Forces will require continuing emphasis on the physical and dental health of those forces that the Department of Defense (DOD) is addressing. An increasing proportion of deployments now include coalition forces, which require a great deal of medical and support capability from U.S. forces and in which the composition and capabilities of those forces is quite heterogeneous and often different from U.S. forces. Increasing use and dependence upon DOD contractor personnel will require an assessment of the characteristics of these additional personnel deployed, such as age, health status, fitness, past medical treatment and records, training proficiency, and possible stress level associated with separation.

The disease non-battle-injury rate (DNBI) in the Desert Shield and Desert Storm operations was the lowest recorded in history and continued a trend for U.S. forces in major deployments. However, there were major special circumstances (no alcohol use and extremely limited contact with the local population) associated with that deployment, and thus the low DNBI rate is unlikely to be repeated in future deployments. An excellent and extensive report of this experience appears in the Institute of Medicine (IOM 1996) publication on the *Health Consequences of Service in the Persian Gulf War*.

In yet-to-be-published data on the Bosnia-Herzegovina deployment, where surveys and data were collected on 10,000 deployed troops and some 170,000 environmental samples were taken, a low 8.1 medical encounters per 100 soldiers per week was reported. The most frequently cited causes for visits to medical facilities paralleled the Desert Storm experience in spite of considerably different geographical and climatic conditions: injuries and orthopedic conditions (27%), respiratory disease (26%), miscellaneous "other" medical conditions (13%), dermatological disorders (12%), and dental disease (10%). Interestingly, perhaps because of controlled food and water supplies, the incidence of gastrointestinal disease was lower than that found in Desert Storm (2%). With the added emphasis on physical conditioning and the use of mechanized equipment and improved repair procedures, routine industrial injuries continued their downward trend, with sports injuries providing the largest portion of musculoskeletal injury (21.0%). Battle injuries in the future, as in the past, will be directly related to the intensity of the conflict, the geography of the site of deployment, and the capability and size of the opposing force.

In Bosnia-Herzegovina, there were very serious concerns about the environmental hazards for our forward-deployed troops. At this time, more is known about Bosnia-Herzegovina, from a toxicological or an environmental health point of view, than is known about most U.S. military bases. Environmental health specialists, based at a forward-deployed laboratory that was almost as sophisticated as most laboratories in the United States collected over 170,000 specimens of air, water, and soil. A very sophisticated clinical laboratory was also forward-deployed. Enormous apprehension about the environment and very substantial efforts by the command structure to protect U.S. personnel from environmental and other hazards resulted in the net effect of a DNBI rate in Bosnia significantly below that for U.S. garrison troops stationed in the United States.

This level of very considerable attention and effort requires an enormous effort on the part of the command structure and the line commanders, not the medical staff, to maintain the level of awareness and sensitivity. If you had 20 to 30 such deployments under way across the world, it would become very difficult.

PSYCHOLOGICAL EFFECTS

Modern telecommunications technologies have added a new element to the deployed experience, at least at fixed positions and on ships, with the availability of instant access to the news of the day in living color from sources such as CNN. Additionally, readily available telephone service and video teleconferencing with loved ones keeps the deployed force bonded to the home environment. Although on the surface these technologies are advantageous to troop morale and well being, they can also have the opposite effect and be an additional source of anxiety and depression. Access to these telecommunications technologies will certainly be easier and more common in future deployments.

In general, U.S. forces are psychologically prepared to deploy and fight. They are further prepared by knowing the objective of the deployment and the estimated length of the engagement. Troops react differently, however, when the goals and objectives of the deployment change, they do not engage the enemy upon arrival in the deployed area, and they have an open-ended or changing term of deployment. This was observed in Desert Shield where boredom and separation from family took its toll on morale and the combat edge of the deployed forces during the last few months of Desert Shield.

Smaller dispersed units, increased utilization of technology, information overload, and less reliance on massed forces will all change the psychological environment and stress the psychological state of the deployed force in spite of intense prior operational training. Urban combat, terrorism, sniper activity, 360-degree threats, industrial pollution, and the handling of civilian (noncombatant) populations will further stress the ground force. The perceived and actual limits of medical support and reliance on one's self and buddy care will tend to increase combat stress. As such, in the immediate future there will be unprecedented psychological and physical stresses on deployed troops, particularly in units deployed in OOTW, that might have significant short- and long-term effects on deployed forces. A predeployment study of the Bosnia-Herzegovina activities identified individuals in the survey who had psychological conditions, which prevented their deployment. This in-depth, predeployment psychological screening, initiated for the Bosnia-Herzegovina deployment, will be an important and effective tool in the prevention of long-term psychological diseases.

LONG-TERM AND REPRODUCTIVE EFFECTS

All wars and engagements have resulted in long-term physical and psychological health effects. The most recent major deployment, the Desert Shield and Desert Storm operations, was no exception with reports of unusual and unexplained illnesses documented in the IOM (1996) report. Reproductive difficulties following deployments, however, have had little emphasis until recently when the press reported on numerous problems with birth defects and miscarriages in couples in which one of the pair served in the desert operations. Although these claims were later proven to be within expected limits for the population at risk and, thus, not related to the deployment as such, a lack of baseline data in the deployed forces, and the general population for that matter, makes the conclusion somewhat less than completely satisfactory.

The same is true for studies of unexplained physical and psychiatric illness. What has not been documented, until recently, is the mental and physical health of the deployed force prior to deployment. DOD has aggressively initiated programs to correct this deficiency, not only as a basis for further study, but to have the data to use as a baseline for follow-on care and compensation when necessary. Specifically and significantly missing in the predeployment survey required in the December 4, 1998, Joint Chiefs of Staff *Memorandum on Deployment Health Surveillance and Readiness*, however, are any questions relative to the reproductive history of the deploying member or his or her spouse. To be of any value in post-deployment studies to identify injury or degree of compensation for injury, these questions must be asked in great depth and the data preserved to protect privacy. In a predeployment survey of the type required, the military procedure of only having the deploying member fill out a form will not be satisfactory.

Overseas Clearance Forms, used for years in the military system, have been notorious for their inaccuracy and lack of data. Depending upon the individual's motivation for the assignment, the forms were filled out to provide the best situation for the individual's deployment agenda. (Even the term "normal" was not well defined. An example is an individual who arrives overseas with a Down's Syndrome child and asks for special schooling and medical care. When reviewing the Overseas Clearance Form, the health of the child was checked as normal—normal in the view of the deploying member for a child with Down's Syndrome.) Therefore, every deploying member should have to have an in-depth interview with a skilled health professional to get reliable reproductive history for a baseline. Only then can comparative pre- and post-deployment studies be of any value. However, until further data prove otherwise, there is no indication that the risks for reproductive health in future deployments will be any greater than those found today.

Post-deployment health studies for forces known to be at risk from a known specific agent, such as that of the Ranch Hand group that studied the effect of dioxin and related compounds on troops in Vietnam, will continue to be utilized in specialized and routinely deployed forces.

CHARACTER OF DEPLOYED FORCES

Although the current armed forces do not represent the ethnic, racial, and gender mix of the general population (approximately 32% minorities and 14% women), a condition exacerbated by the end of the military draft and the institution of the all-volunteer force, it is debatable whether there will be much movement to bring forces closer to the racial and ethnic mix of the nation in future deployments. Major players in this situation will be the nation's economy and employment opportunities as well as the associated training and educational benefits resulting from military service. The recently announced considerations by Congress to markedly improve veterans' benefits, including a college education and stipend after 4 years of service, will play an important role in the mix of future deployed forces.

There is general agreement on one trend. As the relative supply of young men decreases in society, women will increasingly be brought in to the battlespace and play increasingly more important roles in combat and OOTW. With the exception of additional supply requirements for female deployed forces (birth control, female specific medications, and feminine hygiene supplies) and their different reactions to deployment stresses, women have proven that they are effective personnel and easily integrated into a well-commanded unit. The use of women in deployed forces will, nonetheless, continue to require major special considerations in future operations relative to their unique health risks, not the least of which is the potential for, or actual, pregnancy. Again the predeployment health assessment must play a significant role. Women in deployed forces must have easy access to the supplies mentioned above, as well as the means by which to detect pregnancy while deployed. Depending upon the type of deployment, its location, and the potential for operations in hazardous chemical or industrial environments, policies for the evacuation or movement of pregnant personnel out of the risk area must be developed, clearly enunciated, and strictly enforced.

CONCLUSIONS

The future battlespace will most likely be characterized by considerable structural and industrial damage, force dispersion, smaller tailored force structures, new personal equipment, data links to the individual soldier, an urban environment, a 360-degree threat, and a nontraditional enemy force structure. Nontraditional weapons, particularly chemical and biological agents, and weapons developed from future technological advances are likely, and the location of the deployment will not have been planned for in any detail. In spite of rapid and significant changes in technology, equipment, operational tempo, operations, and force size, disease non-battle injury and psychological stresses will remain as the most important threats to future deployed forces in all scenarios. The long-term effects of: toxic and subtoxic levels of chemicals; unknown or evolving bacteria and viruses; the potential for misuse of evolving biologicals and therapies; new weapon technologies; training symposia and techniques; and, the psychological effects of stresses in the deployment and in combat will need continued emphasis and research to provide for prophylaxis prior to deployment, study following the deployment, and treatment, when needed, upon return to garrison or civilian employment. It will be only through this type of research that deployed forces might be protected from all the potential dangers of the future battlespace.

REFERENCES

IOM (Institute of Medicine). 1996. Health Consequences of Service During the Persian Gulf War: Recommendations for Research and Information Systems. Washington, DC: National Academy Press.

JSC (Joint Chiefs of Staff). 1998. Deployment Health Surveillance and Readiness. MCM-251-98. Office of the Chairman, Washington, D.C. (Dec. 4).

ADDITIONAL REFERENCES (NOT CITED)

Antisense 98. 1998. Work in progress. Nature Biotechnology. 16:1319-1321.

Beiting, J. 1993. Defending against an unseen enemy. Mil. Med. Technol. 3:8-11.

Binder, S., and A. Levitt. 1998. Preventing Emerging Infectious Diseases: Strategy for the 21st Century. Report prepared for the Centers for Disease Control and Prevention.

Blanck, R.R., and W.H. Bell. 1991. Special reports: Medical aspects of the Persian Gulf War. N. Engl. J. Med. 324:857-859.

Broad, W.J., and J. Miller. 1998. The threat of germ weapons is rising. Fear, too. The New York Times. (Dec. 27).

Centobene, S. 1998. The future is now. Airman. (Dec.)

Chrousos, G. 1992. The concepts of stress and stress system disorders: Overview of physical and behavioral homeostasis. JAMA. 267:1244-1252.

Cigrang, J., E. Carbone, S. Todd, and E. Fiedler. 1998. Mental health attrition from air force basic military training. Mil. Med. 163:834-838.

Clauw D.J., and G.P. Chrousos. 1997. Chronic pain and fatigue syndromes: Overlapping clinical and neuroendocrine features and potential pathogenic mechanisms. Neuroimmunododulation. 4:143-153.

Correll, J. 1999. On course for global engagement. Airforce Magazine. 82:22-33.

Cowan, D.N., R.F. DeFraites, G.C. Gray, M.B. Goldenbaum, and S.M. Wishik. 1997. The risk of birth defects among children of Persian Gulf War veterans. N. Engl. J. Med. 336:1650-1656.

Directorate of Office of the Special Assistant for Gulf War Illnesses. 1998. Depleted Uranium in the Gulf. Draft. Investigation and analysis. Directorate of the Office of the Special Assistant for Gulf War Illnesses.

Dohrenwend, B. 1997. A psychological perspective on the past and future of psychiatric epidemiology. Am. J. Epidemiol. 147:222-231.

Dohrenwend, B. 1983. Psychological implication of nuclear accidents: the case of Three Mile Island. Bull. N. Y. Acad. Med. 59(10):1060-1076.

Ember, L. 1998. Surviving stress. C&EN. (May 25):12-24.

Engle, C, M. Roy, D. Kayanan, et al. 1998. Multidisciplinary treatment of persistent symptoms after Gulf War service. Mil. Med. 163:202-208.

EPA (Environmental Protection Agency). 1992. Guidelines for Exposure Assessment. (Feb. 7).

Fortune. 1998. Wired Warrior. 21:184-185.

Garland, F.C., C.D. Garland, and E.D. Gorham. 1998. The Association of Unplanned Pregnancy, Marital Status and Age with Adverse Reproductive Outcomes and Elective Abortions in U.S. Navy Women. NHRC Publication 98-7.

Headquarters United States Air Force. 1999. Global Engagement: A Vision for the 2st Century Air Force. Online. Available: http://www.xp.hq.af.mil/xpx/21/nuvis.htm.

Hobfoll, S.E., C.D. Spielberger, S. Breznitz, C. Figley, S. Folkman, B. Lepper-Green, D. Meichenbaum, N.A. Milgram, I. Sandler, I. Sarason, et al. 1991. War-Related Stress. Addressing the stress of war and other traumatic events. Am. Psychol. 46(8):848-855.

Hyams, K., S. Wignall, and R. Roswell. 1996. War syndromes and their evaluation: from the U.S. Civil War to the Persian Gulf War. Ann. Int. Med. 125:398-405.

Hybridon, Inc. 1999. What Is Antisense? Online. Available: http://hybridon.com/graphic_version/antisense/antisense.html.

IOM (Institute of Medicine). 1996. Interactions of Drugs, Biologics and Chemicals in U.S. Military Forces. Washington, DC: National Academy Press.

IOM (Institute of Medicine). 1999. Chemical and Biological Terrorism: Research and Development to Improve Civilian Medical Response. Washington, DC: National Academy Press.

Joseph, S. 1995. DOD News Briefing. (Aug. 1).

Knoke, J.D., G.C. Gray, and F.C. Garland. 1997. Lack of Association of Testicular Cancer With Persian Gulf War Service. NHRC Publication 97-7.

Lombardi, W., and S. Wilson. 1999. Wellness intervention with pregnant soldiers. Mil. Med. 164:22-29.

Marlowe, D., K. Wright and R. Gifford. 1991. Key Desirable Leader Actions and Behaviors in Final Preparation of Small Units and Small Groups for Combat. Report prepared for Chief of Staff of the Army and Vice Chief of Staff of the Army. (Jan.14).

Marlowe, D., K. Wright, and R. Gifford. 1991. Some Considerations On the Human Issues in Troop Return after Operation Desert Storm. Report prepared for: Chief of Staff of the Army and Vice Chief of Staff of the Army. (Feb. 8).

Martin, S., J. Gambel, J. Jackson, et al. 1998. Leishmaniasis in the United States Military. Mil. Med. 163:801-807.

McEwen, B. 1998. Protective and damaging effects of stress mediators. N. Engl. J. Med. 338:171-179.

McKee, K., M. Kortepeter, and S. Ljaamo. 1999. Disease and Non-Disease Battle Injury Among United States Soldiers Deployed in Bosnia-Herzegovina During 1997: Summary Primary Care Statistics for Operation Joint Guard.

Nelson, D. 1999. Core competencies. Airman. XLIII:2-56.

Nice, D.S., R.L. Calderson, and S.M. Hilton. 1997. Reproductive Outcome in the U.S. Navy: Experience of 33,130 Hospitalized Pregnancies During 1982-1992. NHRC Pub. 97-16.

Parker, J. 1998. Maximizing Human Performance in the Military Environment. 2nd SAF Military Medicine Conference.

Pincus, S. 1998. Operational stress control in the former Yugoslavia: A joint endeavor. Mil. Med. 163:358-362.

Sternberg, E. 1997. Neural-immune interactions in health and disease. J. Clin. Invest. 100(11):2641-2647.

Stretch, R.H., and K.H. Knudson. 1998. Psychological health and trauma in male and female soldiers. Mil. Med. 163:363-367.

The Associated Press. 1999. Study Confirms Gulf Illness Claims. (Jan. 15).

Stuempfle, A.K., S.J. Howells, and C.A. Boulet. 1996. Final Report of International Task Force 25 Hazard From Industrial Chemicals.

USACHPPM (U.S.Army Center for Health Promotion and Preventive Medicine). 1999. The Medical NBC Battlebook. Department of Defense. Online. Available: http://chppm-www.argea.army.mil

USACHPPM (U.S.Army Center for Health Promotion and Preventive Medicine). 1999. Short-Term Chemical Exposure Guidelines for Deployed Military Personnel. TG230A. Draft. Aberdeen Proving Ground, Edgewood, MD. (March).

U.S. Army. 1998. Risk Management. Field Manual No. 100-14. Department of the Army, Washington, D.C. (April 23).

U.S. Medicine. 1991. U.S. Medicine in Gulf War. 27:1-113.

U.S. Navy. 1998 Department of the Navy Posture Statement.

Verton, D. 1998. Marines take it to town. Federal Computer Week 7:18.

Wolfe, J., S. Proctor, J. Davis, et.al. 1998. Health symptoms reported by Persian Gulf War veterans two years after return. Am. J. Ind. Med. 33:104-113.

The Nature of Risk Assessment and Its Application to Deployed U.S. Forces

by Joseph V. Rodricks[1]

ABSTRACT

An analytical framework applicable to the assessment of the wide range of risks to health and safety potentially encountered by U.S. forces deployed to unfamiliar environments is presented as a guide to experts involved in the evaluation of diverse information on specific hazards. Adherence to the guidance should ensure that risk assessment results are clearly and consistently presented, and that they are suitable for practical, risk management decision-making. The analytical framework presented is that first described by the National Research Council in 1983 and long in use for assessing risks of hazardous conditions, substances, and agents (referred to collectively as "stressors"). This paper attempts to describe how the analytical framework can be applied in diverse situations, and to many types of stressors (pathogens, toxic chemicals, physical hazards, etc.). The framework for risk assessment, as originally conceived by the NRC, is a guide to the organization and evaluation of information and its attendant uncertainties, and does not require specific methodologic approaches; the methodologies used should be those appropriate to the relevant scientific disciplines (e.g., toxicology, microbiology, etc.). The framework offered in the paper includes a means for reduction of complex information to usable formats. It recognizes that the purpose of the risk assessment process is not to set standards that can be used for "yes-no" decision-making. Rather, in the current context its purpose is to allow DOD decision-makers sufficient information to examine a range of risks that might arise in rapidly changing deployment conditions, and to balance competing risks so that overall risks to deployed forces can be minimized.

INTRODUCTION

The National Research Council (NRC) is undertaking a project with the objective of providing advice to the Department of Defense (DOD) regarding strategies to protect the health of military

[1] The Life Sciences Consultancy, 750 17th Street, NW, Suite 1000, Washington, D.C., 20006.

personnel when they are deployed to unfamiliar environments. Such deployments might result in the exposure of U.S. forces to chemical and biological agents of war, and to other substances released by enemy forces with the intention of causing harm. Moreover, U.S. forces might also become exposed to a variety of infectious agents, environmental contaminants, and conditions of stress not necessarily arising from battle but nonetheless associated with the environments to which they are deployed.

Protection of deployed forces requires an understanding of the risks of disease and injury they face and the development and implementation of strategies to mitigate those risks. The necessary understanding of health risks arises out of the process of risk assessment. Development and implementation of strategies to mitigate risks falls within the domain of risk management. This paper offers a description of the conceptual and scientific basis for risk assessment, the types of knowledge and data necessary for its conduct, the accommodation of scientific uncertainties within its conduct, and the various ways in which risk-assessment results can be used in risk-management decision-making. In addition, the paper describes the specific problems encountered in the application or risk-assessment methodologies to the evaluation of risks faced by deployed forces. The overall purpose of the paper is thus to provide a broad, analytical framework for the assessment of the wide range of health risks potentially encountered by forces deployed to unfamiliar environments. The framework is expected to serve as a guide to experts involved in the organization and evaluation of diverse information on specific threats. The purpose of having such a guide is to ensure that risk-assessment results are clearly and consistently presented, and that their means of presentation are suitable for practical, risk-management decision-making. It is noted here, and discussed more fully below, that the analytical framework for risk assessment to be presented is not intended to replace the scientific evaluations and judgments of experts in the specific technical areas coming under discussion. Rather, it is only to serve as a guide for the systematic organization and evaluation of technical information and uncertainties, so that clarity, consistency, and practicality are achieved in the manner in which risk-assessment results are presented.

The paper is concerned with risk management only to the extent that it offers a discussion of how risk-assessment results might be used to achieve various degrees of health protection. Issues such as the options available for achieving risk-management objectives are outside the scope of this paper. Guidance documents for risk management have been developed by several branches of the DOD (Naval Safety Center 1996; Department of the Air Force 1998; Department of the Army 1998). The concepts and terms adopted in those various documents are broadly consistent with those used in this document.

The basic analytical framework presented in this paper is one long in use for assessing health risks of hazardous conditions, substances, and agents (NRC 1983, 1994). It will be seen, however, that under this framework, risk-assessment results might be expressed in different ways. Because risk assessment is a tool for practical decision-making, the specific means for describing results should be those most helpful to the ultimate users of the information, the risk managers. This paper proposes an approach that would seem to be suitable for decision-making in the context of troop deployments, but it would be recognized that alternative approaches, under the same analytical framework, exist. It is expected that some modifications in the approach offered here are expected as the NRC project develops, and as alternative risk-management options come under review.

GENERAL NATURE OF RISK ASSESSMENT

Basic Definitions and Concepts

Risk is the probability that adverse effects will occur under specified conditions. In the context of risks to human health, adverse effects manifest themselves as specific diseases or as injuries to the structure or function of the human organism. The nature and magnitude of the risks associated with substances in the environment vary both with the nature of the substance and with the conditions of exposure to it. The conditions of exposure that determine risk usually include the magnitude, duration, and frequency of exposure to the substance, and often also includes the route of entry into the body. In the present context, and for ease of exposition, the term "stressor" will be used to describe any and all chemical, biological, and physical entities in the environment that might, singly or in combination, pose risks to deployed forces.

Risk assessment is the process through which an understanding of risks is acquired (NRC 1994). The term might be used in two somewhat different contexts. First, it might be used to describe an actual scientific investigation of a group of individuals exposed to a specific stressor for the purposes of determining whether the individuals are at excess risk and, if so, the magnitude and nature of their risk. Second, it might be used to describe the attempt to predict risks in individuals that are not the subject of study, but who might become exposed to stressors that, under other conditions, are known to pose risks. Predictive risk assessment, which is the subject of the present paper, necessarily involves the use of risk information collected under one set of conditions (including information collected in experimental settings), together with a number of science-based inferences, to describe risks that might exist under other conditions (e.g., under conditions expected to be experienced by deployed forces). Predictive risk assessment is necessary if the goal is to protect human health. It is the only means available to describe the conditions of exposure that should be avoided if human health is not to be put at significant risk, or to understand the nature and magnitude of the risks created when exposures become excessive. Human health protection can be achieved only if knowledge of these conditions is acquired in advance of exposure (Rodricks 1994).

Risk management is the term used to describe all activities involved in the development and implementation of risk-mitigation strategies. It involves decisions regarding risk acceptability and trade-offs in specific circumstances, risk avoidance goals, and the technical means for achieving them. Risk management relies upon the results of risk assessments, but involves consideration of other factors, including new risks that might arise when decisions are made to avoid certain risks (risk trade-offs). Risk management is a very large subject, and a complete discussion of it requires detailed understanding of the circumstances under which specific populations (in this case, deployed U.S. forces) might face risks. As such, it is largely outside the scope of this document.

These definitions and concepts were first proposed in 1983 by a committee of the National Research Council, which issued a report entitled *Risk Assessment in the Federal Government: Managing the Process* (NRC 1983); another committee of the NRC, in a report issued in 1994, *Science and Judgment in Risk Assessment*, reaffirmed these concepts. The definitions and concepts are now widely recognized in the risk-assessment community, and, as will be shown, are applicable to the problem at hand.

Framework for Systematic Organization and Evaluation of Knowledge and Data

Risk assessment, in its predictive mode, does not create new data and knowledge. Rather, it is the attempt to organize existing information and knowledge in useful and clear ways, so that inferences regarding risk can be made. It draws upon knowledge and data developed within the basic scientific and technical disciplines—epidemiology, toxicology, pathology, microbiology, medicine, and biostatistics, and also all of the disciplines involved in evaluating human exposures to environmental agents—and seeks to organize that information in systematic ways, consistent with the standards of those disciplines. Scientific evaluation of that organized information is left to experts in the relevant disciplines, although risk assessment requires that the bases for conclusions reached regarding the available data be explicitly justified and described. Risk assessment also requires that all significant scientific uncertainties in the available information be described and accounted for.

Risk assessment does not require any specific methodological approach to data evaluation, but it does require explicit justification of data choices, methodologies, and of the treatment of scientific uncertainties (NRC 1994). Most of the remaining sections of this paper are devoted to a discussion of how these goals can be achieved, drawing upon precedents established in other areas in which risk assessment has been used in decision-making, but with due consideration of the special needs of the present context.

General Content of Risk Assessment

As described by the NRC (1983, 1994), all risk assessments, irrespective of the stressors and situations to which they are to be applied, contain the same types of information and analysis. The NRC also proposed that, for the sake of clarity, the information should be organized in a specific way. Thus, all risk assessments involve, as a first step, a careful description of the specific stressors of concern, and the specific groups of individuals that might become exposed to those stressors. Once the stressors and population groups that are the subject of the risk assessment are specified, information is collected regarding the following questions (see Figure 1):

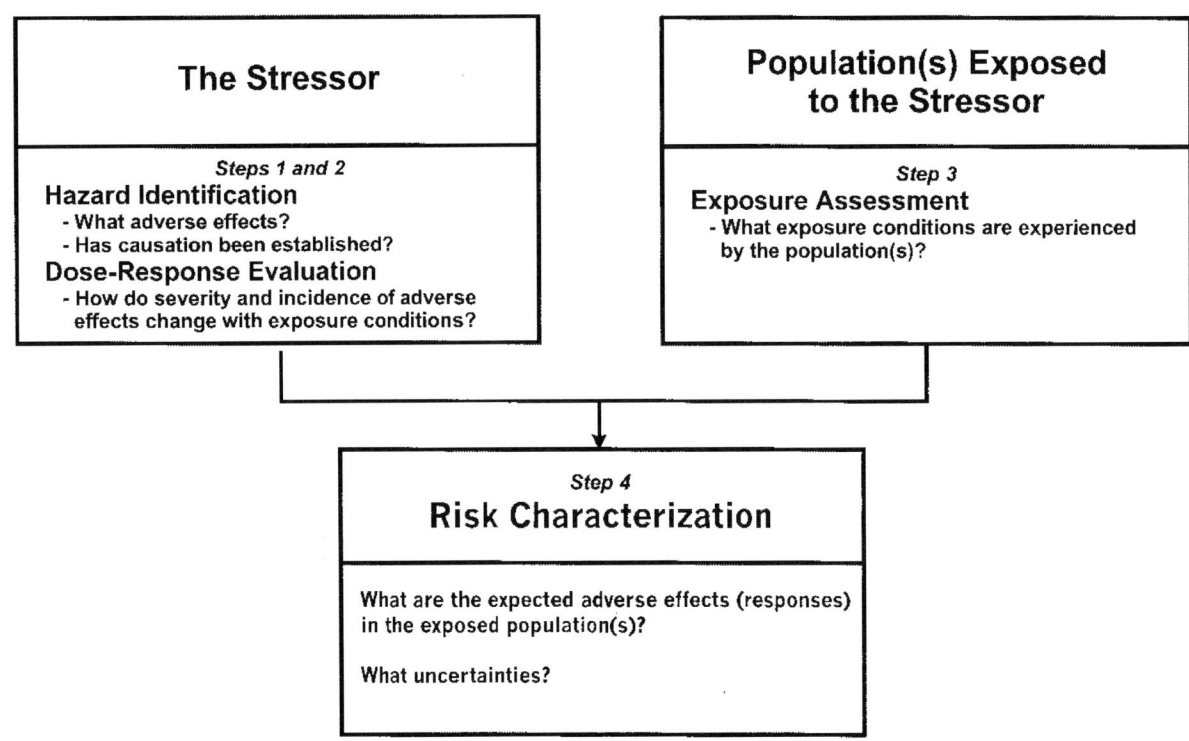

FIGURE 1 Risk assessment involves systematic organization and evaluation of data.

Step 1: Hazard Identification. What types of adverse effects have been shown to be associated with exposure to the stressor? For each effect, how well has a causal association been established? If hazards have been identified in experimental (animal) models, are the findings likely to be relevant to humans?

Step 2: Dose-Response Evaluation. For each type of adverse effect (hazard) associated with exposure to the stressor, how do the severity and incidence of those effects (responses) change as the conditions of exposure (dose)[2] to the agent change?

Information regarding these first two steps is specific to the stressor, and is typically to be found in the scientific and medical literature. The results of the hazard identification and dose-response evaluations are then integrated with the results of:

Step 3: Human Exposure Assessment. Under what conditions are the individuals of concern exposed or potentially exposed to the stressor? "Conditions" includes consideration of those factors (dose size, duration, frequency, route of entry) that, based on Step 2, are known to relate to response.

The result of the integration of results from Step 3 with those from Steps 1 and 2 is a description of the risks of adverse effects in the exposed population—the nature, severity, and incidence (probability) of adverse effects expected in the population under its actual or expected conditions of exposure. The NRC chose to label this fourth step in the assessment process as a risk characterization, because this term best reflects the fact that accurate and precise quantitative estimates of risk, though desired, are rarely achievable because of limitations in knowledge and data (NRC 1983). The NRC envisioned that risks would be described quantitatively, when possible, but always accompanied by qualitative descriptions of factors not readily quantifiable. Indeed, in some cases only qualitative characterizations of risk will be possible.

Although all assessments contain these four steps, they need not proceed in the order shown in Figure 1. This matter will be further discussed in connection with the discussion of the uses of risk-assessment results.

Need to Deal with Scientific Uncertainties

Although the logic in the organization of information for risk-assessment purposes is apparent, the difficulties encountered in attempts to complete a risk assessment are often formidable. Indeed, many of the questions that need to be considered to complete an assessment cannot be completely answered with available knowledge and information. Typical questions include the following:

1. How do hazard and dose-response data collected in one population group apply to population groups having a different range of susceptibilities to the agent?

2. How do hazard and dose-response data collected in experimental systems apply (if at all) to human populations?

3. How do hazard and dose-response data collected over a given period of exposure, or a given route of exposure, apply to populations exposed over different time periods or exposure routes?

4. Is it possible to predict response (risks) at doses that are lower than the minimum dose at which risks can be measured? (All risk measurement systems have limited detection power, and cannot detect many small-to-moderate-sized risks.)

---

[2] The NRC, and now common usage, refers to this step as a dose-response evaluation, but it is clear that the term "dose" is intended to be applied broadly, to include all measure of exposure relevant to the response. A more descriptive term might be "exposure-risk evaluation."

5. What measures of dose (what conditions of exposure) provide the most accurate prediction of response (risk)?

6. How can population exposures be described based on data limited to discrete segments of the population, or limited to specific points in time?

It is often the case that well-documented answers to questions such as these are not available. Because it is not possible to complete risk assessments without providing answers to such questions, it must be recognized that risk-assessment results are necessarily uncertain, and specific assessments are uncertain in rough proportion to the number of unanswered questions that arise in the course of their conduct (Bogen 1990; Finkel 1990).

The NRC (1983) has emphasized that any attempt to provide answers to questions for which there is limited empirical support must be recognized as at least partially based on what was called a "science policy" choice. The NRC committee promoted the use of science policy choices, as long as the specific choices to be used were explicitly described, and used consistently in all risk assessments; such choices thus become "default options," to be used when knowledge or information is highly limited.

Regulatory agencies such as the U.S. Environmental Protection Agency (EPA) have prepared guidelines for risk assessment that describe the defaults to be used. Some critical regulatory defaults are presented in Text Box 1 (Barnes and Dourson 1988; EPA 1996). Many of the defaults presented in Text Box 1 are used by agencies such as EPA and the Food and Drug Administration (FDA), when their concern is the general population. For occupational groups, additional considerations enter the picture and often lead to somewhat difference choices (discussed later).

The insertion of specific factors to account for uncertainties—such as the factors of 10 used to deal with variability in responses to toxicity (Defaults 4 and 5, Text Box 1)—has become common practice in risk assessments. These uncertainty factors, and the criteria for their selection, are critical components of any risk assessment (Barnes and Dourson 1988), and they will require considerable discussion within the context of risks to deployed forces. The examples given in Text Box 1 are not all relevant to the risk questions posed in this paper, and are presented only to make clear the need to consider such factors. A final point on the issue of uncertainty in risk assessments is that the regulatory defaults listed in Text Box 1 are offered in the absence of data relevant to specific stressors. Thus, in all specific cases, actual data, when sufficient, override defaults (also discussed later).

TYPICAL USES OF RISK-ASSESSMENT RESULTS

General Nature of Decision-Making Based Upon Risk-Assessment Results

Heretofore most decision-making based on risk-assessment results has taken place in the context of the regulation of chemical and radiation risks. Both the general population and occupational populations have been the subjects of such regulations. In most cases risk-management decisions have resulted in some type of numerical standard, usually limiting the allowed concentration of an agent in a specific environmental medium. With respect to the use of risk-assessment results in such regulatory standard-setting, the process is generally the following (NRC 1983):

1. Risks under current exposure conditions are estimated.
2. A risk-reduction goal is established.
3. The exposure level that corresponds to the risk goal is estimated.
4. The level estimated in Step 3 is the maximum level of exposure allowed in the population to be protected.

TEXT BOX 1

Some Defaults Used by Regulatory Agencies for Toxicological Risk Assessments.

1. In the absence of data demonstrating their irrelevance, animal toxicity data will be used to estimate human risk.
2. In the absence of data demonstrating their irrelevance, data from the most sensitive animal model will be used.
3. Human data are preferred to animal data for purposes of human risk assessment, but only if those data are adequate (i.e., sufficient to establish causation, and sufficient to provide quantitative dose-response data).
4. In the absence of data suggesting another factor, average humans will be assumed to be ten-fold more sensitive than experimental animals (not used for carcinogens, see below).
5. In the absence of data suggesting another factor, the "most sensitive" humans will be assumed to be ten-fold more sensitive than the "average" human.
6. All forms of toxicity other than carcinogenicity will be assumed to exhibit thresholds.
7. In the absence of data to the contrary, all carcinogens will be assumed to pose risks at all nonzero exposures, and their risks will increase in direct proportion to cumulative lifetime dose.

Descriptions are those of the author. Many defaults listed here are meant to apply to the general population, not to occupational populations. (See text for references.)

---

5. Standards, expressed as concentrations in air or water or food or soil, or in all of these media, are calculated so that the maximum allowable exposure level is not exceeded in populations exposed via these media. (Discussions of how these goals are to be achieved, and how compliance with them is measured, are outside the scope of this paper.)

It can be seen that the first two steps—the conduct of the risk assessment and the risk-reduction goals—are the critical components of this process. In the context of regulations, it is possible to make certain generalizations about these two steps. First, risk assessments for the general population have often involved different uses of available data and different default assumptions than have risk assessments directed at occupational groups (NRC 1994). It has been assumed that, because they generally involve healthy adults and do not include the most vulnerable segments of the general population, occupational populations are likely to display less variability in response to hazardous agents than do members of the general population. Second, with respect to risk-reduction goals, regulators have sought to ensure that none of the adverse effects of the agent will occur in the populations to be protected and accordingly, have sought to reduce risks to levels thought to be negligible or insignificant (Rodricks 1992). Finally, in many cases, the selection of risk-reduction goals is influenced by considerations other than public health protection—technical feasibility, costs—that are dictated by the requirements of applicable laws.

The model for using risk-assessment results described above is not the only possible one, and is probably not the most useful one for decision-makers who are asked to protect the health of deployed forces.

Model I (NRC 1983)	Model II (Alternative)
Assess risks of current exposures. ↓ Determine whether risk is excessive. If yes, identify risk-reduction goals. ↓ Estimate maximum allowable exposure levels, based on identified risk reduction goal. ↓ Establish standards (limiting concentrations) so that maximum allowable exposure levels are not exceeded	First, Anticipate exposure to identified stressor. ↓ Conduct hazard and dose-response evaluation ↓ Record hazard, dose-response evaluation in readily usable format. Second, Estimate expected dose[a] of stressor in population. ↓ Compare dose estimate to hazard, dose-Response information recorded above. ↓ Determine risk expected in population. ↓ If relevant, compare risks of different actions. ↓ Determine action to be taken to minimize overall risk.

[a]Dose is short hand for all conditions of exposure expected to determine risk.

FIGURE 2 Two models of risk-based decision-making.

Alternative Decision-Making Models Based on Risk-Assessment Results

The model for decision-making described above is applicable when populations are already exposed to a source of risk, and a determination is made that current risks are excessive and need to be reduced to insignificant levels, that is, levels that are likely to protect against any of the adverse effects of a stressor. An alternative model is designed to deal with anticipated, not current, exposures. In such circumstances (which arise in some regulatory contexts in which premarketing approvals for certain products are required), the hazard identification and dose-response evaluation steps of a risk assessment are completed for the agent of concern. These steps of the assessment yield a description of the nature of the adverse effects associated with exposure to the agent and the relationships between the severity and incidence of those effects (response) and the dose (conditions of exposure).

This information can be presented to risk-management decision-makers. These decision-makers are then presented information on the conditions of exposure experienced by the populations of concern: their exposure conditions might be estimated based on anticipated modes of contact with the agent, or based on actual data pertaining to such contact. Faced with information on conditions of exposure (either anticipated or actual), risk-management decision-makers can refer to the hazard and dose-response assessments and determine the nature and extent of risk to be incurred by the population they are charged with protecting. At this stage, decision-makers might then evaluate various options for risk mitigation, and (in the ideal case) choose that which provides the greatest degree of health protection, given the circumstances in which the decision needs to be made.

The two models for risk-based decision-making are outlined in Figure 2. As discussed in the next section, it is the second model (Model II, Figure 2) that would appear to be the most applicable to the problem of risks to deployed forces.

RISKS TO DEPLOYED U.S. FORCES: OVERVIEW OF PROPOSED ASSESSMENT AND MANAGEMENT FRAMEWORKS

Forces deployed to unfamiliar environments might face a range of battle-related risks, including those related to chemical and biological warfare agents, and additional risks of infectious disease, exposure to chemical contaminants in air, water, food, and soil, and a variety of physical threats, including those associated with accidents and explosions, and with certain forms of ionizing radiation, and with excessive heat, cold, and noise. Even certain medical treatments designed to protect forces from certain risks might, themselves, pose other kinds of health threats (Medical NBC Battlebook, U.S. Army Center for Health Promotion and Preventive Medicine). Forces might be exposed to some of these sources of risk only infrequently but in other cases might be exposed continuously through the period of deployment. Several sources of risk might be experienced simultaneously. Actions taken to avoid certain sources of risk might result in exposure of forces to other sources. The situation is complex, and can be managed effectively only if suitable risk-based decision models are in place and their characteristics understood by decision-makers.

The risk-assessment framework described in the foregoing is, it will be suggested, suitable for organizing and evaluating all of these many types of health threats to deployed forces. It will also be suggested that Model II of risk-based decision-making, described in Figure 2, will be most useful for the protection of deployed forces.

Following is a broad overview of how the risk-assessment framework and decision-making model might be applied to each of the types of threats that might be encountered by deployed U.S. forces. Later sections will detail each of the steps outlined here. In outline form, the proposed framework is as follows:

1. Identification of all stressors of possible concern, and elaboration of their sources and pathways to deployed forces.

2. Development of hazard and dose-response information for each stressor, and presentation of information in a usable format.

3. Development of methods for estimating doses[3] of stressors anticipated for or incurred by deployed forces.

4. Estimation of risks to deployed forces and application of decision-making criteria developed with the goal of maximizing health protection, consistent with the circumstances under which risks are encountered.

The guidance offered here pertains to the requirements of risk assessment, and does not deal with specific methodologies that properly fall within the fundamental scientific disciplines upon which risk analyses depend. The emphasis in risk assessment is on clarity and completeness of presentation, explicit consideration and accommodation of scientific uncertainties, and usable presentation of risk

---

[3] As in the earlier text, the term dose is used for ease of exposition. In the context of discussions of specific stressors, its characteristics are influenced by whatever measures of exposure are relevant to the risk being assessed.

results. The guidance is thus offered to ensure consistency, explicitness, and usability; the quality of the underlying scientific information and knowledge, and the appropriate methods for evaluating it are judgments reserved for experts in their particular, relevant disciplines. Those experts, it is hoped, will not see risk assessment as a rigid methodology requiring specific methods of scientific evaluation, but rather as a systematic framework for organizing information and for forcing a high degree of explicitness in the treatment of that information and the uncertainties in it, and for producing usable results.

STRESSORS OF CONCERN AND THEIR SOURCES AND PATHWAYS TO DEPLOYED FORCES

Definition of Stressors

For ease of exposition, stressor has been adopted to apply to all entities and environmental conditions that might threaten deployed forces. No single term is clearly appropriate to describe all such entities and conditions, but this term is arbitrarily selected for convenience. A list of the types of agents of concern as potential threats to deployed forces is presented in Table 1. The types of hazards usually associated with each stressor are also listed; further descriptions of the process of hazard identification, the first step of the proposed risk-assessment framework, is offered in the following section. Implementation of the risk-assessment strategy proposed here requires a listing of all specific stressors of concern, and not simply the broad categories listed in Table 1.

Sources of Stressors and Pathways of Human Exposure

Under the risk-assessment framework presented here, complete evaluations of how and to what extent deployed forces might become exposed to these types of stressors are conducted within the exposure assessment step, described more fully later. It is important, however, that some characterizations of the sources of these stressors, the possible pathways by which deployed forces might become exposed, and the nature of their expected exposure accompany their initial listing. It is also advisable to list stressors in approximate order of the frequency with which deployed forces are expected to encounter them, and in order of their degrees of danger. This initial listing is a useful guide to the hazard and dose-response evaluations. It can be used to set priorities for the conduct of hazard and dose-response evaluations, so that efforts at information gathering and analysis are first directed at what will likely be the highest risk stressors and exposures.

In addition, these initial characterizations of exposure will assist in identifying the types of hazard and dose-response information most relevant to the expected conditions of exposure. Thus, for example, little effort need be devoted to inhalation toxicity data for chemicals that are likely to reach deployed forces only through drinking water, and little effort need be expended researching for chronic hazard information for stressors that forces are likely to encounter only rarely and for very limited periods of time.

DOD has already assembled much information regarding stressors, their sources, and the ways in which forces might encounter them (The Medical NBC Battlebook, The U.S. Army Center for Health Promotion and Preventative Medicine). This information is no doubt the appropriate starting point for the proposed risk assessment. As steps are taken to complete the hazard identification and the dose-response evaluation, it becomes necessary to ensure that risk-assessment criteria for organizing and drawing inferences from data are met.

TABLE 1 Types of Stressors That May Pose Health and Safety Risks to Deployed U.S. Forces

Stressors[a]	Hazards to be Considered
Chemicals	Toxicity, flammability, explosivity, radiation
Pathogens	Infections, infectious diseases
Toxins[b]	Toxicity
Medicines	Side effects
Physical structures	Traumatic injuries from accidents
Moving vehicles	Traumatic injuries from accidents
Environmental conditions	Physical, psychological stresses

[a]The term "stressors" is the author's, used for convenience (see text).

[b]Toxins are chemicals produced by microorganisms, plants, and animals and are typically large (and often not very stable) molecules such as peptides and proteins; it might be necessary to treat them separately from other chemicals, because of the pathways by which they might reach deployed forces.

Source: The Medical NBC Battlebook, The U.S. Army Center for Health Promotion and Preventive Medicine.

HAZARD IDENTIFICATION

Definition

Under the risk-assessment framework proposed here, the hazard identification step involves a description and critical scientific review of the available data concerning the types of adverse health effects (diseases or injuries) that have been associated with exposures to the stressor under consideration. All stressors in the environment can, under some conditions, cause harm to health (i.e., pose hazards) and most can cause different types and degrees of hazard as exposures change. Whether one or more of the hazardous properties of a stressor will be expressed in groups of deployed forces can be ascertained only after the remaining steps of a risk assessment are completed. The purpose of this first step is to describe and catalog for each stressor of interest the types of hazards that have been associated with it, under any conditions; such a thorough catalog ensures that no hazard potentially relevant to risk assessment will be overlooked.

The Problem of Causation

The ease with which a causal relationship between a stressor and a particular health hazard can be established depends upon many factors, including the nature of the stressor (whether it is a well-characterized single substance or a complex mixture), the nature of the hazard (whether it is one that appears immediately after an exposure, or only after a long delay), and the extent and nature of scientific investigation it has received (whether information derives from case reports, from epidemiological studies, or from experimental studies). A few stressors have received significant and intensive study, most have received limited study, and some have not been studied at all. All of these factors are to be considered in judgments regarding the evidence for causation.

Many scientific disciplines are involved in the study of the wide variety of stressors of potential concern to deployed forces: epidemiology, clinical medicine and toxicology, experimental toxicology, microbiology, physiology, psychology, and pharmacology, among others. Within these various disciplines, there are ordinarily agreed-upon criteria used to assemble relevant literature and to evaluate it, and to ascertain whether causal relationships have been adequately documented. In many cases, causal relationships might have been well established in experimental systems (e.g., in laboratory animals), and judgments will need to be made regarding the relevance to human causation (Calabrese 1983). Similarly, in the case of data from epidemiological studies, professionals usually apply certain criteria to the available evidence (e.g., The Hill Criteria, [Hill 1965]) to establish the likelihood of causation.

It is not the purpose of this paper to establish or suggest criteria for causation, but rather to ensure that each hazard identification that is undertaken conclude with a discussion of causation for each of the hazards that have been associated with the stressor. The criteria applicable to the disciplines relevant to the particular stressor under review are to be applied by experts in those disciplines. Associations that might not satisfy causation criteria should also be described.

Sources of Information

Most information pertaining to hazard identification comes from case reports, epidemiological studies, and laboratory studies. Depending upon the disciplines involved, and precedents established therein, differing weights might be given to these different sources of information. In many cases, detailed investigations of the biological mechanisms underlying the production of disease or injury might be available; information from such investigations might often aid in the establishment of causation, or of the relevance of animal data to humans (EPA 1996).

The specific sources of information relevant to stressors of concern to deployed forces include the publically available scientific and medical literature, and information developed by the DOD and other governmental agencies. The means for collecting this information is not within the scope of this paper, but it is suggested that search strategies that ensure comprehensiveness be developed and applied.

Content of Hazard Identification Narrative

The successful application of the risk-assessment framework proposed here requires that all available hazard information for each stressor be systematically assembled, and that a narrative description of that information be prepared. To be maximally useful, it is advisable that narratives for all stressors be organized in approximately the same way. The structure shown in Text Box 2 is suggested, although there are other useful ways to organize data, and discussions among future participants might lead to alternative structures. It is suggested that a relatively uniform approach be developed for all stressors.

Generally, the hazard identification narrative and the final hazard characterization section (Text Box 2) will include an extensive discussion of the specific conditions of exposure under which specific types of hazards are produced. It is critical that all such information be captured in the hazard identification step, and that it be summarized, preferably in an easily usable, tabular form. Such information will be necessary for completion of the next step in the risk assessment. In the context of risks to deployed forces, it is particularly important to note any data suggesting delayed effects. Such effects might be those coming long after exposure, or they might occur only after long-term repeated exposures.

Data Limitations and Gaps

It is seen in Text Box 2 that the final section of the proposed narrative format concerns data gaps. All data characterizing hazards are expected to have limitations, and their elucidation should be contained within the critical components of the hazard narrative. Data gaps are different. The phrase as used here is intended to apply to exposure conditions for which there are no usable data concerning hazards.

> **TEXT BOX 2**
>
> Proposed Organizational Structure for Hazard Identification Narrative
> 1.0 Identification of stressor
> 2.0 Chemical and physical properties
> 3.0 General description of conditions under which deployed forces may come into contact with stressor
> 4.0 Routes of entry into body or modes of contact with body
> 5.0 Behavior in the body
> 6.0 Case reports relating to hazards
> 7.0 Epidemiological studies
>   7.1 Acute exposures
>   7.2 Repeated exposures, up to __ days
>   7.3 Repeated, chronic exposures
> 8.0 Experimental studies
>   8.1 Acute exposures
>   8.2 Repeated exposures, up to __ days
>   8.3 Repeated, chronic exposures
> 9.0 Data available concerning interactions among stressors
> 10.0 Mechanisms of disease or injury
> 11.0 Characterization of hazards: tabulation, critical discussion, causation
> 12.0 Gaps in available data

When such circumstances are encountered, it could mean that there is no identifiable hazard associated with a specified condition of exposure, or it might mean that no attempt has been made to identify the hazard. In any case, all such data gaps should be noted; some might be highly relevant to deployed forces, and might thus seriously hinder attempts to assess risk, whereas others might be only marginally relevant. Elucidation of data gaps is a helpful guide to research, as is elucidation of other data limitations.

Mixtures and Interactions

Data relevant to the combined effects of two or more stressors of concern to deployed forces should be included in the hazard identification narratives of each of the stressors involved. Such descriptions should include the conditions of exposure under which interactions can occur, the likelihood that such conditions could occur under the conditions experienced by deployed forces, any evidence that the adverse effects are simply additive, or that they arise out of some different type of interaction (antagonistic or synergistic) (see paper by Yang in these proceedings).

DOSE-RESPONSE EVALUATION

Definitions of Dose and Response

The second step of the risk-assessment framework is the dose-response evaluation. This phrase arose out of the fields of epidemiology and toxicology, where its meaning is generally understood. It is, however, not a fully descriptive phrase, and might seem awkward for some of the stressors of concern to deployed forces. For purposes of the present discussion, the phrase conditions of exposure is more apt. This phrase encompasses one or more of the following:

- the magnitude of exposure to the stressor;
- the frequency and duration of such exposure; and
- the routes of such exposure (i.e., inhalation, ingestion, dermal, other).

In some cases the physical or chemical forms of the stressor might vary (e.g., amphorous versus crystalline silica), and these variations might affect its hazardous properties; when these forms are important they are also components of the conditions of exposure. As in the use of the term stressor, the term dose will be used in the following as a convenient shorthand for conditions of exposure.

Response is the term used to describe the hazards produced at various doses. The response is thus a description of the risk. Response (risk) generally includes:

- a description of the nature of the disease or injury;
- a description of its severity;
- a discussion of whether the disease or injury is reversible, and, if so, the typical rate of reversibility;
- a description of the incidence of disease or injury; and
- a discussion of whether the hazard is immediate or delayed.

The dose-response evaluation thus entails the development of a description of the relationship between dose of stressor and response, over a range of doses.

Measures of Dose

The doses of the wide variety of stressors of concern to deployed forces are measured in many different ways. Under the criteria for sound risk assessments, it is recommended that whatever measures of dose are used, they should be those measures that are known to relate to response. It is important that the dose-response evaluation include a discussion of the reasons for the selection of specific measures of dose.

The ultimate evaluation of risk will require that the doses likely to be incurred by deployed forces be measured and expressed in ways that are directly relevant to the measures of dose that are determinants of response (risk). The means for ensuring that proper measures of dose are used will be discussed in the next section. In some cases it will be possible to express dose measures quantitatively, but in other cases it might not be possible to do so. It is expected, for example, that environmental conditions leading to excessive physiological or psychological stress will be described in largely qualitative ways; such descriptions are encompassed within the broad definition of dose within the risk-assessment framework proposed here.

The risk-assessment framework described here allows for evaluations of the risks of physical trauma and injury from accidents, explosions, fires, floods, and for evaluations of physical and psychological stress. The use of the term dose is no doubt awkward for these types of risk, and might not be well received by experts in these subjects. It is not a significant defect in the risk-assessment framework proposed here that its terms of reference are not readily adaptable to these types of risk. Experts in the relevant disciplines, using suitable descriptive terms, will nevertheless be asked to arrive at some usable description of the conditions (dose) under which deployed forces are likely to be at risk from these various stressors.

It is generally useful, and in fact convenient, to present dose-response evaluations separately for different exposure durations. It is proposed here to use three categories of exposure duration: acute, intermediate, and chronic. The term acute is used here in its conventional sense of a one-time exposure, although it is recognized that, for different agents, the one-time exposure might extend from a few minutes to many hours. In the field of chemical toxicology, acute is often subdivided into periods of 15 minutes, 1 hour, 8 hours, and 24 hours, because the magnitudes of exposure that produce adverse effects, and the severities of those effects, can, for some agents, vary considerably with these relatively small changes in exposure duration. Acute exposures might occur more than one time in the life of an individual; exposures are to be considered acute only if they are sufficiently separated in time to ensure that any effects produced are not additive or cumulative (NRC 1986).

The terms intermediate and chronic are more ambiguous in meaning, and there appears to be no single definition involved in the evaluation of the wide range of stressors of interest here. The three categories of acute, intermediate, and chronic exposure durations will be used here with the recognition that precise and consistent definitions can be identified only after all participants in the risk assessment are able to discuss these usages and their appropriate definitions.

Response Measures and Their Relationship to Dose

Responses to various doses of hazardous stressors come in many forms. These responses will have been tabulated, discussed, and critically reviewed in the hazard identification step. Out of the information set forth there, dose-response profiles can be developed for acute, intermediate, and chronic exposure conditions.

There are many ways in which responses can be expressed. For present purposes, it is proposed that four categories of response be developed and their relationships to dose described as mortality; severe, irreversible (or slowly reversible) injuries or diseases; minor, readily reversible injuries; and no adverse effects (Table 2).

Other categories can be envisioned and, within each of the above categories, information concerning the incidence of these effects within a population might also be included. It is suggested, however, that these four categories, together with the further categorizations of doses as of acute, intermediate, and chronic duration, will provide sufficient and readily usable information for risk-management purposes. The information proposed here, together with the information to be provided about doses to be incurred by deployed forces in different circumstances, will allow risk managers to determine whether deployed forces are at risk (will incurred doses exceed the maximum no-effect dose?). Methods to be considered in the development of these types of dose-response profiles for stressors of concern to deployed forces will now be considered. It is recognized that adjustments might need to be made in the proposed approach for different categories of stressors, but it is suggested that the general goals of the evaluation, and the framework into which it fits, should not need to be significantly altered.

The Presentation of Dose-Response Information

It is proposed that, for each stressor of concern, a tabular presentation of dose-response information be developed; the suggested format is shown in Table 2. The tabular presentation should be accompanied by a narrative description of its basis, synthesized from the hazard identification narrative, and with an additional description of the reliability and representativeness of the data available relating to dose-response. Extensive discussion will follow later, on the development of the dose information.

The notes to Table 2 define the Ds consistently with the descriptions given previously. With Table 2, risk managers can, for example, see that for the particular stressor reviewed, acute exposures from zero up to D1A are likely to be without adverse effects; doses in the range from D1A to D2A are likely

TABLE 2 Suggested Format for Presentation of Dose-Response Information for Each "Stressor" of Concern to Deployed Forces

Responses (Adverse Effects, Immediate & Delayed)	Doses (for different exposure durations)		
	Acute (A)	Intermediate (I)	Chronic (C)
Mortality	D3A	D3I	D3C
Serious, Irreversible	D2A	D2I	D2C
Minor, Reversible	D1A	D1I	D1C
No Effect Likely	D=0	D=0	D=0

Notes

1. Ds are the doses at which adverse effects, either immediate or delayed, are expected to occur. Generally, D3>D2>D1 and DA>DI>DC.

2. D3 = min. dose for mortality; D2 = min. dose for serious, irreversible effect; and D1 = min. dose for the most minor effect.

3. Some Ds can be expressed only qualitatively, as a set of conditions (e.g., conditions leading to physical or psychological stress). The Ds are expressed in the terms or units that are relevant to the responses.

4. Ds are derived by considering the nature of the data upon which they are based, the nature of the population whose risk is being assessed, and sources of variability and uncertainty in the data and the population under assessment.

5. Table to be accompanied by narrative description of its scientific basis.

6. In the typical regulatory use of this framework, health protection standards fall somewhere between D=0 and D1.

to cause only minor, reversible effects (e.g., irritation of the eyes, airways, or skin); and doses above D2A might be highly hazardous; and doses above D3A are likely to be lethal. Again, the measurement of dose will vary according to the stressor.

For some stressors, to which deployed forces might be exposed by more than one route, it might be necessary to develop a separate dose-response profile for each route. The risk assessor will need to determine whether specific responses are restricted to a specific route (in which case doses incurred by that route are to be considered independent of doses incurred by other routes) or whether doses from all relevant routes are to be combined. If the latter is the case, some means will have to be found to limit the allowable Ds by each route, so that combined exposures by several routes do not exceed the total allowable D. Finally, it should be emphasized that for some stressors, the Ds can be expressed only qualitatively, or semi-quantitatively, as a set of environmental conditions. Some means will have to be found to define such Ds in usable ways—a simple, narrative statement for example—that can be included as footnotes to the table.

Considerations in the Development of Dose-Response Information for Table 2

Thresholds

For many if not most of the stressors of concern, there will be some dose (broadly defined to include all relevant conditions of exposure) that must be exceeded before even minimal adverse effects are produced. The so-called threshold dose will vary among stressors, with different effects of the same stressor, and will also vary among individuals in a population. The doses labeled D1 in Table 2 are intended to represent minimum-effect doses, and thus will lie just above the threshold dose. Just as threshold doses will vary among members of a population, according to their individual sensitivities, so will the D1s and all the other Ds in the dose-response table. One challenge for risk assessment is the problem of estimating Ds for populations having the characteristics of deployed forces, when the data from which they are to be estimated derive from different human populations or from experimental animals (Dourson et al. 1996).

The Possibility That Some Stressors Do Not Display Thresholds

It might be the case that some stressors, particularly biological and chemical agents designed as weapons of war, have threshold doses and minimum effective doses that are so small that it is practically impossible to avoid seriously harmful exposures. For such stressors, it might be that all doses are to be considered harmful, and the critical assessment of risks comes only in the exposure assessment step, where the probability of exposure becomes the determinant of risk.

Some chemical carcinogens and forms of radiation are thought to pose risks at all nonzero exposures (NRC 1994, EPA 1996). In the regulatory context, described earlier, it was seen that carcinogenic chemicals and radiation are assumed to pose risks at all exposures greater than zero, and that their risks increase in proportion to dose. The adoption of linear, no-threshold models to describe low-dose risks for carcinogenic substances is based in part on biological evidence and in part on science policy assumptions and public health dictates that involve the precautionary principle (NRC 1994).

It should be emphasized that with respect to such carcinogenic agents, it has not been considered necessary to reduce exposures to zero (to ban products) to protect public health. Rather, the approach has been to reduce exposures to those corresponding to low levels of risk (as estimated using linear, no-threshold models). The Occupational Safety and Health Administration (OSHA) and the Nuclear Regulatory Commission have, in a relatively large number of decisions, not forced lifetime risks for occupational carcinogens to levels below about 1 in 10,000 (Rodricks 1992, 1994). Standards for carcinogens established by these agencies are, it should be noted, often accompanied by warnings to workers and other protections to ensure that excessive exposures do not occur, or occur only rarely.

It is likely that some of the stressors to be encountered by deployed forces will be carcinogenic. In many, if not most cases, these exposures will be limited in duration and will often occur only intermittently. The occupational groups of concern to the OSHA and the Nuclear Regulatory Commission are usually exposed every working day, and for a working lifetime. It is possible that exposures to carcinogens of the type expected for deployed forces will pose little or no risk because of their limited duration. Some such stressors (e.g., those that are direct-acting, genotoxic substances) might pose risks of cancer even after a few exposures (EPA 1996).

Other mechanistic considerations enter the picture. It is now widely recognized that not all carcinogens operate by the same mechanisms, and that, irrespective of the exposure duration, some of these carcinogens are likely to operate by threshold mechanisms, and so their dose-response evaluation might proceed as it does for other threshold stressors (see paper by Rozman in these proceedings).

Judgments regarding the appropriate approach of low-dose risk assessment for such stressors, in the context of the exposures to be experienced by deployed forces, will have to be left to experts in toxicology and carcinogenicity, and case-by-case decisions will have to be made. If threshold and minimum effect doses (Ds) can be identified and justified, then their estimation will proceed as with other threshold stressors. If there are some stressors that are thought to present risks at all nonzero exposures, then a decision will have to be made regarding the level of risk that is to be considered minimal. Precedents from the OSHA and the Nuclear Regulatory Commission might be useful to guide such decisions (Rodricks 1992).

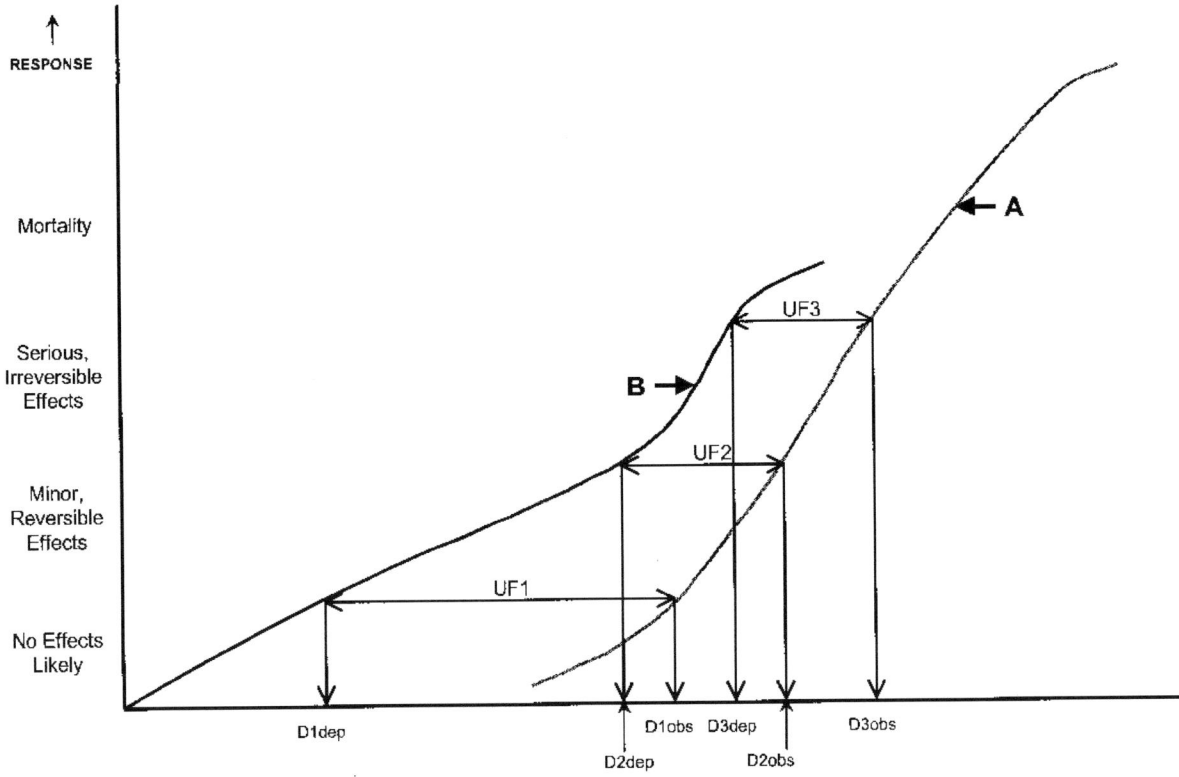

FIGURE 3 Hypothetical dose-response relationships for exposure to a hazardous stressor. Curve A is a composite relationship derived from the available date relating to D*obs* to response. In most actual cases, information for different portions of Curve A will derive from different studies or sources. Curve B is the relationship intended to apply to deployed forces. UFs are uncertainty factors applied to deal with uncertainties in the observed data. UFs vary as a function of the nature, quality, and representativeness of the observed data. The Ds are expressed in whatever units or terms are relevant to the response for the particular agent under review. D1*dep*, D2*dep*, and D3*dep* are transferred to table format in Table 2.

Estimating Critical Risk Doses (Ds) for Deployed Forces

Figure 3 displays two hypothetical dose-response curves for a stressor of concern. The response axis is divided into the four categories of adverse effects already discussed. Along the dose axis are a range of increasing doses expressed in units or terms appropriate to the stressor. Curve A represents the dose-response relationship for the agent and, as discussed earlier, one curve will be developed for acute exposures, another for intermediate exposures, and a third for chronic exposures. It can be seen that the available evidence suggests that no effects are expected until the dose labeled D1*obs* is reached, and that effects become increasingly serious as the dose is increased to D2*obs* and D3*obs*.

This observed dose-response relationship might not, indeed is likely not, to come from any single study. It is more likely to represent a composite of data from several studies, some involving human subjects and some involving experimental animal subjects. For some stressors, data might not be available to describe such a relationship in full; in fact, incomplete data are likely in many cases. For the present, it will be assumed that the evidence will allow estimation of a relationship approximating Curve A in Figure 3.

It must now be considered that the data supporting Curve A will in most cases be derived from studies in population groups that might or might not represent the range of sensitivities expected in the population of deployed forces. Moreover, in many cases, the observed data will have been derived from animal studies. As in all areas of risk assessment, it must be decided how well the observed dose-response data represent the population—in this case deployed forces—that is the subject of the risk assessment.

It is the general practice in risk assessment to evaluate potential differences in response between the subjects studied and those that are the subjects of the risk assessment (NRC 1994; Dourson et al. 1996). As a starting point, deployed forces represent a segment of the human population that is generally the healthiest and, therefore, the least vulnerable to the adverse effects of environmental stressors. In this respect, they are like many other occupational cohorts—children, the aged, the infirm, and individuals with debilitating health conditions are generally excluded. The importance of these observations lies in the fact that not only are deployed forces likely to be less sensitive or vulnerable to the adverse effects of stressors in the environment, but the range of variability in response is also likely to be much smaller than it is for the general population.

Deployment is, it should be emphasized, an unusual situation that most individuals never have to face. It is possible that normally healthy individuals, who should be the most resistant to the effects of environmental stressors, might, under conditions of deployment, become more vulnerable than would ordinarily be expected. This subject requires more review and analysis by participants in the risk-assessment process. It should probably not be assumed, without further investigation, that deployed forces are no more vulnerable to environmental stressors than are ordinary occupational cohorts.

Within the context of risk assessment, it is necessary that experts make some judgment regarding how well the population studied represents the population of deployed forces. Once this judgment is made, uncertainty factors (UFs) are introduced to estimate critical doses applicable to deployed forces. These are noted in Figure 3 as D1*dep*, D2*dep*, and D3*dep*, and Curve B represents an approximation of the dose-response relationship for deployed forces. No particular UF is to be inferred from Figure 3, although UFs of differing magnitude, including UFs of magnitude 1, are possible, depending upon the nature of the database used to develop the composite Curve A.

Text Box 1 presented some UFs commonly used by regulatory agencies for assessing variability in thresholds for toxic chemicals among humans and differences in response between experimental animals and humans. It should be emphasized that the specific UFs listed in Text Box 1 are intended to apply to the general population, in which more individuals of greater sensitivity will be present than in the population of deployed forces, and in which a wider range of sensitivities is expected. No similar standardized UFs have been established for occupational groups; rather, case-by-case judgments have been made. It is expected that such case-by-case judgments will also have to be made in the context of risks to deployed forces, taking into account the ways in which such populations might differ from their ordinary occupational cohorts.

It should also be pointed out that there are often uncertainties other than those related to variabilities in response between experimental animals and humans and variabilities among members of the human population. UFs have been used to compensate for other types of data limitations (e.g., for the absence of data relating to chronic exposures, or for the absence of data on the minimum effective dose [D1]). Within the field of toxicological risk assessment, it is accepted practice to introduce UFs, in the manner described above, as long as some justification is given for their use. It is not clear that such precedents exist in other areas of risk assessment, so that further discussion of this important issue will be needed before appropriate methodologies can be described.

Creating Dose-Response Tables and Narratives

The derivations of estimated critical doses for each stressor and for each of the three different exposure durations, as depicted in Figure 3, lead to the estimates necessary to create Table 2. It is proposed that Table 2 be accompanied by a narrative statement of its basis. With this table and statement, the hazard identification and dose-response steps of the risk assessment will be complete.

Relationships to Existing Standards

OSHA, EPA, the American Conference of Governmental Industrial Hygienists, and other organizations have published chemical and biological exposure guidelines for many chemical and some biological stressors. Several compilations of recommended exposure limits for short-term exposures are also available for some chemicals (USACHPPM 1999; see references therein). These various recommended exposure limits were developed in a variety of contexts, and for a number of reasons might not be directly applicable to the risk-assessment goals presented here. Some elaboration of this point is necessary.

First, it should be recognized that most existing occupational exposure guidelines are intended to be applied as lines of demarcation between safe (risk free) and unsafe (risky) exposures. They were derived to provide risk managers with a simple yes-no decision model. (Although the developers of these various limits recognize that occasional excursions above them are not necessarily harmful, they are nevertheless applied as if such excursions should be avoided.) This yes-no approach is suitable for situations in which risk mangers are in a position, through careful planning, to control exposures (in a regulatory context), and to ensure that when (in the case of accidents) exposures cannot be controlled, individuals can be removed from affected areas. The yes-no model is most useful in circumstances such as these.

The circumstances in which deployed forces might become exposed are often not controllable in the same way, and in many cases some degree of harm will not be avoidable. The type of information on risk proposed here, as expressed in Table 2, provides decision-makers far more information on the likelihood, magnitude, and seriousness of the risks that might arise under different conditions.

Most existing occupational and general population standards are also intended to represent exposures that are not likely to pose any discernible risk. They thus fall somewhere in the no-effects-likely zones of Table 2 and Figure 3. Their relationships to the minimum-effective dose (D1) is ascertainable by reference to the data upon which those standards are based, but cannot otherwise be known. In the context of exposures incurred by deployed forces, it is not sufficient for decision-makers simply to be aware of the no-likely-risk exposure, but rather it is necessary that such decision-makers have knowledge of the exposure at which adverse effects are first expected (D1), and the levels at which serious effects are likely to occur (D2 and D3). (It is recognized that recent efforts by EPA and the NRC are directed at developing the type of dose-response information for acute exposures that is proposed here, although with the intention that they be applied to the general population.)

Other differences between available occupational standards and those to be developed for deployed forces need to be considered. For example, occupational standards are generally applicable to workers exposed 8 hours a day and 5 days a week, for a working lifetime. Deployed forces might be exposed to some stressors for 24 hours a day, and on every day, but are not likely to be exposed for a working lifetime. Some stressors for which there are inhalation occupational standards might be present as contaminants of the food or water of deployed forces. For these several reasons and more as well, great care must be taken in using available occupational standards, and certainly in using standards developed by EPA or FDA to protect the general population, without considering their relevance to the nature of the population of deployed forces and their applicability to the risk-assessment requirements depicted in

Table 2. No doubt some of the information used to develop available occupational standards can be used for assessing risks to deployed forces, but wholesale adoption of such standards without critical review will lead to a wholly different and far less useful risk-assessment model. The earlier point, that deployed forces might not be similar in sensitivity to ordinary occupational cohorts, needs also to be considered.

The U.S. Army Center for Health Promotion and Preventive Medicine (ACHPPM) has developed in an undated draft form, a set of *Short-Term Chemical Exposure Guidelines for Deployed Military Personnel*. These guidelines were developed for air and water contaminants, and are intended to cover a range of exposure durations, from 1 hour to 14 days (air), and from 5 days to 2 weeks (water). Considerable effort and thought has gone into the development of the guidelines, and ACHPPM has drawn from the work of the NRC and other expert regulatory and scientific authorities. The guidelines are, however, conceptually similar to regulatory standards, and do not present the more thorough dose-response and long-term exposure information envisioned herein. It is, however, a possibly usable model for yes-no decision-making.

ASSESSMENT OF EXPOSURES OF DEPLOYED FORCES

Using the Results of the Hazard and Dose-Response Evaluations (Table 2)

Referring to Figure 2, and the model proposed herein for decision-making (Model II), it can be seen that it is now necessary to discuss the problem of assessing the exposures to stressors expected or incurred by deployed forces. Health risks to be expected or incurred can be identified only if such an exposure assessment can be completed. In effect, the purpose of the exposure assessment step is to estimate the doses (Ds) of the stressor to be expected or incurred by forces under the circumstances of deployment. Such estimates will allow risk managers to understand the extent and severity of the expected health risk by reference to the proposed dose-response (Table 2). A discussion of some of the issues that need to be resolved to develop adequate exposure information for use in risk assessment, as well as a discussion of the various options for risk-management decision-making, follows.

Measurement or Estimation of Doses

For some stressors of concern, analytical methods are or will be available to measure directly the doses to which deployed forces might be exposed. In other cases, methods are or will be available to measure concentrations of stressors in the various environmental media to which deployed forces might be exposed; these measurements of concentrations might or might not be direct measurements of the relevant doses, and means will have to be developed to convert concentration information to dose information. The subject of the availability of reliable analytical methods for measuring stressor doses or concentrations is not discussed in this paper. It is assumed that such methods are or will become available. Without such methods, it will not be possible to understand the nature or magnitude of the risks expected or incurred by deployed forces.

This paper is concerned, instead, with the methods for evaluating exposure information for purposes of use in risk assessment. Two approaches to acquiring relevant dose estimates are available:

1. Estimation of doses expected to be incurred under various deployment scenarios, in advance of deployment; and

2. Measurement of doses during deployment (real time measurement).

Both of these approaches have value. The first can be used for planning purposes, and can guide risk management on the stressors expected to be of greatest concern during specific deployments. The second can provide direct measurement data during deployment; by quick reference to the dose-response information, immediate knowledge of potential health risks can be acquired.

As previously discussed, there are some stressors that are so extremely hazardous that there might be no practical means to ensure health protection of exposure were it to occur. For such stressors, the exposure assessment would take the form of an estimation of the probability of exposure expected under various deployment scenarios; the availability of such estimates would allow appropriate safeguard planning in advance of deployment. The use of this approach for some stressors falls within the framework for risk assessment proposed in this paper; it simply recognizes the fact that exposures to certain extremely dangerous stressors must be prevented if health is to be protected, and uses projected estimates of the probability of exposure as a guide to risk management.

The Need for Commensurate Measurement of Dose

For each stressor it is necessary that the measurement of dose expected or incurred by deployed forces be the same as that in which its risk information is presented in Table 2. Thus, the experts involved in the estimation or measurement of doses need to have knowledge of the requirements for risk assessment. In many cases there will be little difficulty meeting these requirements. Risk doses for chemical contaminants of air, for example, will ordinarily be expressed in units of air concentration times duration ($c \times t$); analytical methods for such contaminants can readily provide the same data for deployed forces. Similarly, the dose information for risks of contaminants of drinking water can be expressed as drinking-water concentrations, based on the incorporation of knowledge of the daily water consumption rates of deployed forces.

Food contamination presents a somewhat more difficult problem, because it might be difficult to predict the specific dietary component that will become contaminated with a given stressor. Rates of consumption of different components of the diet vary greatly, so that contamination of a greatly consumed component at a given concentration of a stressor will result in a larger dose than does contamination (at the same concentration) of a little-consumed item. The most conservative approach for food is one that assumes that each component of the diet constitutes the total daily diet, but such an approach might lead to large overestimates of risk in many situations. Further discussion of the question of the appropriate expressions of dose for food contamination will be necessary before the problem can be resolved.

The greatest exposure assessment difficulty arises when a given stressor might contaminate all environmental media. In those instances in which the dose-response evaluation demonstrates that risks by one route of exposure are different from and independent of risks resulting from other routes, then the problem is somewhat simplified, in that air exposures can be evaluated separately from exposures through food and water (and possibly soil), as can dermal exposures. Even in this simplified case, it will still be necessary to express risk doses as concentrations in food and water (and perhaps soil) to ensure that the total oral dose from all sources can be estimated. Thus, data or assumptions regarding relative rates of consumption of food and water will have to be incorporated into the evaluation. Clearly, if risks are additive across all exposure routes, the problem is even more difficult. The problem can be at this time only pointed out, but it cannot be resolved without discussions among the risk-assessment experts during the evaluation of specific stressors (Lioy 1997).

Risk Characterization and Decision-Making

Completion of the exposure assessment step for deployed forces provides the information necessary to assess risks. At this stage, estimated Ds incurred by deployed forces are evaluated by reference to Table 2 that is applicable to the stressor of concern. In the ideal, risk managers would have an understanding of each of the risks faced by deployed forces in a given deployment situation and would also have an understanding of the new risks that might arise should various actions be taken to alter the circumstances of deployment. The availability of all this risk information would presumably allow the best possible decisions, given the deployment circumstances and the alternatives available, to minimize overall risks to health. The risk-assessment framework proposed here, although identical to that ordinarily used in regulations, is not intended to yield results that are used only to establish standards. Rather, they are intended to give DOD decision-makers sufficient information to examine a range of risks that might arise in rapidly changing deployment conditions, and to balance competing risks. It recognizes that a simplistic yes-no decision-making model is inadequate to deal with the circumstances under which forces are deployed, and that in many cases some risks will have to be incurred. The framework offered here provides decision-makers sufficient understanding of the range of exposures over which risks of differing severity might occur (Table 2), and thus maximizes the likelihood that the most serious hazards can be avoided.

REFERENCES

Barnes, D.G., and M. Dourson. 1988. Reference dose (RfD): description and use in health risk assessments. Regul. Toxicol. Pharmacol. 8:471-486.

Bogen, K.T. 1990. Uncertainty in Environmental Health Risk Assessment. New York, N.Y.: Garland Pub.

Calabrese, E. 1983. Chapter 1. In: Principles of Animal Extrapolation. New York, N.Y.: John Wiley and Sons.

Department of the Air Force. 1998. Pp. 91-215. In: Operational Risk Management (ORM) Guidelines and Tools. Air Force Pamphlet 91-215. Department of the Air Force, Washington, D.C. (July).

Department of the Army. 1998. Risk Management. Field Manual No. 100-14. Department of the Army, Washington, D.C.

Dourson, M.L., S.P. Felter, and D. Robinson. 1996. Evaluation of science-based uncertainty factors in noncancer risk assessment. Regul. Toxicol. Pharmacol. 24:108-120.

EPA (U.S. Environmental Protection Agency). 1996. Proposed Guidelines for Carcinogen Risk Assessment. Office of Research and Development. Fed. Register 51:33992-34003.

Finkel, A. 1990. Confronting uncertainty in risk management: A guide for decision-makers. Washington, D.C.: Center for Risk Management. Resources for the Future.

Hill, A.B. 1965. The environment and disease: Association or causation? Proc. R.l Soc. Med. 58:295-300.

Lioy, P.J. 1997. Exposure analysis and its assessment. Pp. 39-50. In: Comprehensive Toxicology. Vol I: General Principles, I.G. Sipes, C.A. McQueen, A.J. Gandolfi, and J. Bond, eds. Pergamon.

Naval Safety Center. 1996. Draft Reference Guide for Operational Risk Management. DSN 564-3520 x7277. Online. Available: http//:safetycenter.navy.mil/

NRC (National Research Council). 1983. Risk Assessment in the Federal Government: Managing the Process. Washington, D.C.: National Academy Press.

NRC (National Research Council). 1986. Criteria and Methods for Preparing Emergency Exposure Guidance Level (EEGL), Short-term Public Emergency Guidance Level (SPEGL), and Continuous Exposure Guidance Level (EGL) Documents. Washington, D.C.: National Academy Press.

NRC (National Research Council). 1994. Science and Judgment in Risk Assessment. Washington, D.C.: National Academy Press.

Rodricks, J.V. 1992. Assessing risk. Pp.180-201. In: Calculated Risks, Understanding the Toxicity and Human Health Risk of Chemicals in Our Environment. Cambridge, Mass.: Cambridge University Press.

Rodricks, J.V. 1992. Managing. Pp. 202-223. In: Calculated Risks, Understanding the Toxicity and Human Health Risk of Chemicals in Our Environment. Cambridge, Mass.: Cambridge University Press.

Rodricks, J.V. 1994. Risk assessment, the environment, and public health. Environ. Health Perspect. 102:258-264.

USACHPPM.(U.S. Army Center for Health Promotion and Preventive Medicine). 1999. The Medical NBC Battlebook. Department of Defense. Online. Available: http://chppm-www.argea.army.mil

USACHPPM (U.S. Army Center for Health Promotion and Preventive Medicine). 1999. Draft. Short-Term Chemical Exposures Guidelines for Deployed Military Personnel. T6-230A. Aberdeen Proving Ground, Edgewood, MD. (March.)

Future Health Assessment and Risk-Management Integration for Infectious Diseases and Biological Weapons for Deployed U.S. Forces

by Joan B. Rose[1]

ABSTRACT

The health of the United States armed forces has been viewed as a critical component of the strength, readiness, and effectiveness of the military's ability to meet various degrees of threats to peace, human rights abuses, and other global disasters in the United States and the world. Compared with any other country or entity in the world, the U.S. military has one of the best surveillance and monitoring systems for assessing the risk of infectious disease globally. The monitoring is broad-based, specific for a large list of pathogenic agents, but includes generic symptomology that might be due to a multitude of current, emerging, or reemerging microorganisms; the monitoring is also timely. Gastrointestinal illness and respiratory and skin infections remain a problem for deployed troops.

It is now well known that microbial infections can result in chronic outcomes associated with heart, neurological, and immunological disorders. Therefore, hospitalization data will no longer suffice as the sole measure of severity and lost effectiveness to the troop force at large. Better assessment of antibiotic-resistant bacteria, coxsackieviruses, and Legionella and an evaluation of the underdiagnosis and underreporting of protozoa such as Cryptosporidium are needed. New microorganisms are being reported every year that might be associated with many of these illnesses, and prospective surveillance might be needed using new techniques to better understand the infection rates and asymptomatic infections.

Risk-assessment methods can now be used to quantify the risk of microbial infections and to address exposure and potential outcome from naturally occurring microorganisms and biological weapons. Hazard identification includes the identification of the microbial agent as well as the spectrum of human illnesses ranging from asymptomatic infections to death. The host response to the microorganisms with regard to immunity and multiple exposures should be addressed here, as well as the adequacy of animal models for studying human impacts. Endemic and epidemic disease investigations, case studies, hospi-

---

[1]Department of Marine Sciences, University of South Florida, 140 7th Ave., S., St. Petersburg, FL, 33701; email: jrose@seas.marine.usf.edu.

talization studies, and other epidemiological data are needed to complete this step in the risk assessment. The variables need to be carefully defined and the data quantified as ratios. The dose-response assessment is the mathematical characterization of the relationship between the dose administered and the probability of infection or disease in the exposed population. Dose-response assessments have been referred to as probability-of-infection models, which are developed from mostly human volunteer studies. The exposure assessment determines the size and nature of the population exposed, the route, concentrations, and distribution of the microorganisms, and the duration of the exposure. The description of exposure includes not only occurrence based on concentrations but also the prevalence (how often the microorganisms are found) and distribution of microorganisms in space and over time. Exposure assessment is determined through occurrence monitoring and predictive microbiology. Quantitative risk characterization should estimate the magnitude of the public health problem, and demonstrate the variability and uncertainty of the hazard, using four distributions: (1) the spectrum of health outcomes; (2) the confidence limits surrounding the dose-response model; (3) the distribution of the occurrence of the microorganism; and (4) the exposure distribution. Assessments of occurrence and exposure can be further delineated by distributions surrounding the method of recovery and survival (treatment) distributions.

The risk-assessment framework already fits into the Department of Defense's (DOD's) programs associated with risk management. The critical need will be the development of databases that can be used in the decision and management process. Although health outcomes and morbidity and mortality statistics are available from numerous databases and surveillance programs, the data lacking are often the long-term assessments and chronic outcomes. The exposure assessment, particularly during deployment, is more suspect to uncertainty, especially in terms of quantitative evaluations. Geographic, climatic, seasonal, dose-response, and exposure scenarios can be used to develop tools for setting priorities for assessment of predeployment risks. Risk models can be evaluated for plausibility during outbreak investigations or disease surveillance operations. Exposure and health outcomes must be better assessed.

The use of quantitative assessments allows one to begin to build exposure scenarios in which thresholds associated with ineffectiveness in the troops in a given time frame can be determined for specific agents. For biological weapons, dose-response models should be developed and time and concentration exposure and consequence scenarios should be built and evaluated.

Finally, the formal expansion of DOD's mission on emerging infectious diseases in June 1996 by Presidential Decision Directive NSTC-7 now includes global surveillance, training, research, and response. One of the major assets in implementing this new directive is the overseas research laboratory system that is currently in place: the DOD Infectious Disease Research Laboratories. At a minimum, each laboratory staff should be trained in risk-assessment methods, should have molecular capabilities (polymerase chain reaction [PCR]), and be trained in the use of the global information system (GIS) for maintaining and analyzing the databases.

INTRODUCTION

The health of United States armed forces has been viewed as a critical component of the strength, readiness, and effectiveness of the military's ability to meet various degrees of threats to peace, human rights abuses, and other global disasters in the United States and the world. Much effort has gone into the development of frameworks for addressing the hazards that the military might face, particularly when deployed to hostile and foreign environments. A deployment of U.S. troops is defined as a "movement resulting from a Joint Chiefs of Staff /unified command deployment order for 30 continuous days or greater to a land-based location outside the United States that does not have a permanent U.S. military medical treatment facility" (Memorandum for Under Secretary of Defense for Personnel and Readiness, Office of the Chairman, The Joint Chiefs of Staff, December 4, 1998).

There has been a tremendous change throughout the twentieth century in the types of health risks that the armed forces might face, and in the ability to identify and monitor these risks and to manage or control them. Health surveillance has improved and there is an enhanced ability to monitor the environment for hazardous exposures. Despite these gains, as the twenty-first century nears, the world is faced with the emergence and reemergence of infectious diseases. Disease surveillance at the global level has identified, in addition to endemic levels of diarrhea and respiratory disease, new bacteria, parasites, and viruses. These have been identified through dramatic outbreaks such as Legionnaire's disease from the bacterium *Legionella* and hemorrhagic fevers associated with the Hanta virus and other types of viruses; specific studies associating peptic ulcer disease and *Helicobacter*; epidemic levels of bloodborne and sexually transmitted HIV; and outbreaks of *Cryptosporidiosis* from drinking water and *Escherichia coli* 0157:H7 from food (Lederberg 1997). In addition, antibiotic resistance has emerged, causing a threat to the control of old-world killers such as tuberculosis.

There is currently a greater appreciation of the diversity, adaptability, and evolutionary complexities associated with infectious diseases, and much of this appreciation has been gained through research and studies with new molecular techniques. The technological advances in the study of microbiology, infectious disease, and molecular biology have also paved the way for a potential increased risk associated with the development and use of biological weapons.

Force Health Protection (FHP) is a framework that describes procedures for assessing the types of hazards, the exposure and populations at risk, and the monitoring of the health of all personnel deployed. FHP and other force protection plans have adapted various versions of the National Research Council's (NRC's) risk-assessment paradigm and integrated this assessment into management strategies to address the health of troops before, during, and after deployment and to protect defense personnel from hazardous chemicals and toxic materials. The use of this type of framework for biological and infectious agents is relatively new.

Risk-assessment methods following the NRC paradigm were initially used on a limited scale for judging waterborne pathogenic microorganisms (Haas 1983; Gerba and Haas 1988; Regli et al. 1991; Rose and Gerba, 1991; Rose et al. 1991; Haas et al. 1993). Haas (1983) was the first to look quantitatively at microbial risks associated with drinking water based on dose-response modeling. Rose et al. (1991) used an exponential model with quantitative risk assessment in the development of the Surface Water Treatment Rule to address in particular the performance-based standards for the control of *Giardia* as part of the requirements under the Safe Drinking Water Act (EPA 1989). Currently, risk assessment is being used for assessing food protection programs.

In a study for the U.S. Army, Cooper et al. (1986) attempted to quantify the risks of water-related infection and illness to Army units in the field. They reviewed the literature on infectious dose and clinical illness for potential waterborne pathogens. Using this information, the probability of infection was assessed using logistic, beta, exponential, and lognormal models. A generalized model was then developed incorporating expected pathogenic concentrations, consumption volume, and risk of infection for different military units. The study attempted to incorporate organism concentrations, effective treatment, and risk of infection. This attempt, however, was hampered by a limited existing database on microbial concentrations and infectious dose.

Quantitative microbial risk assessment (QMRA) has now gained wide acceptance in the evaluation of waterborne and foodborne disease. Methods and databases for development of QMRA for microbial agents associated with airborne, vectorborne, and dermal exposure have received less attention. However, the data on health, exposure, and dose-response, although limited, might be sufficient for undertaking preliminary risk assessments. The development of QMRAs along with improved methods for environmental monitoring will likely lead to more effective management and prevention strategies for U.S. deployed troops.

The purpose of this report is to:

- summarize the emerging infectious diseases and microbiological contaminant risks that U.S. deployed troops might face currently and in the future;
- briefly examine the various health disease databases that are available; and
- address quantitative research and data needs for integration of the microbial and biological risks into DOD risk-assessment and risk-management frameworks.

REVIEW OF PAST INCIDENCES AND FUTURE RISKS

Disease and Non-Battle-Injury Reports

Health promotion and disease prevention in the field are seen as critical to deployed troops, because illness can significantly compromise the objectives of the mission. Surveillance of infectious disease risks are determined by measured rates, usually as the number of people who have disease X per 1,000 or 10,000 people per some unit of time. In U.S. health databases, the rates are usually reported on an annual basis per 10,000 or 100,000 people. It is important to understand that most infections and diseases are underreported because of the failure of individuals to seek medical attention, laboratories to conduct proper tests, and the reporting system.

The identification of disease (or illness) is made by one of several methods (Table 1). The difference between disease and illness is minor in some cases. Disease is defined as the process or mechanism that ultimately results in an illness or a condition that impairs vital functions. An individual could have a disease without initially having any symptoms. Symptoms are effects of the illness that can be described by the individual who is ill, also known as self-reporting (e.g., headache, diarrhea, stomach cramps, vomiting, fatigue). Clinical assessment of the illness is generally defined by a measurable description of the illness (e.g., fever, bloody stool). Infection is colonization of the microorganism in the body and might result in disease and symptoms, which is the initial step in the microbial disease process. However, this can also result in asymptomatic, or subclinical, infections. Symptoms and clinical descriptions (fever, rash, inflammation) can be very specific, as with measles, which is associated with one specific agent, or they can be generic, as with diarrhea, which is associated with many different types of microorganisms.

The second means of identification is clinical diagnosis, which is the detection of the specific microorganism in a host specimen (e.g., laboratory identification in a liquid stool of an enteric pathogen). This requires the collection of a specimen (sputum, feces, blood, biopsy) and a specific diagnostic test (specific growth, biochemical tests, stains, genetic or protein markers, microscopic identification). This also means that there is some understanding of the agents that might be responsible for the disease symptoms and the process of disease resulting in the infection of specific cells or organs in the body. Infection without the individual reporting symptoms (an asymptomatic infection) can be detected by clinical diagnosis.

The final method of identification is associated with the response of the host system to infection that elicits an antibody response that can be detected in blood or, in some cases, saliva. This antibody response might be associated with past or current exposure, and in some cases, depending on the type of antibody and amount, one can determine the approximate timing of the exposure and infection. Expo-

TABLE 1 Methods for Diagnosing Infections and Disease

Method	Approach	Advantages and Disadvantages
Symptoms and clinical descriptors	Based on individual's feelings (headache) and measurable impacts (fever, rash).	Can easily diagnose, or identify individuals; however is not generally agent specific but more generic (e.g., diarrhea).
Clinical diagnosis	Based on testing specimens (sputum, feces or blood) for presence of the agent.[a]	Can specifically identify agent; however individual must deliver a specimen and there must exist a test method for the agent.
Antibody response (serological testing)	An indirect test (blood or in some cases saliva) for the presence of antibodies that the body produces as a result of infection.[b]	Is specific to the agent and in some cases might be able to determine the timing of the exposure and infection. Test method must exist.

[a]Asymptomatic infections can be detected.
[b]Antibody response may or may not be protective from subsequent exposure and infection and does not usually occur without infection.
Source: Haas et al. 1999.

sure without infection rarely causes an antibody response, except in the case of repeated exposure to very high concentrations of the agent, such as occurs with some vaccinations.

The Disease and Non-Battle-Injury (DNBI) reporting system is a tool used at the unit level to assess the "vital signs of the unit." This system is set up to evaluate the health of individuals predeployment, during deployment, and post-deployment. The primary function of the DNBI reports is to bring immediate attention to unacceptable high rates of illness, and thus to provide better prevention, treatment, and intervention in a timely manner.

During predeployment, health is evaluated on self-reporting of symptoms; only a few specific tests are undertaken. Blood samples were rarely collected until the Bosnia deployment. Readiness is addressed through education and management approaches and immunizations:

• Health assessment undertaken based on self-reporting of symptomology. Testing for specific type of microbial agent only with referral.
• Specific tests: HIV (within 12 months) and tuberculosis skin test (within 24 months).
• Education on known biological, chemical, and physical hazards (providing known countermeasures, e.g., insect repellant).
• Immunizations: Required are tetanus-diphtheria, influenza, hepatitis A virus (HAV), measles-rubella/measles-mumps-rubella (MR/MMR), and polio. Others might include yellow fever, hepatitis B virus (HBV), typhoid, and plague.

During deployment, the DNBI reports are made weekly. The tracking of disease is summarized weekly and reported at measured rates in percentages based on the number of patients seen divided by the average troop strength deployed. These reports are based on self-reporting illnesses of a serious enough level to require a visit to the medical staff. Primary complaints and final diagnoses are included in the report, as well as days of light duty, lost work days, and admissions. Text Box 1, from the Memorandum for Under Secretary of Defense for Personnel and Readiness, Office of the Chairman, The Joint Chiefs of Staff, December 4, 1998, has the list of infectious agents that are reportable.

> **TEXT BOX 1**
> **Tri-Service Reportable Medical Event List**
>
> Amebiasis
> Anthrax
> Biological Warfare Agent Exposure
> Botulism
> Brucellosis
> Campylobacter
> Carbon Monoxide Poisoning
> Chemical Agent Exposure
> Chlamydia
> Cholera
> Coccidioidomycosis
> Cold Weather Injury (All)
>   Frostbite
>   Hypothermia
>   Immersion Type
>   Unspecified
> Cryptosporidiosis
> Cyclospora
> Dengue Fever
> Diptheria
> E.coli 0157:h7
> Ehrlichiosis
> Encephalitis
> Filariasis
> Glardiasis
> Gonorrhea
> H. Influenzae, Invasive
> Hantavirus Infection
> Heat Injuries
>   Heat Exhaustion
>   Heat Stroke
>
> Hemorrhagic Fever
> Hepatitis A
> Hepatitis B
> Hepatitis C
> Influenza
> Lead Poisoning
> Legionellosis
> Leishmaniasis (All)
> Leishmaniasis.
>   Cutaneous
> Leishmaniasis.
>   Mucocutaneous
> Leishmaniasis.
>   Unspecified
> Leishmaniasis. Visceral
> Leprosy
> Leptospirosis
> Listeriosis
> Lyme Disease
> Malaria (All)
>   Malaria. Falciparum
>   Malaria. Mmalariae
>   Malaria. Ovale
>   Malaria. Unspecified
>   Malaria. Vivax
> Measles
> Meningococcal Disease
>   Meningitis
>   Septicemia
> Mumps
> Pertussis
> Plague
> Pneumococcal Pneumonia
>
> Poliomyelitis
> Q Fever
> Rabies, Human
> Relapsing Fever
> Rheumatic Fever, Acute
> Rift Valley Fever
> Rocky Mountain Spotted Fever
> Rubella
> Salmonellosis
> Schistosomiasis
> Shigellosis
> Smallpox
> Streptococcus. Group A, Invasive
> Syphilis (All)
>   Syphilis. Congenital
>   Syphilis. Latent
>   Syphilis. Primary/ secondary
>   Syphilis. Tertiary
> Tetanus
> Toxic Shock Syndrome
> Trichinosis
> Trypanosomiasis
> Tuberculosis. Pulmonary
> Tularemia
> Typhoid Fever
> Typhus Fever
> Urethritis. Non-gonococcal
> Vaccine, Adverse Event
> Varicella, Active Duty Only
> Yellow Fever
>
> Source: Memorandum (MCM-251-98) from Chairman of the Joint Chiefs of Staff dated 04 December 1998.

Suggested reference rates are rough general guidance numbers (acceptable limits); rates above these rates might indicate a problem. Expert judgment is used to make final decisions regarding the immediacy of the risks and the actions to be taken in further assessment and control. Temporal trends of illness are also tracked. Table 2 shows suggested limits for categories of general illnesses.

Upon post-deployment, health evaluations are again made by self-reporting of symptoms. Positive responses are followed up. However, no testing is undertaken routinely.

It is generally accepted that surveillance systems greatly underestimate the level of disease in any given community and, although providing a picture of past risk, thus might not accurately reflect future risk. This becomes problematic for emerging pathogens for which there is no established procedure for testing patients, and surveillance systems rarely address the various exposure or transmission pathways.

TABLE 2 Weekly DNBI Report for Category of Illness and Suggested Acceptable Levels

Category	Suggested Reference Rate[a]
Combat/operational-stress reactions	0.1% (1/1,000)
Dermatological	0.5% (5/1,000)
GI, infectious	0.5%
Gynecologic	0.5%
Heat/cold injuries	0.5%
Injury: recreational/sports	1.0% (10/1,000)
Injury: motor vehicle accidents	1.0%
Injury: work/training	1.0%
Injury: other	1.0%
Ophthalmologic	0.1%
Psychiatric, mental disorders	0.1%
Respiratory	0.4% (4/1,000)
STDs	0.5%
Fever, unexplained	0.0%
All other medical and surgical	
Total DNBI	4.0% (40/1,000)

[a]Time frame is weekly assessment.
Source: Memorandum (MCM-251-98) from Chairman of the Joint Chiefs of Staff dated 04 December 1998.

TABLE 3 Advantages and Limitations of the DNBI Report

Advantages	Limitations
1. Reports on generic symptoms (GI, respiratory).	1. Excludes *Helicobacter* and most enteric viruses.
2. Large number of agents that are reportable (Textbox 1).	2. Relies primarily on self-reporting; clinical diagnosis might not be routine (e.g., are all diarrhea specimens examined for *Cryptosporidium*?) and antibody assessments (seroprevalence data) are not routinely included (only in specialized reports).
3. Weekly reporting.	
4. Severity data recorded (days lost, hospitalization).	3. Report is indication of past exposures and might not indicate the route of exposure.
	4. Data on the unknown etiologies category are not included in the sum total.

In addition, outcome might be assessed by mortality in the extreme case or without identification of consequence (e.g., severity of the illness, number of days sick, medical care).

The advantages of the DNBI reporting system over most systems are in the broad scope of the specific and generic assessments made and the timeliness of the reporting. The DNBI systems might then identify unknown pathogens or microorganisms that cause more than one type of symptom in those exposed. There are a few limitations; for example, ulcers from the gastrointestinal infections are excluded, although it is now recognized that *Helicobacter* is a cause of this type of illness (Taylor and Blaser 1991). In addition, because most illnesses are exhibited after an incubation time ranging from 1 day (bacteria), 7 days (parasite), to 21 days (HAV), the DNBI record is a record of past exposures (Table 3).

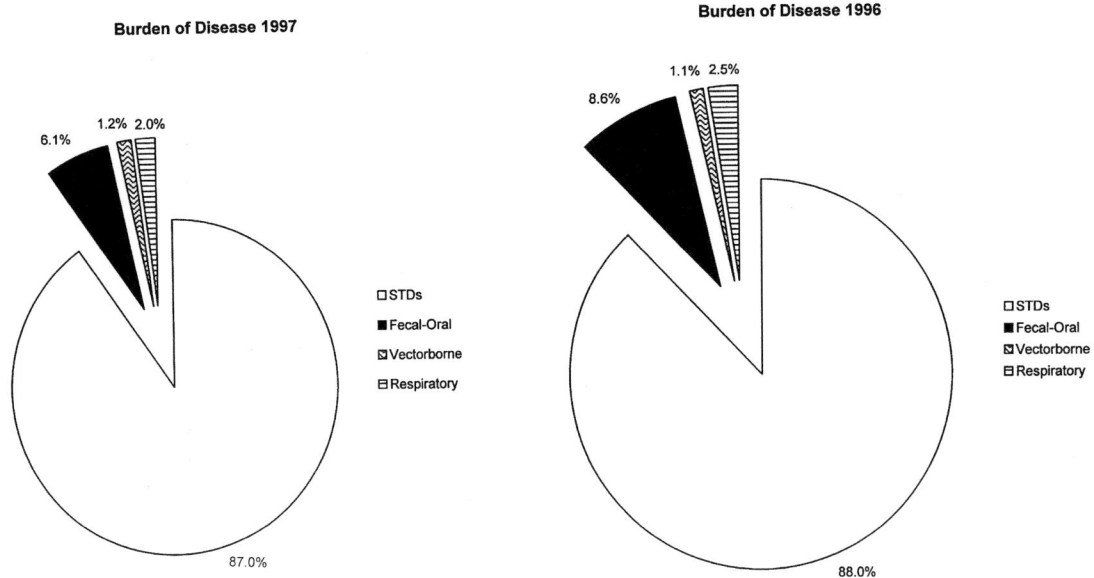

FIGURE 1 Conditions reported by the Defense Medical Surveillance System, Jan.-Dec., 1996 and 1997 (MSMR 1997a, 1998a).

The Defense Medical Surveillance System reports all DNBI data on a monthly basis. The following is a brief review of the cumulative 1997 and 1998 reports, followed by some summaries and conclusions.

Figure 1 shows the disease reports for 1996 and 1997 within the military for four main categories of illnesses by route of transmission (sexually-transmitted disease [STD], fecal-oral, vectorborne, and respiratory). These data come from 7,061 case reports in 1996 and 10,007 case reports in 1997. STDs accounted for 88% and 87% of the cases in 1996 and 1997, respectively (chlamydia, gonorrhea, urethritis, herpes, and then syphilis). Fecal-oral agents were second, contributing to 8.6% and 6.1% of the cases for the two years, respectively. Included in the top four in descending order were *Salmonella, Campylobacter, Shigella,* and *Giardia* in 1996, and *Salmonella, Shigella, Campylobacter,* and *Giardia* in 1997. Guillain-Barré syndrome, a neurological complication associated with *Campylobacter* infections was reported in both years (3 and 4 cases, respectively). This outcome has also been related to reactions to immunizations (Medical Surveillance Monthly Report (MSMR) 1995). Viral meningitis could likely be due to enteric viruses and should be considered fecal-oral (41 and 92 cases, respectively). Respiratory illness contributed to 2.5% and 2.0% in 1996 and 1997, respectively, with varicella contributing to most other cases, followed by influenza and tuberculosis. Vectorborne diseases were associated with 1.1% and 1.2% of the cases for 1996 and 1997, respectively. Malaria, leishmaniasis, and Lyme disease were the top microbial pathogens in this category.

Hospitalization records and days lost from effective work were used to evaluate the severity of the outcomes. When muscular and joint problems were excluded (which are the number one cause of reported hospitalizations) the top five causes of hospitalizations were diseases of the digestive system, followed by respiratory diseases, genitourinary diseases, infectious and parasitic diseases, and diseases of the skin and subcutaneous tissue (Figure 2).

These data are for all troops stationed in the United States, Europe, Pacific, and other regions (e.g., Korea). No discernable differences were noted geographically for the STDs. Although STDs are

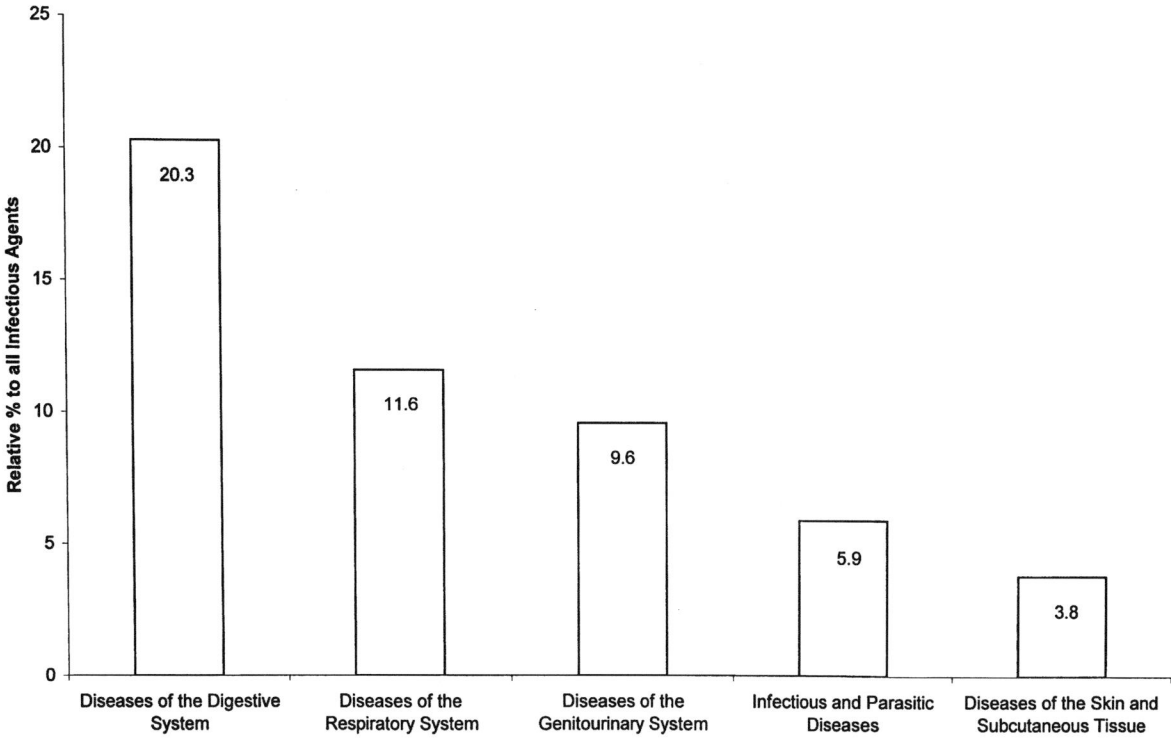

FIGURE 2 Severity based on active-duty hospitalization rates, U. S. Army (MSMR 1998b).

problematic, the attendance by a physician, diagnosis, and reporting are likely much greater than many of the other types of infections; thus, the infectious disease risks based on this reporting system appear skewed. These data might be particularly misleading regarding the risk for deployed troops outside the United States. The completeness of reporting is dependent on the etiological agent; for example, for the two militarily important tropical infectious diseases, malaria and leishmaniasis, reporting was 67% and 81% complete. Reporting of varicella and Lyme disease was 20 to 25% complete. For diseases such as hepatitis, dengue, and campylobacteriosis, 0% were reported of those that were reportable. Therefore, underreporting is likely a problem for many of the fecal-oral and respiratory agents.

Respiratory disease is one that continues to plague the troops. Recruits, trainees, and those upon initial deployment appear to be at greater risk. Immunizations are available for adenovirus Type 4 and Type 7 and the influenza viruses (Table 4). However, outbreaks of influenza continue to occur due to the variety of subtypes that exist throughout the world. In an outbreak of influenzalike illness in an aviation squadron in Hawaii, the efficacy of the vaccine for preventing the illness was only 16.7% (MSMR 1998c). Therefore, use of year-round vaccination and treatment has been able to reduce the respiratory disease but has not been able to eliminate it.

The military's surveillance program for respiratory disease includes 14 sentinel bases (seven foreign bases, Germany, Guam, two in Japan, Korea, Turkey, and United Kingdom, and seven U.S. bases, Alaska, California, Colorado, Mississippi, New Jersey, and two in Texas). Throat swabs are obtained from those who meet a case definition; therefore, asymptomatic cases are not detected.

Transmission of respiratory agents can be person to person through hands (thus handwashing can facilitate prevention) or through contaminated fomites (surface disinfection might prove useful for

TABLE 4 Results of the 1995-1996 Respiratory Surveillance Program

Microorganism	Number Isolated	Treatment/Vaccine	Comments
Streptococcus A Beta hemolytic	86/1,071 8%	Benazthine Penicillin Chemoprophylaxis	
Total viruses	512/1,634 31.8%		
Influenza A	358/1,634 22%	Vaccines	Nov.-Jan. peak
Influenza B	56/1,634 3.4%	Vaccines	Mar.-May peak
Enteroviruses	~52 3.2%	None	
Adenoviruses	~27 1.6%	Vaccine for Types 4 and 7	
Parainfluenza Types 1, 2, and 3	~12 0.7%	None	
Herpes simplex virus	~8 0.5%	None	

Source: MSMR 1996a.

prevention), and enteroviruses (coxsackieviruses) might account for some of the dramatic spread of infections through troops. Respiratory transmission (aerosolization) is the final route, although in some cases the pathway is not very well defined. Interestingly for Group A streptococci, Ferrieri et al. (1972) have proposed a sequence of spread from skin infections to the nose and throat (Figure 3). This bacterium is one of the major causes of impetigo and has been associated with infections after scratches and bites from insects, which can be controlled to some extent through the use of antibacterial lotions applied to the abrasions. The seasonality of diseases such as influenza has been hypothesized to be a result of animal reservoirs and survival potential of the pathogenic agent.

For those on active duty, coming from field sites, Adult Respiratory Distress Syndrome (ARDS) apparently is common. Studies have reported on individual cases of ARDS (MSMR 1997b); however, the etiologies, trends, and rates have not been reported, although studies are under way. Therefore, unknown respiratory illnesses are likely the majority of the reported cases of ARDS.

Fever of unknown origin (FUO) is a term described for those experiencing elevated temperature that could not be ascribed to any specific agent. Studies on the more severe cases (those hospitalized for 1 day or more) reported a rate of 2.68/100,000 (0.03/1,000) per month. Of these cases, 45% were diagnosed upon primary assessment as FUOs and in 12.7% that was the only diagnosis (total of 1,437 hospitalizations from 1990-1997 (MSMR 1998d). Vaccine reactions were found to be contributing to 5.3% of these FUOs, and other types of unknown infections, throat (7.4%), respiratory (2.1%), and gastrointestinal (4.9%), accounted for much of the remainder. Infantry men more than any other military occupational group were found to be at a greater risk among those hospitalized three days or longer where vaccine reactions were eliminated. The diagnosis and reporting of FUOs has been inconsistent for those FUOs of shorter duration (1 to 2 days); trends and unusual occurrences are more difficult to ascertain due to the high variability. The more severe illness, which lasts for more than 3 days, shows much less variability.

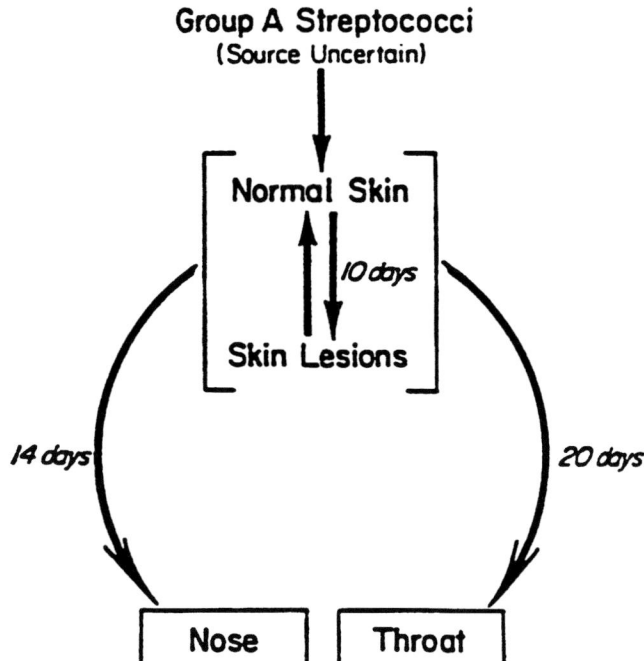

FIGURE 3 Concept of the sequence of spread of Group A streptococci among different body sites (Ferrieri et al. 1972).

Reports on deployment surveillance have shown that gastrointestinal and respiratory risks are the most significant cause of immediate acute outcomes associated with clinic visits and hospitalizations. Trends also demonstrate a decrease in the number of cases with time. Therefore, the greatest burden of illness is reported early on in deployment.

Gastrointestinal illness was the leading cause of morbidity among U.S. troops in the Persian Gulf deployment during 1990-1991 (Hyams et al. 1995). Parasitic infections were not found to be a significant cause of disease. Although *Escherichia coli* and *Shigella sonnei* were the primary pathogens identified, of great concern was the high level of antibiotic resistance identified (20 to 80% of the isolates were resistant). Outbreaks of the Norwalk virus and other unknown etiologies likely to be viruses were common. Serological investigations (antibody testing) found 6% of the combat units might have been infected with the Norwalk virus. The source of the diseases was associated primarily with vegetables and fruits imported from neighboring countries. It is clear from the identification of the *Shigella* and Norwalk agents that human fecal wastes and perhaps untreated sewage were the cause of much of the contamination.

Diarrheal disease was also quite high in an exercise in Thailand, and risks there were also associated with consumption of indigenous foods (MSMR 1998e). Gastrointestinal outbreaks have been associated with both food and water. A United Nations deployment to Haiti in June 1995 experienced a suspected waterborne outbreak due to the consumption of unapproved bottled water. The rate ranged between 15 to as high as 94 cases per 1,000 per month, with a high weekly rate seen in the third month (40/1,000/wk).

Common cold and upper respiratory complaints were common during deployment. Studies found that troops living and working in tightly constructed air conditioned buildings were at greatest risk. Possible causes of this, such as *Legionella*, were not investigated.

Comparing hospitalizations with clinic visits demonstrates that the level of disease in a force is likely to be 50 to 100 times greater than what is reported by hospitalization rates. This has been shown

TABLE 5 Examples of DNBI and Hospitalization Rates Associated With Deployments

	GI	Respiratory	Time Frame
Bosnia hospitalization trends	8.76/1,000	2.85/1,000	Cumulative incidence (48 weeks)
Gulf War outpatient visits	1 to 39/1,000[a]	1 to 22/1,000[b]	Range of weekly rates of outpatients in 40,000 troops (31 weeks)
Thailand clinic visits	12/1,000	9/1,000	Average visits per week

[a]Highest rates seen in the fourth to fifth week associated with fresh fruits and vegetables.
[b]Highest rates seen in the first two weeks and a second peak seen during U.S. Marine Expeditionary Forces deployment.
Sources: Hyams et al. 1995; MSMR 1997c, 1998e.

in numerous outbreaks where hospitalizations and case data were compiled (see following section on building databases). Although mild diarrhea might not affect the individual's activities to any great extent, it is more than likely that 1 to 3 days of effective time were lost. Table 5 shows some examples of DNBI and hospitalization rates associated with deployments (Hyams et al. 1995; MSMR 1997c; MSMR 1998e). Notice that the rates during the Bosnian deployment for the severe cases are reported over the complete time frame, whereas the rates for the Persian Gulf and Thailand deployments are reported for a range and an average of weekly clinic visits. It is most appropriate to report both visits and hospitalizations for comparisons over the time of the deployment. The disease levels from one deployment to another need to be examined in light of exposure tied to sources, season, and geographic locale, as well as changes in policies that factor in decreasing the risks.

Vectorborne diseases have also been shown to emerge during deployment. During Operation Desert Shield/Storm in eastern Saudi Arabia, 12 cases of viscerotropic and 20 cases of cutaneous leishmaniasis were identified (697,000 allied soldiers deployed; cumulative rate of 0.017/1,000 and 0.03/1,000 cases, respectively; 4.3/1,000 cases of cutaneous leishmaniasis seen in the Colombian Army) (Martin et al. 1998). The parasite is transmitted through bites from the sand fly. Domesticated animals can serve as reservoirs, and in Italy two cases of this disease in children of active-duty members might have been due to the high prevalence of the disease (15-50%) in dogs (MSMR 1998f). Attack rates of the disease in other deployments have been as high as 60%, with exposures of only 6 hours.

Physical protection, such as using nets, DEET lotion, and treating bedding and clothing, is seen as paramount to control. Education and predeployment training as well as better entomological surveillance will provide better preparedness. Clearly one of the lessons learned during Operation Desert Storm was that previous reports on the geographic areas at risk had missed this part of Saudi Arabia. In addition, chronic effects that might be exhibited post-deployment as a result of such exposures will need to be considered.

A combined U.S.-Australian military operation in Queensland, Australia, in March 1997 exhibited the successful approach that is used by the military for control of vectorborne diseases (MSMR 1997d). Arboviruses were endemic to the region and the exercise corresponded to the seasonal peak of transmission of the Ross River virus (RRv). Entomological surveys found RRv in four mosquito species. Out of the 9,000 troops who were engaged in ground operations, six cases of the disease were confirmed through serological testing and clinical manifestations (0.67/1,000 cases). The use of personal measures that protect against the mosquito were reinforced, and in fact it was found that protective measures were not adhered to by those who became ill.

Twelve cases of malaria associated with those who had served in Korea were reported, and seven cases of leptospirosis, all in children, were reported in the Pacific region (MSMR 1997e; MSMR 1996b; MSMR 1998g). Malaria is caused by a mosquitoborne protozoan and leptosporosis is spread through contact with water contaminated with urine from infected animals.

Emerging Infectious Agents

Worldwide, the leading cause of death remains the variety of infectious diseases that plague human beings. In the United States, the risk of dying from an infectious disease rose from fifth place to third place just in the last decade due to emerging and reemerging microorganisms. It is also clear that acute end points of disease are inadequate to describe the risks, and many chronic diseases, heart disease, neurological disorders, and cancer are due to microbial infections (Table 6). New microorganisms are identified each year and well-recognized pathogens have reemerged (Figure 4). Health outcomes and the ability to diagnose diseases as well as the potential for exposure will ultimately influence the assessment of these microbial agents.

Fecal-Oral Agents

Fecal-oral agents can be transmitted through person to person contact and contaminated water and food, as well as through surface contact. Zoonotic potential is a critical issue and in some cases transmission through the food chain, such as *Salmonella enteritis* in eggs, needs to be identified as the key risk. Microorganisms are excreted in feces in high numbers, survive in the environment, are resistant to many conventional treatment processes, and cause infections at low exposure levels. Given that most of the world fails to treat human and animal wastes prior to discharge in water, the risk of exposure remains significant.

Enteric Viruses

There are several hundred enteric viruses that have been identified and new types are being reported. Some of the key concerns with these viruses includes issues regarding health outcome and exposure assessment include:

- New viruses are being discovered (picobirnaviruses).
- Chronic health outcomes are now known.
- Groundwater contamination and potential exposure is high.
- Survival during cooking has been documented (e.g., shellfish).

Hepatitis A virus is considered to be endemic in most Latin American and Caribbean countries (Craun 1996). Although the risk of exposure is high, there is a vaccine available. The symptoms of hepatitis A include fever, nausea, anorexia, and malaise, often with mild diarrhea. The liver cells are ultimately infected causing cytologic damage, necrosis, and inflammation of the liver. Illness usually lasts from 1 to 2 weeks but might last several months. A new and emerging concern worldwide is other types of viral hepatitis.

Devastating waterborne disease outbreaks of the hepatitis E virus (HEV) have occurred in some parts of the world but not in others. In Kanpur, India, in 1991, there were 79,000 cases of HEV due to sewage contamination of the drinking water. Children are often asymptomatic and the mortality rate is between 0.1 and 4% (Grabow et al. 1994). In pregnant women in their third trimester, the mortality rate

TABLE 6 Acute and Chronic Health Effects Associated With Various Microorganisms

Agent	Acute Effects	Chronic or Ultimate Effects
Bacteria		
E. coli O157:H7	Diarrhea	Adults: death (thrombocytopenia)
		Children: death (kidney failure)
Legionella pneumoniae	Fever, pneumonia	Elderly: death
Helicobacter pylori	Gastritis	Ulcers and stomach cancer
Vibrio vulnificus	Skin and tissue infection	
Campylobacter	Diarrhea	Death: Guillian-Barré Syndrome
Salmonella	Diarrhea	Reactive arthritis
Yersinia	Diarrhea	Reactive arthritis
Shigella	Diarrhea	Reactive arthritis
Cyanobacteria (blue-green algae) and other toxins	Diarrhea	Potential cancer
Leptospirosis	Fever, headache, chills, muscle aches, vomiting	Weil's Disease, death (not common)
Aeromonas hydrophila	Diarrhea	
Parasites		
Giardia lamblia	Diarrhea	Failure to thrive
		Severe hypothyroidism
		Lactose intolerance
		Chronic joint pain
Cryptosporidium	Diarrhea	Death in immunocompromised host
Toxoplasma gondii	Newborn syndrome	Dementia and/or seizures
	Hearing and vision loss	
	Mental retardation	
	Diarrhea	
Acanthamoeba	Eye infections	
Microsporidia (Enterocytozoon and Septata)	Diarrhea	
Viruses		
Hepatitis viruses	Liver infection	Liver failure
Adenoviruses	Eye infections, diarrhea	
Caliciviruses (small round structured viruses, Norwalk virus)	Diarrhea	
Coxsackieviruses	Encephalitis	
	Aseptic meningitis	
	Diarrhea	
	Respiratory disease	Heart disease (myocarditis), reactive insulin-dependent diabetes
Echoviruses	Aseptic meningitis	

Source: CDC 1997.

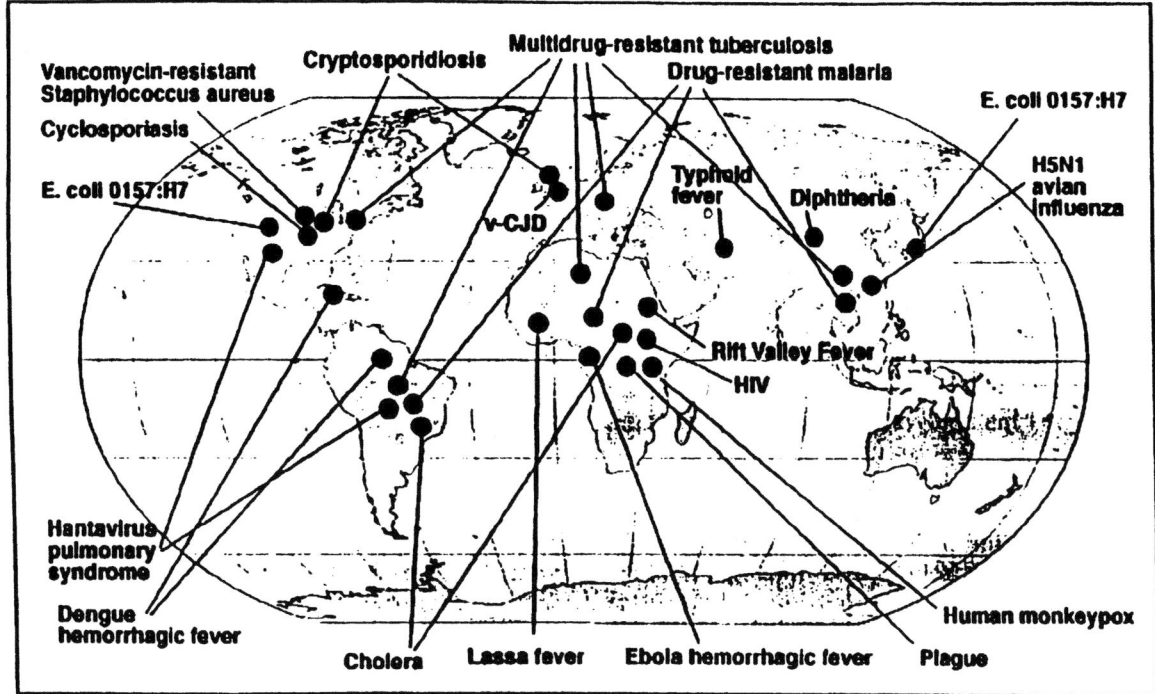

FIGURE 4 Examples of new and reemerging diseases (Fauci 1998).

can exceed 20% (Gust and Purcell 1987). There has been speculation HEV is endemic in various parts of the world, and subclinical cases might be contributing to the spread of the disease.

The coxsackieviruses now need to be considered separately as one of the enteroviruses that might be related to more significant risks (Bendinelli and Friedman 1988).

Diarrhea has been one of the risks associated with many of the enteric viruses such as Norwalk virus, but more serious chronic diseases have now been associated with viral infections and these risks need to be better defined. Studies have now reported that coxsackie B virus is associated with myocarditis (Klingel et al. 1992). In other recent studies, enteroviral RNA was detected in endomyocardial biopsies in 32% of patients with dilated cardiomyopathy and 33% of patients with clinical myocarditis (Kiode et al. 1992). In addition, there is emerging evidence that coxsackie B virus is also associated with insulin dependent diabetes, and infection with this virus might contribute to an increase of 0.0079% of these diabetes cases (0.079/1,000) (Wagenknecht et al. 1991).

Coxsackieviruses should be diagnosed serologically and clinically. Clinical conditions are associated with many systems including:

- Respiratory
- Central nervous system
- Cardiovascular
- Muscle and joints
- RE system and glands
- Gastrointestinal

Symptoms can include everything from general fatigue, headaches, and diarrhea to a fever.

Other concerns associated with coxsackieviruses are:

- Asymptomatic infections can lead to chronic outcomes (myocarditis).
- A multitude of symptoms can be seen in a population after exposure (heterogeneous outcomes).
- Coxsackie B viruses are commonly found in sewage.
- Concurrent exposure to the virus and other contaminants (e.g., metals) has demonstrated increased risk.

New viruses are continually being discovered and characterized, such as astroviruses, toroviruses, and small round structured viruses all associated with fecal-oral transmission and diarrhea. Although at one time the viruses were thought to be host-specific, the potential for zoonotic transmission from animals does exist. The picobirnaviruses (PBV) are unique double-stranded, bi- or tri-segmented RNA viruses, and are found in people and animals, including chickens (Chandra 1997). They have been shown to be a cause of acute diarrhea in children (Cascio et al. 1996) and prevalence in human stools was 9 to 13% with and without symptoms (Gallimore et al. 1995). Reports of PBVs have come from Italy; Caracas, Venezuela; and the United Kingdom, and it is likely that they have worldwide distribution.

Contamination of groundwater with viruses is of great concern due to the resistant nature of the viral structure and the colloidal size (20 to 80 nm), which makes this group of microorganisms easily transported through soil systems. Viruses also survive up to months in groundwater and are more resistant to water disinfection than are the coliforms (Yates and Yates 1988; Gerba and Rose 1990). Studies in the United States have found viruses in 20 to 30% of the groundwater where coliforms were not predictive of viral contamination (Abbaszadegan et al. 1999). New techniques using polymerase chain reaction (PCR) have shown that there is much more contamination than previously recognized (Table 7). There are no data on the occurrence of viruses in groundwater in most other parts of the world.

Protozoan Parasites

Cryptosporidium was first diagnosed in humans in 1976. Since that time, it has been well recognized as a cause of diarrheal illness (Dubey et al. 1990). Reported incidences of *Cryptosporidium* infections in human populations range from 0.6 to 20%, depending on the geographic locale. There is a greater prevalence in populations in Asia, Australia, Africa, and South America. *Cryptosporidium* is the most significant waterborne disease in the United States today. The occurrence of *Cryptosporidium* in surface waters has been reported in 4 to 100% of the samples examined at levels between 0.1 to 10,000/100 L, depending on the impact from sewage and animals (Lisle and Rose 1995). Groundwater, once thought to be a more protected source, has shown between 9.5 and 22% of samples positive for *Cryptosporidium* (Hancock 1998). In North America, there have been 12 waterborne outbreaks of *Cryptosporidium*. It has also been associated with drinking water outbreaks in the United Kingdom, Japan, and Holland. The largest outbreak in the United States occurred in Milwaukee, Wisconsin, in 1993 where 400,000 people became ill and 100 died due to contamination of the water supply (MacKenzie et al. 1994).

Cyclospora cayetanensis (previously called a cyanobacterium-like body) is a single-cell coccidian protozoan that has been implicated as an etiologic agent of prolonged watery diarrhea in humans (Ortega et al. 1993). The organism was first described as early at 1977 (Ashford 1979) and has been reported with increased frequency since the mid-1980s. *Cyclospora* has been described in patients from

TABLE 7 Virus Detection in Groundwater in the U.S. by Various Methods

Virus	Method	Percentage of Samples Positive
Culturable enteric viruses	Cell culture	6.8 (12/176)
Enteroviruses	PCR[a]	30
Hepatitis A virus	PCR	7
Rotavirus	PCR	13
Total viruses	PCR	39.3 (53/135)

[a]PCR, nucleic acid amplification for detection of the internal components of the virus, PCR may detect non-viable viruses.
Source: Abbaszadegan et al. 1999.

North, Central, and South America, Europe, Asia, and North Africa; however, the true prevalence of this parasite in any population is unknown (Soave and Johnson 1995).

Cyclospora is now known to be an obligate parasite of immunodeficient and immunocompetent humans (Ortega et al. 1993). In an immunocompromised person the parasite can cause profuse, watery diarrhea lasting several months. The infection is much less severe in immunocompetent patients. Symptoms can range from no symptoms to abdominal cramps, nausea, vomiting, and fever lasting from 3 to 25 days (Goodgame 1996).

Although *Cryptosporidium* appears to be predominantly waterborne, *Cyclospora* has been related more often to transmission through contaminated produce from a world market. The differences between the protozoa and their transmission might be due to their biology and structure, size of the oocysts, need for sporulation, and presence of animal reservoirs (Table 8).

Microsporidia are obligate intracellular spore-forming protozoa that are capable of infecting both vertebrate and invertebrate hosts. Their role as an emerging pathogen in immunosuppressed hosts is being increasingly recognized. The prevalence of microsporidiosis in studies of patients with chronic diarrhea ranges from 7 to 50% worldwide (Bryan 1995). It is unclear whether this broad range represents geographic variation, differences in diagnostic capabilities, or differences in risk factors for exposure to microsporidia. Typical symptoms of infection include chronic diarrhea, dehydration, and significant weight loss (>10% of body weight). Other symptoms include keratitis, conjunctivitis, hepatitis, peritonitis, myositis, central nervous system infection, and renal disease. Treatments are available for certain species of microsporidia; however, some species remain resistant to therapy.

In the United States there is currently a lack of data to suggest widespread occurrence of human strains of *Microsporidia* in surface waters. *Microsporidia* species that live in humans and animals have been detected in all water and wastewater (Dowd et al. 1998). However, because *Microsporidia* spores are excreted from infected individuals into wastewater, there is the potential for their occurrence in sewage contaminated waters. Animal hosts for *Microsporidia* also enhance the possibility that the organisms could be amplified and deposited into water supplies at high levels. *Microsporidia* spores have been shown to be stable in the environment and remain infective for days to weeks outside their hosts (Shadduck and Polley 1978; Waller 1979; Shadduck 1989). Because of their small size (1 to 5 µm), they might be difficult to remove using conventional filtration techniques, and there is a concern that these organisms might have an increased resistance to chlorine disinfection similar to *Cryptosporidium*.

Toxoplasma gondii is considered a tissue protozoan of cats and other felines that become infected mainly from eating infected rodents or birds, or from feces of infected cats. The disease has flu-like

TABLE 8 Comparison of *Cryptosporidium* and *Cyclospora*

Attribute	*Cryptosporidium*	*Cyclospora*
Taxonomy	Intestinal coccidian	Intestinal coccidian

Infective unit	Oocysts 4–5 μm
	    Immediately infectious upon excretion
		Oocysts 8–10 μm
		    Requires sporulation[a] in the environment, not immediately infectious upon excretion

Animal reservoir	*C. parvum* found in most mammals, can cross species barriers	*C. cayetanensis* documented only in humans
Foodborne disease	4 outbreaks in the U.S.	5 Large clusters in U.S. and Canada seen 1995, 1996, and 1997, involving >3,000 cases; primary transmission associated with fruits and vegetables
Waterborne disease	12 Waterborne outbreaks in North America since 1985, 17 in United Kingdom, 2 in Japan; primary transmission	1 Outbreak in Chicago, 1 in Nepal

[a]Sporulation is a process by which the oocysts undergo maturation in the environment before becoming infectious.
Source: Rose and Slifko, 1999.

symptoms, with swollen glands in the neck, armpits, or groin area. Most people recover without treatment. In the immunocompromised, the infection might cause severe disease, and infection during pregnancy might lead to fetal infection, chronic chorioretinitis, or death.

Foodborne transmission has been a source of toxoplasmosis; however, two outbreaks of the disease have been associated with contaminated surface water. In 1979, 600 U.S. soldiers attended a 3-wk training course in a jungle in Panama. Within 2 weeks of their return to the United States, 39 out of 98 soldiers in one company came down with a febrile illness. Serological testing revealed 31 confirmed cases of acute toxoplasmosis. The outbreak was attributed to the ingestion of contaminated water while on maneuvers in the jungle (Benenson et al. 1982).

In March 1995, the Capital Regional District of Victoria, British Columbia, identified 110 cases of toxoplasmosis. The outbreak was attributed to a single drinking water source for the area. The number of newly identified cases of toxoplasmosis declined sharply after the drinking water reservoir suspected of contamination was shut down. An estimated 3,000 people (1% of the population) might have been infected by the municipal drinking water contaminated with toxoplasmosis (Canadian Water Works Assoc. 1995).

Bacterial Pathogens

Epidemics of cholera have devastated Europe and North America since the early 1800s. A lack of sanitation and an increasing population, often with limited access to clean water, has brought about numerous disease outbreaks. A total of 1,076,372 cases and 10,098 deaths due to cholera in the Americas were reported by June 1995 according to the Pan American Health Organization (PAHO). In 1994, non 01 cholera was detected for the first time from the Bug River (freshwater) in Poland, and recently, Hong Kong has reported two outbreaks of cholera (Lee et al. 1996). Although the cause of the Hong Kong outbreaks was not clearly identified, increasing pollution of coastal waters has been implicated. Further concern over the cholera epidemic stems from the discovery of a new strain of *Vibrio cholera* 0139, which has resulted in increased mortality rate (Lee et al. 1996). Inadequate disinfection or the lack of disinfection has contributed significantly to the spread of cholera throughout Africa and Latin America. Water, seafood, and rice are common vehicles for spreading the disease.

Helicobacter pylori has been cited as a major etiologic agent for gastritis and has been implicated in the pathogenesis of peptic and duodenal ulcer disease (Taylor and Blaser 1991). It has also been associated with the development of gastric carcinoma (Eurogast Study Group 1993). The mode of transmission of *H. pylori* is not well characterized. Recent studies suggest that some gastrointestinal dissemination might be due to vomiting in childhood (Axon 1995). Persons living in low socioeconomic conditions have consistently been shown to have a high prevalence of *H. pylori*, and the organism has also been found routinely in the feces of children living in endemic areas (Thomas et al. 1992). Klein et al. (1991) reported that in Peru, the water source might be a more important risk factor than socioeconomic status in acquiring *H. pylori* infection. Children whose homes had external water sources (without piped water, use a water container and bring water from a central water system to the home) were three times more likely to be infected than those whose homes had internal water sources (piped through a distribution system). Among families with internal water sources, there was no difference in *H. pylori* infection associated with income. Children from high-income families whose homes were supplied with municipal water were 12 times more likely to be infected than were those from high-income families whose water came from community wells. These findings show that substandard municipal water supplies might be important sources of *H. pylori* infection.

Escherichia coli O157:H7 is an enteropathogenic strain of *E. coli*. Infection with the organism can cause severe bloody diarrhea with abdominal cramping. In small children and the elderly, fluid replacement is of the utmost importance for a full recovery. A common more serious complication of infection with *E. coli* O157:H7 is hemolytic uremic syndrome (HUS), which causes a loss of red blood cells and kidney failure. In severe cases, HUS can cause permanent kidney damage or death. *E. coli* O157:H7 has been shown to survive similarly to typical *E. coli* strains under routine drinking water conditions. There have been two documented outbreaks of waterborne disease caused by *E. coli* O157:H7. In the 1990 Cabool, Missouri outbreak, there were 243 cases, with 32 hospitalizations and 4 deaths (Geldreich et al. 1992; Swerdlow et al. 1992). The second documented waterborne outbreak of *E. coli* O157:H7 took place in Scotland, with 496 cases (272 laboratory-confirmed cases) and 19 deaths (Dev et al. 1991). Foodborne disease appears to be more common and outbreaks affecting 700 in the western United States and 8,000 cases in Japan have occurred (Meng and Doyle 1998). Cattle (up to 57% are infected) and other ruminants are the major reservoirs; however, the pathogenic *E. coli* have been isolated from dogs, horses, swine, and cats. Contamination during slaughtering and inadequate storage and cooking are associated with the disease. Contaminated hamburger (15-40% of the lots tested) has been shown in the United States, Canada, the United Kingdom, and the Netherlands.

Salmonella typhimurium DT104 has emerged in the United Kingdom, Germany, France, Austria, Denmark, and the United States (Meng and Doyle 1998). This bacterium carries with it antibiotic resistance to ampicillin, chloramphenicol, streptomycin, sulphonamides, and tetracyclines. The number of cases has been increasing. The infection is characterized by enterocolitis (8 to 72 hours latency period) with nonbloody diarrhea and abdominal pain usually within 5 days. Hospitalization has been reported at 36% of the cases. Chronic outcomes include reactive arthritis, Reiter's syndrome, and ankylosing spondylitis. This bacterium, like other *Salmonellae*, is associated with many different foods and has been found in sheep, cattle, pigs, goats, chickens, turkeys, and domestic pets.

Campylobacter has recently been identified as the number one agent of foodborne disease. This bacterium, which can come from chickens and other animals, is prevalent in the United States and United Kingdom, according to recent surveys. This might likely be due to better diagnostics and reporting. Guillain-Barré syndrome (GBS) is a major cause of neuromuscular paralysis in the United

States, with an estimated 2,628 to 9,575 cases each year; between 20 to 40% of the cases were caused by infections with *Campylobacter* (Buzby et al. 1997). The health outcomes associated with *Campylobacter*-associated GBS have been estimated at <1% developing GBS, 20% of those requiring ventilation and 10% of those dying.

Prions

Prions are protein-based agents that are able to self-replicate and cause disease. The two that have been identified are Creutzfeldt-Jakob disease (CJD) and bovine spongiform encephalopathy (BSE). These agents cause neuropathology and death. The agents are highly resistant to heat. BSE was reported at epidemic levels in cattle in the United Kingdom with a peak of 1,200 cases per month in 1992-1993. Transmission occurs through the consumption of BSE-contaminated meat products and animal feed associated with organ supplements. CJD cases might also occur through the diet; however, the cases are rare and risk to humans has been estimated to be very low (Gale 1998; Gale et al. 1998).

Respiratory Agents

Influenza

Avian H5N1 influenza in Hong Kong served to remind the medical community of the on-going challenge in the control of influenza. Vaccine development and application will always be behind the disease curve. Although transmission from bird flocks to humans has been documented on occasion, the exact nature of the initial transmission into a community is ill-defined. Thus, exposure-prevention methods have not been readily implemented. The strong seasonality of influenza should be further investigated with regard to environmental and climatic conditions that enhance the spread of the disease. Attack rates for influenza can be high, 20 to 140/1,000, and the disease can spread quickly among contacts. An additional complication is that Guillain-Barré syndrome following influenza immunizations has been documented by the Vaccine Adverse Event Reporting System. Forty-four cases were reported in 1994 to 1995; the rate is unknown because the total number vaccinated was not reported (MSMR 1995).

A new virus in the family Paramyxoviridae in pigs has been recently described in Sydney, Australia (Philbey et al. 1998; Chant et al. 1998). Respiratory and reproductive effects in pigs were noted. Two workers in the area had an influenzalike illness with rash and serological testing showing no alternative cause, and both were seropositive for the newly described virus. Zoonotic transmission is likely, but the details of the exposure pathway have not been delineated.

Legionella

Legionella bacterium causes a severe pneumonia known as Legionnaires disease and a mild respiratory infection known as Pontiac fever. It is spread through the waterborne respiratory route; no person-to-person transmission occurs. The bacterium is usually found naturally in surface and groundwater. Surveillance data from England and Wales suggests that approximately 40% of Legionnaires cases are community-acquired and the remainder are associated with travel (Figure 5). Urinary antigen detection could be a promising new diagnostic tool that could help identify and eliminate the risk. Diagnosis and reporting are poor, particularly for mild cases. This might be an unknown and unrecognized risk for troops.

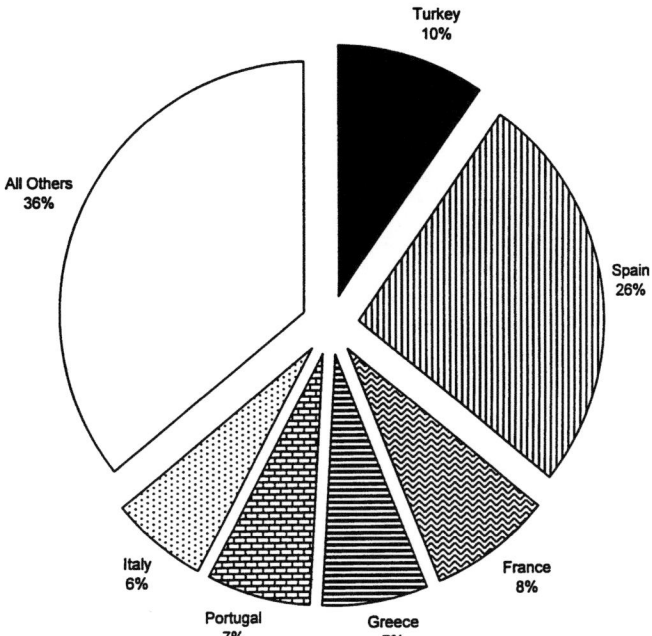

FIGURE 5 Distribution of *Legionella* cases by country visited (Joseph et al. 1998).

Skin Infections

Primary skin infections are associated with impetigo, ecthyma, folliculitis, furuncle, carbuncle, sweat gland infections, erysipelas, and erythrasmas. Impetigo accounts for 78% of all infections, generically referred to as atopic dermatitis. The major cause of skin infections are due to transient bacteria, Group A streptococci and resident bacteria, *Staphylococcus aureus,* and *Staphylococcus epidermidis*. Hypersensitivity has been identified in some cases, and vancomycin-resistant staphylococci have also emerged (Fauci 1998).

Vectorborne Agents

Perhaps more than any other category of disease, more progress has been made in understanding vectorborne diseases: the ecology of the host-parasite interactions, spread of disease, development of vaccines, and measures to prevent exposure to the vector. The worldwide spread of the vectors, the difficulty in implementing control measures, and newly identified resistant strains are challenges that continue to present themselves to deployed troops. Table 9 summarizes some of the key vectorborne diseases.

Hanta Viruses

Hanta viruses include 14 different viruses and are found throughout the world causing hemorrhagic fever and renal (HFR) syndrome in the Eurasian land mass and adjoining areas. Hanta virus pulmonary syndrome can also be found in the Americas (Schmaljohn and Hjelle 1997). Various types of rodents have been identified as vectors (mouse, rat, vole, and lemming). The viruses are transmitted to humans through inhalation of rodent excreta that contain the virus. Exposure occurs when the virus-associated excreta from soil and dust are aerosolized through indoor and outdoor activities. The diseases, previ-

TABLE 9 Major Vectorborne Diseases

Vector	Disease	Vaccine Available Or Under Development (D)
Mosquitoes	Malaria	Vaccine
	Filariasis	
	Dengue	Vaccine (D)
	Encephalitis	Vaccine
	Yellow fever	Vaccine
Ticks	Lyme disease	
	Rocky Mountain spotted fever	
	Tularemia	
Fleas	Plague	Vaccine (D)
	Endemic typhus	
Sand flies	Leishmaniasis	
Black flies	River blindness	
Bed Bugs	Chagas disease	
Rodents	Hanta virus	Vaccine (D)
	Leptosirosis	

ously known as Korean hemorrhagic fever or endemic hemorrhagic fever, have been recognized for centuries. It was not, however, until the 1950s that the western world began addressing these viral syndromes, partly as a result of 3,200 cases in United Nation forces in Korea (Gajdusek 1962).

Key characteristics in Hanta virus exposures include:

- Occurrence of outbreaks in ports-of-call.
- High virus loads in rodent population, along with increased numbers or density of rodents associated with higher risks.
- Outdoor exposures through farm work, threshing, sleeping on the ground, and indoor exposures associated with rodent infestations and inadequate cleaning.

New viruses and rodent vectors are constantly being identified. Worldwide, about 200,000 cases of HFRs involving hospitalization are reported, with the majority in China, Russia, and Korea. Mortality can be significant, ranging from 1 to 15% to as high as 40%. Given the wide distribution of rodents and their respective viruses, there appears to be a great potential for disease and continued outbreaks.

Dengue

Dengue is a severe viral illness that is spread by the mosquito *Aedes aegypti*. First described in the 1950s in Southeast Asia, the disease had, by the 1970s, emerged in the Americas in tropical and subtropical regions. This could be an emerging threat to troops that are stationed in more urban areas. It is transmitted from people to vector to people without an animal reservoir involved, and it is estimated that between 250,000 and 500,000 cases occur worldwide annually. The severity of the disease is related to sequential infection by two serotypes (Halstead 1988). Characteristics of this disease are high attack rates (70 to 80%) and high mortality rates (40 to 50%) if untreated (with appropriate treatment, mortality is 1 to 2%) (Beneson 1995; Gubler and Clark 1995).

Malaria

Malaria affects worldwide populations more than any other vectorborne disease. Up to 500 million people a year are thought to be infected; 2.1 billion are at risk (Nchinda 1998). Mortality is estimated at 1.5 to 2.7 million deaths a year. The disease is caused by the protozoan *Plasmodium* and is transmitted by the *Anopheles* mosquito. Malaria has been a concern in Africa, the Pacific, and Asia. The increasing number of cases has been related to a number of factors:

- Approximately 20 to 30% of the strains of the protozoa are resistant to chloroquine (one of the major therapies), and this is spreading.
- Population changes due to high birth rates, migration, and conflicts increases the susceptible population.
- Environmental changes in rainfall, agriculture, and urban development have led to changes in breeding habitats.
- Vector evolution and biting habits have changed.

Biological Weapons

Biological agents used as weapons will be spread through similar transmission routes as naturally occurring infectious agents. Fecal-oral microorganisms will likely be spread by contaminating the food or water supply. Indeed two incidences of intentional food contamination with *Salmonella* and *Shigella* have been reported (Kolavic et al. 1997; Torok et al. 1997). Although inhalation might be a common route of exposure for agents like anthrax, the potential to infect a large number of people by contaminating the water supply and the resistance of the spores to conventional disinfection practices should not be overlooked.

Respiratory exposure with dispersion through aerosols, using spray tanks, biological bombs, and other dispenser systems, is one of the most likely routes of transmission (Franz et al. 1997). An excellent review of biological weapons has been presented by Franz et al. (1997) (Table 10). The U.S. Army Medical Research Institute of Infectious Diseases has also published the third edition (July 1998) of the *Medical Management of Biological Casualties* (Fitzen et al. 1998) with comprehensive descriptions of agents, symptoms, diagnosis, vaccines, prophylaxis, and treatment available. Although incubation times, clinical features, and mortality rates have been described for these agents, a full quantitative assessment has not been undertaken. For example, mortality (or lethality) has been described as moderate or high without quantitative rates reported. Infectious dose is reported, incubation times, and duration of illness, but no dose-response modeling or outcome modeling has been undertaken. Vaccines are available; however, the efficacy and availability might be limited. Although certain measures can be taken to prevent biological weapon attacks, the outcome if such an attack occurs needs to be carefully evaluated so that action plans can be developed.

One of the main differences between natural and biological weapons (BW) exposures will occur in the dose, because it is likely that higher concentrations would be employed. A complete risk assessment would include the development of dose-response models from animal feeding studies (see following section on building databases). The use of dose-response models could be used directly in quantitative exposure estimates associated with the likely type of delivery systems, concentrations, and time of exposure to better predict outcomes of various BW attacks. These will be agent-specific and the effects from various attack scenarios could be examined. Plausibility evaluation, if the models could be tested, could be carried out against actual incidences in which biological weapons were used, such as the anthrax release in the Soviet Union in 1979.

TABLE 10 Some Biological Agents Used as Weapons

	Route of Exposure	Secondary Transmission	Comments
Bacterial Agents			
Anthrax spores	Respiratory, ingestion, contact	No	High mortality, 65-80% Vaccine
Brucellosis	Respiratory, ingestion, contact	No	No vaccine
Plague	Respiratory	Yes	Moderately communicable Vaccine
Q fever	Contact respiratory	No	Vaccine
Tularemia	Contact, vectorborne, respiratory	No	Moderate mortality Vaccine
Viral Agents			
Encephalitis	Respiratory	No	
Hemorrhagic fevers	Vectorborne	No	Some with moderate mortality
Small pox	Respiratory, contact	Yes	Not readily communicable Moderate to high mortality Vaccine
Toxins			
Botulinum	Respiratory, ingestion	No	High mortality Vaccine
Staphylococcal enterotoxin B	Respiratory, ingestion	No	
Plant toxin: Ricin		No	High mortality

Source: Franz et al. 1997.

One of the major concerns is the availability of vaccines in the future for agents with high mortality. These BW agents should be targeted as a priority for dose-response modeling and quantitative microbial risk assessment. Although the infectious dose and clinical outcomes have been well described, these will not be sufficient for developing the risk rankings that are needed. On the exposure side, one BW might be delivered at a greater dose for a greater duration than another. The longevity of the contamination and potential for subsequent exposure (e.g., soil) after delivery should also be accounted for. On the human health side, the ability to quickly diagnose and treat the disease, availability of vaccines, and the swiftness and consequence of the impact (morbidity and mortality) need to be considered.

Multiple Exposure Issues

In exposure assessment and dose-response modeling, single contaminant experiments and evaluations have been the primary focus of most studies. It has long been recognized that one of the major deficiencies in the application of risk-assessment protocols is the failure to consider exposure to mixtures or multiple stressors. The Gulf War syndrome has brought this issue to the forefront, and it will be necessary to address this complexity.

Exposure to multiple stressors could affect either the dose-response relationship or the health outcome. Feeding studies with enterobacteria and pseudomonads have demonstrated an increased infectivity (lower dose-response curve) associated with individuals taking bicarbonates or antibiotics. In theory, the neutral-

TABLE 11 Infectious Oral Dose for 50% of the Mouse Population for *Pseudomonas aeruginosa* (Streptomycin-Resistant Strain) Given Different Antibiotics

Antibiotic	Infectious Dose for 50% of the Population, CFU
Untreated	9.1×10^8
Ampicillin	1.7×10^7
Clindamycin	1.2×10^7
Metronidazole	3.0×10^8
Kanamycin	1.3×10^6
Streptomycin	9.1×10^4

Source: Hentges et al. 1985.

ization of stomach acids or decrease of microflora of the gut allows for infectivity to take hold, avoiding some of the nonspecific immune functions that humans employ to ward off infection.

Hentges et al. (1985) showed that antibiotics decreased the resistance of mice to intestinal colonization when inoculated orally with 10^8 colony forming units (CFUs) of *Pseudomonas aeruginosa* (Table 11). Of the mice that did not receive antibiotics, 20% still passed *P. aeruginosa* in the feces on day 14 as compared with mice treated with ampicillin (90%), clindamycin (70%), and metronidazole (50%). Buck and Cooke (1969) examined the colonization of healthy human volunteers with *P. aeruginosa* and reported that an oral dose $>1.5 \times 10^6$ CFU was required. With oral doses of 1.5×10^6 to 2.0×10^8, excretion of *P. aeruginosa* in the feces was detected for up to 14 days if the volunteer was also taking ampicillin. Excretion of the agent was limited to 6 days in volunteers not taking antibiotics. None of the volunteers experienced any disease symptoms from the *P. aeruginosa*.

Poor nutritional habits have also been linked to greater severity of health outcome after infection. The high mortality rate due to cholera in Africa as opposed to South America was, in part, suggested to be influenced by poor nutritional levels in the population.

Not only can stressors affect the infectivity of microorganisms, but invading microorganisms also can affect the absorption of other chemical stressors. Glynn et al. (1998) found that cadmium absorption increased during coxsackie B3 virus infections.

Health outcomes (the severity of illness) are also known to vary, although attack rates and dose-response do not change. Clearly, the host immune system is one of the major influences on outcome. Stressors to the immune system thus might result in more symptomatic as opposed to asymptomatic illness and more severe illness. For example, it is now known that the coxsackieviruses are associated with various forms of heart disease, eye infections, and respiratory disease. Studies in mice have shown an increased virulence (severe outcomes) associated with selenium deficiency (Beck et al. 1994). The epidemic optic and peripheral neuropathy in Cuba affecting 50,000 was associated with infections by coxsackie A9 and B4 viruses (84% of the cases) and was somewhat alleviated by supplements of B complex vitamins, vitamin A, and folate (Mas et al. 1997). Interestingly, infections with coxsackieviruses with exposure to metals has also been demonstrated to be associated with an increased risk of myocarditis (Llback et al. 1994). Toxic heavy metals (cadmium, nickel, and methyl mercury) might also affect the inflammatory character of the infection and enhance the potential for autoimmune diseases such as diabetes and myocarditis.

One of the hypotheses of the Gulf War syndrome was that the combination of vaccinations followed by the other exposures to chemical or biological agents contributed to the health effects that were observed. It is clear that at least some proportion of those vaccinated do have an adverse effect that has been recorded primarily as fever in the Vaccine Adverse Event Reporting System. Autoimmune and neurological maladies have been described with infections from *Campylobacter, Salmonella, Shigella,* and *Yersinia,* and coxsackieviruses. These have been documented with and without symptomology, that is, the outcome is due to the infection and not the level of illness. It is unclear whether infection following immunizations might enhance these outcomes in some antagonistic fashion.

Although most medical professionals (e.g., WHO and CDC) do not prescribe to the association between hepatitis B vaccination and multiple sclerosis, there have been recent court cases that have ruled that the evidence was sufficient to link the two multiple factors involved (Hepatitis Control Report 1998). The strength of the data, the risk-risk trade-off might need to be assessed before the scientifically defensible causality is definitely proven or not proven.

War syndromes from the Civil War, Vietnam War, and the Persian Gulf War have been described and show a remarkable similarity in the health problems found in troops today. The types of symptoms reported included fatigue, shortness of breath, headache, sleep disturbances, impaired concentration, and forgetfulness (Hyams et al. 1996). The other similarity is the high frequency of reported diarrhea. It is possible that this is due to unrecognized chronic syndromes (such as those reported with coxsackieviruses) or exposure to multiple stressors, mentioned above, associated with the enteric bacteria.

The disease surveillance that is currently in place can be used to examine these issues, but better exposure assessment must be undertaken. Animal models with experimentation associated with mixtures need to be developed, including mixtures of microorganisms with antibiotics, vaccinations, metals, and other infections.

RISK-ASSESSMENT AND RISK-MANAGEMENT STRATEGIES

Risk assessment might be viewed by some as a professional process that includes the participation of many established scientific disciplines. As defined in this context, risk assessment is the qualitative or quantitative characterization and estimation of potential adverse health effects associated with exposure of individuals or populations to hazards (materials or situations, and physical, chemical, or microbial agents). Risk assessment is not used in isolation, but is part of risk analysis. Risk analysis includes risk assessment, risk management, and risk communication.

The integration of risk management and risk assessment is seen as a necessary requirement in the development of a workable framework (see Figure 6). Regulatory agencies are now attempting to develop the best approach for undertaking and using microbial risk assessment for policies that will improve water quality, food safety, and public health.

The analysis phase (Figure 7) of risk assessment includes two aspects: human health effects analysis (symptomatic and asymptomatic infection; severity, duration, hospitalization, and medical care; mortality; host immune status; susceptible populations) and exposure analysis (vehicle, amount, route, single exposure versus multiple exposures over time, demographics of those exposed). Exposure analysis also includes occurrence assessment (methods, concentrations, frequency, spatial and temporal variation, regrowth, die-off, and transport). The data that ties the exposure analysis to the health outcomes quantitatively is done through dose-response modeling, with defined studies on exposures to the infectious units of bacteria, viruses, or protozoa. Quantitative information will be needed to undertake a quantitative microbial risk assessment (QMRA).

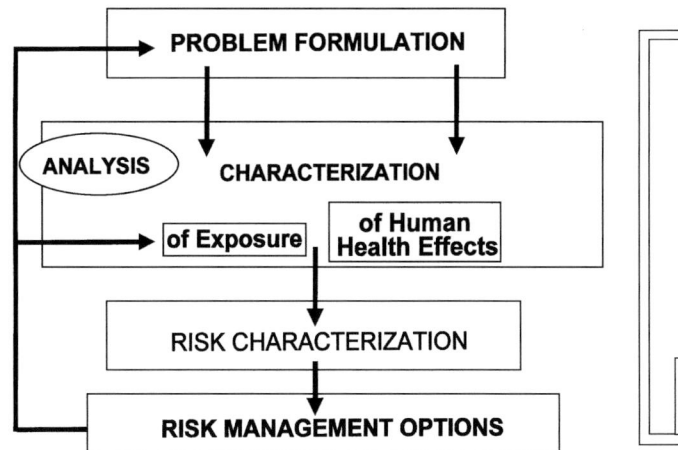

FIGURE 6 Framework for integration of risk management and microbial risk assessment. (Source: Adapted from ILSI 1996.)

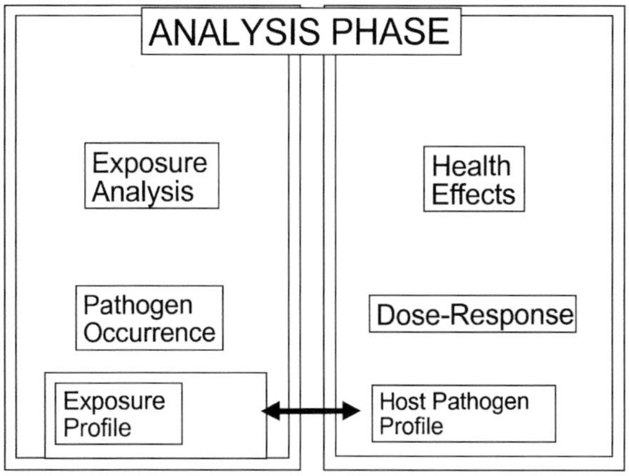

FIGURE 7 Analysis phase for microbial risk assessment (ILSI 1996).

Risk Assessment for Microorganisms

Hazard Identification

Hazard identification includes the identification of the microbial agent as well as the spectrum of human illnesses and disease associated with the specific microorganism. The types of clinical outcome range from asymptomatic infections to death. These data come from the clinical literature and studies from clinical microbiologists. The pathogenicity and virulence of the microorganism itself is of great interest, as well as the full spectrum of human disease that can result from specific microorganisms. The host response to the microorganisms with regard to immunity and multiple exposures should be addressed here, as well as the adequacy of animal models for studying human effects. Endemic and epidemic disease investigations, case studies, hospitalization studies, and other epidemiological data are needed to complete this step in the risk assessment. The transmission of disease is often microbial-specific (e.g., rabies and vectorborne diseases such as malaria or influenza); therefore, in some cases, the transmission (and to some extent the exposure) is tied into hazard identification for microbial risks. Often in these types of studies the variables are not well defined. For QMRAs, these need to be specifically described (see following section on building databases).

Dose-Response Assessment

The dose-response assessment is the mathematical characterization of the relationship between the dose administered and the probability of infection or disease in the exposed population. Dose-response assessments have been referred to as probability-of-infection models. Various doses of specific microorganisms have been given to sets of (in most cases) human volunteers. For most studies, a single dose was administered and the subjects were evaluated. The percentage of individuals infected at each dose was fit to a best-fit curve. The microorganisms were measured in doses that were obtained by counting the specific microbe in the laboratory, such as colony counts on agar media for bacteria, plaque counts in cell cultures for viruses, and direct microscopic counts of cysts or oocysts for protozoa. However, for protozoa, this results in essentially particle counts (nonviable organisms viewed microscopically could be counted in the dose), whereas for bacteria and viruses, the opposite problem exists (viable but nonculturable organisms are not counted). Despite these limitations in estimation of the dose, the methods used are similar to those used to detect these same microorganisms in environmental samples. Natural routes of exposure were used—direct ingestion, inhalation, or contact. Both disease and infection were measured in these studies as the end point. In most cases, less virulent strains of the microorganisms and healthy human adults were used. Multiple exposures should have been evaluated, but in most studies, they were not.

Threshold Issues in Microbial Dose-Response Modeling Risk Assessment

Current scientific data support the independent-action (or single-organism) hypothesis that a single bacterium, or virus, or protozoan can initiate and produce an infection. This concept has also been suggested as providing the explanation for sporadic cases of infectious disease. Although it is clear that the host defenses (immunity at the cellular and humoral level) do play a critical role in determination of which individuals might develop infection or a more severe disease, it has also been suggested that these do not provide the complete explanation (Rubin 1987). In the early literature, it was suggested that many microorganisms were needed to act cooperatively to overcome host defenses to initiate infection. The independent-action theory, however, suggests that each microorganism alone is capable of initiating the infection, but more than one is needed because the probability that a single microorganism will successfully evade host defenses is small (Rubin 1987).

The evaluation of the dose-response data sets also support the independent-action hypothesis because in almost every case the exponential or the beta model provide a statistically significant improvement in fit over the lognormal model that could be used to predict a threshold (Haas 1983). Currently, there are no scientific data to support a threshold level for these microorganisms.

Two risk equations have been described for the variety of microorganisms. For protozoa like *Cryptosporidium* and *Giardia*, the probability of infection $\pi(P_i)$ was defined by the exponential model:

$$\pi(P_i) = 1 - e^{(-rN)}$$

where, r is the fraction of microorganisms that are ingested that survive to initiate infection (which is organism-specific), and N is the exposure. For *Cryptosporidium*, $r = 0.00467$ (95% confidence limits (CL), 0.00195-0.0097) (Haas et al. 1996). The *Giardia* risk assessment model was previously published (Rose et al. 1991) and the value for *Giardia* was $r = 0.0198$ (95% CL, 0.009798-0.03582).

Dose-response for many of the viruses and bacteria, including rotaviruses, HAV, coxsackieviruses, echoviruses, *Salmonella* and *Shigella*, have all been developed from human feeding studies (Haas et al. 1999). In these studies, the best-fit curve was the beta-Poisson model.

$$\pi(P_i) = 1 - \left[1 + \frac{d}{N_{50}}\left(2^{\frac{1}{\alpha}} - 1\right)\right]^{-\alpha}$$

The method of maximum likelihood was used to fit dose-response models to the available experimental data on the particular microorganisms. In this case, two variables, and N_{50} provided an increased goodness-of-fit over the exponential model. N_{50} may be described as the dose that results in 50% infection in the subjects exposed. Known also as the infectious-dose 50, or ID_{50}, this can be used as a comparative measure of infectivity.

Although the human data sets are extensive, they are not exhaustive in terms of answering many of the questions regarding the host-microbe interaction. Many animal data sets exist, but have not been modeled. In the future, more human and animal studies will be needed to further address both hazard identification and dose-response assessment, including virulence, strain variation, immunity, autoimmune reactions, and multiple exposures.

Exposure Assessment

The exposure assessment is aimed at determining the size and nature of the population exposed and the route, concentrations, and distribution of the microorganisms and the duration of the exposure. The description of exposure includes not only occurrence based on concentrations but also the prevalence (how often the microorganisms are found) and distribution of microorganisms in space and over time. This assessment is determined through occurrence monitoring and predictive microbiology.

Exposure assessment depends on adequate methods for recovery, detection, quantification, sensitivity, specificity, virulence, viability, and transport and fate through the environment. For many microorganisms, the methods, studies, and models are not available or have limitations in application or interpretation (e.g., detection of viable and nonviable microorganisms). Often the concentration in the medium associated with the direct exposure (drinking water, food) is not known but must be estimated from other databases. Therefore, knowledge of the ecology of these microorganisms, sources in the environment, and transport and fate are needed, including inactivation rates and survival in the environment, ability to regrow (as in the case of some bacteria) and resistance to environmental factors (temperatures, humidity, sunlight). Finally, the movement through soil, air, water, and vectors should be modeled.

Risk Characterization

Quantitative risk characterization should estimate the magnitude of the public health problem, and demonstrate the variability and uncertainty of the hazard, with four distributions: (1) the spectrum of health outcomes; (2) the confidence limits surrounding the dose-response model; (3) the distribution of the occurrence of the microorganism; and (4) the exposure distribution. Assessments of occurrence and exposure can be further delineated by distributions surrounding the method recovery and survival (treatment) distributions.

It might be possible to group microorganisms in each category by relative similarities, similar health outcomes, dose-response, or potential for exposure. In addition, parts of the risk assessment (health outcomes and dose-response models) might have applicability to many transmission routes and different exposures, particularly for fecal-oral agents (e.g., food versus water).

Setting Priorities Using Health and Exposure Data

The risk assessment framework is a scientifically-based approach that can be used to understand the hazard, define the exposure, evaluate the consequences and relative risk, address controls, and begin to evaluate unknowns and emerging threats. If used as a tool for setting priorities for the various infectious agents apart from the dose-response modeling, the data can be judged in two broad categories: exposure and health outcome.

For exposure data, the ability to control that exposure should be addressed. For health outcome data, the ability to treat the disease or immunize against it needs to be considered (Figure 8).

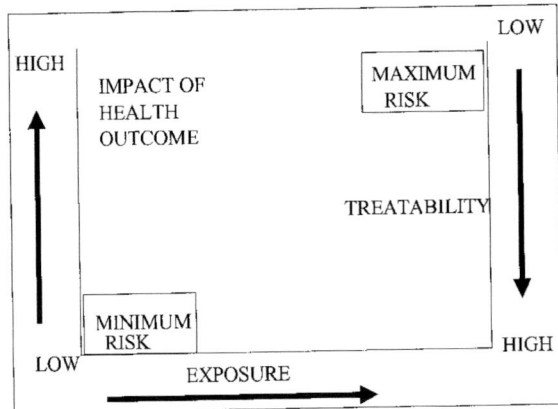

FIGURE 8 Risk matrix for infectious agents.

Thus, the approach for categorizing the risks and setting their priorities would include:

- Exposure and transmission: controls available for preventing exposure.
- Health outcomes: Vaccinations and treatment available for prevention and cure.
- Probability of infection (dose-response modeling).

Certain infectious agents might have attributes that would contribute toward a greater risk. Factors leading to higher risk might include:

- Transmission by more than one route.
- Geographic diversity.
- Zoonotic potential.
- Excretion at high numbers.
- High survival rates (resistance to environmental or engineering controls or stresses).
- Secondary and tertiary transmission.
- Low dose-response (high infectivity at low dose).
- Resistance to drugs, antibiotics.
- Unavailable or limited vaccines.
- Poor diagnostics.
- Producing chronic and acute outcomes.

The priorities would focus on those agents and illnesses (gastrointestinal and respiratory) for which there is the greatest morbidity and severe outcome and for which lack of vaccinations, poor treatment, antibiotic resistance, or poor diagnostics led to limited data. The exposure can be segregated by season, geography, and transmission (fecal-oral, vectorborne, respiratory) and would include those with the greatest potential for exposure.

Decision Frameworks

Many frameworks already exist for analysis of chemical and toxicological hazards. These frameworks, with slight modifications, would be useful for analyzing infectious agents. Figure 9 presents the risk assessment and risk management system used for the NRC toxicological program. The use of decision trees might be useful for gathering critical data to finalize the exposure assessment, even

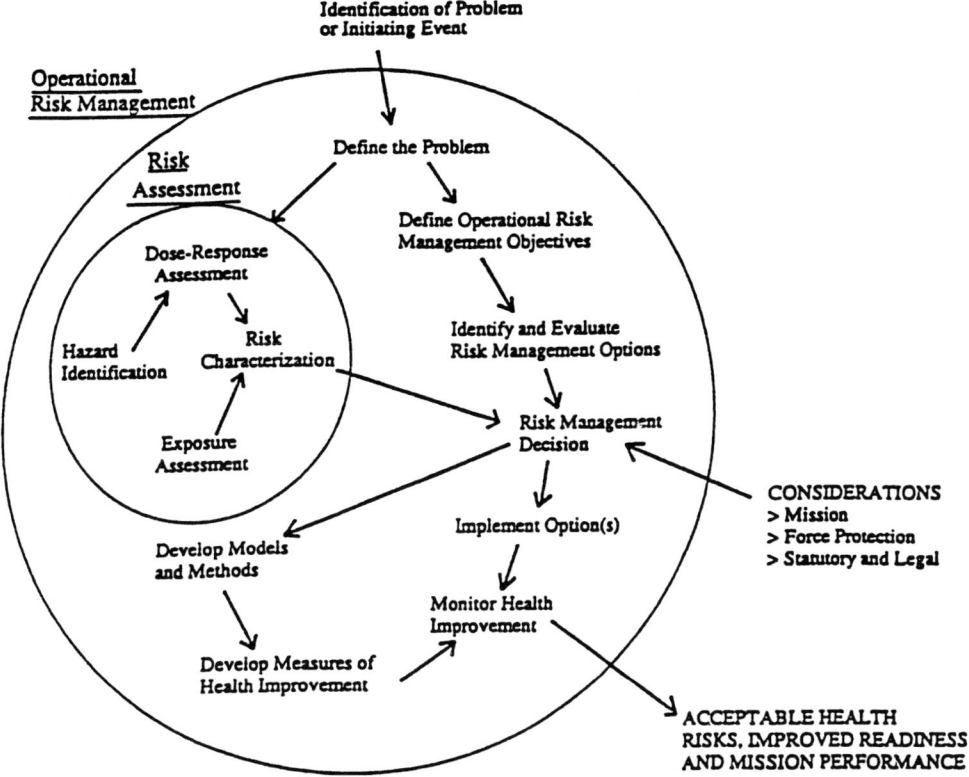

FIGURE 9 NRC risk assessment within the toxicological management scheme (Source: Adapted from NRC 1994).

without full characterization of health effects. Decision trees can be used to set priorities and eventually make management decisions for reducing the potential for exposing the population to microorganisms.

One potential framework has already been used for food safety and has been proposed for water. The hazard analysis critical control point (HACCP) system is aimed at specific operations whose ultimate goal is to ensure food safety. The physical, chemical, or biological hazard is defined, as well as the specification of the control criteria. The point at which the hazard can be controlled to acceptable levels or eliminated is then defined and is known as the critical control point (CCP). In theory, the CCP is the point at which the process or operation can be monitored to meet the performance specified to achieve the level of hazard reduction. In practice, very little has been done to implement this approach.

HACCP, when used for food safety, is food specific; therefore, the hazards and CCP might be different for beef, shellfish, or produce. Often the goal would be to establish a number of CCPs representing the entire food chain from the farm to the table with multiple barriers for protection. HACCP is a management strategy, but has elements of the risk-assessment process inherent to it. This includes some hazard identification and exposure assessment. The system is largely nonquantitative and does not incorporate dose-response or risk characterization. It can be argued that better management decisions regarding the controls, the performance standards, and monitoring can be made if a more thorough risk assessment is undertaken.

Elements in the food supply chain include production, harvest, processing, transport, packaging, storage, and wholesale and retail marketing. Finally, there is preparation in the home or restaurants. If

TABLE 12 An Example of Hazards Defined by Transmission or Exposure Potential and Control Points

Type of General Hazard or Disease By Transmission	Sources	Specific Transmission Risks	Issues to be Addressed
Fecal-oral	Humans	Foodborne	Wastewater treatment
			Agricultural practices
	Animals	Waterborne	Wildlife
			Food supply
	Birds	Person-to-person	Potable and nonpotable water treatment (individual, camp, and recycling of water)
		Fomites	Cross-contamination
			Personal hygiene
Respiratory	Humans	Direct-contact	Personal hygiene
	Birds	Airborne	Wildlife
	Water	Waterborne	Indoor ventilation
			Plumbing and piping
Vectorborne	Insects	Person-vector-person	Geographic distribution of vector and disease
	Rodents	Reservoir-vector-person	Seasonality
			Climate factors
			Behavior of vector, reservoir, and human
Contact	Humans	STDs	Behavior
	Environment (soil & water)	Skin infections: waterwashed	Use of prophylaxis
	Insects	Insect borne	Protective gear, housing clothing

this concept were applied broadly to all microorganisms of concern, then a separate systems assessment that would be hazard- and transmission-specific (e.g., for vectorborne diseases) would need to be established. The CCPs, the monitoring, and controls would also be specific. Several examples can be used to address the risk-assessment process and the relationship to HACCP (Table 12; Figure 10).

BUILDING DATABASES FOR NATURALLY-OCCURRING MICROBIAL HAZARDS AND BIOLOGICAL WEAPONS

Although health outcomes and morbidity and mortality statistics are available from numerous databases and surveillance programs, the data lacking are often the long-term assessments and chronic outcomes. However, the exposure assessment, particularly during deployment, is more suspect to uncertainty, especially in terms of quantitative evaluations.

Assessment of Health Outcome

After exposure to a microorganism and after infection begins (defined by dose-response or attack rates), the number of possible outcomes includes asymptomatic illness, various levels of acute and chronic disease (mild illness to more severe illness to chronic problems to conditions that require hospitalization) and potentially death (mortality).

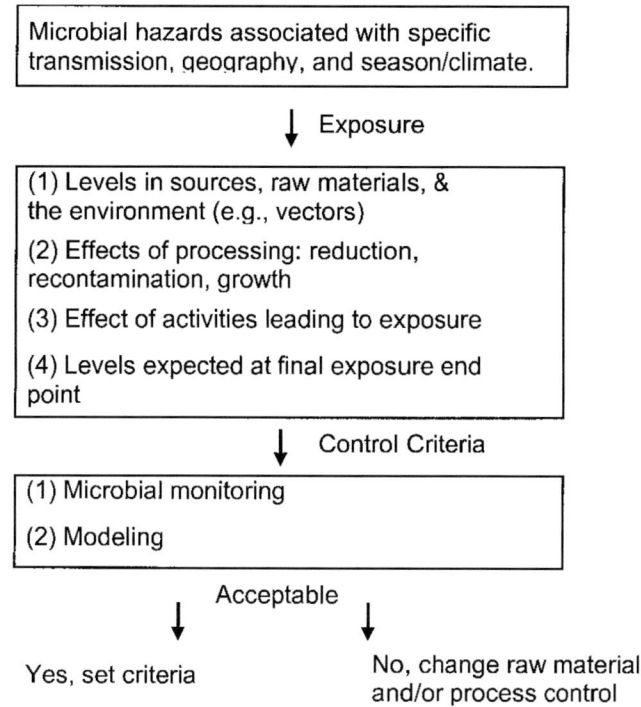

FIGURE 10 Use of risk assessment for setting criteria in HACCP (Source: Adapted from Notermans and Mead 1996).

The cases or measured rates described previously in epidemiological studies or disease surveillance of infectious diseases can be divided into several groups: (1) endemic risks that are the constant low-levels of diseases or infections that are present in a population; (2) epidemic risks that are disease cases in excess of the number of cases normally found or expected, and are constituted as an outbreak if limited to a specific population; and (3) outbreaks that are defined as two or more cases associated with a common exposure in time and place or source. In most cases, these studies rely on routine health surveillance methods, whereby the individuals seek medical attention, submit laboratory samples, and are diagnosed. Often this is done retrospectively, through the examination of records or through personal interviews and recall.

The attack rate is defined by the ratio of cases of an illness that occur relative to the total population exposed. The problem with this ratio is that often the numerator (cases) and denominator (those exposed) are not very well defined. These attack rates are not only subject to the accuracy of the investigation but are also subject to the level of the contamination (which is rarely identified), concentration of the microorganism in the exposure medium, frequency of exposure, and type of microorganism (dose-response). However, it appears that at least in drinking-water outbreaks (perhaps under conditions of lower levels of contamination), it is the microbial hazard that influences these attack rates, which correlate well with the dose-response values for the individual microorganisms (Figure 11). For example, on average, 22% of the populace in the communities exposed developed illness when the drinking water was tainted with *Campylobacter,* and 53% of the populace became ill during waterborne outbreaks of the Norwalk virus.

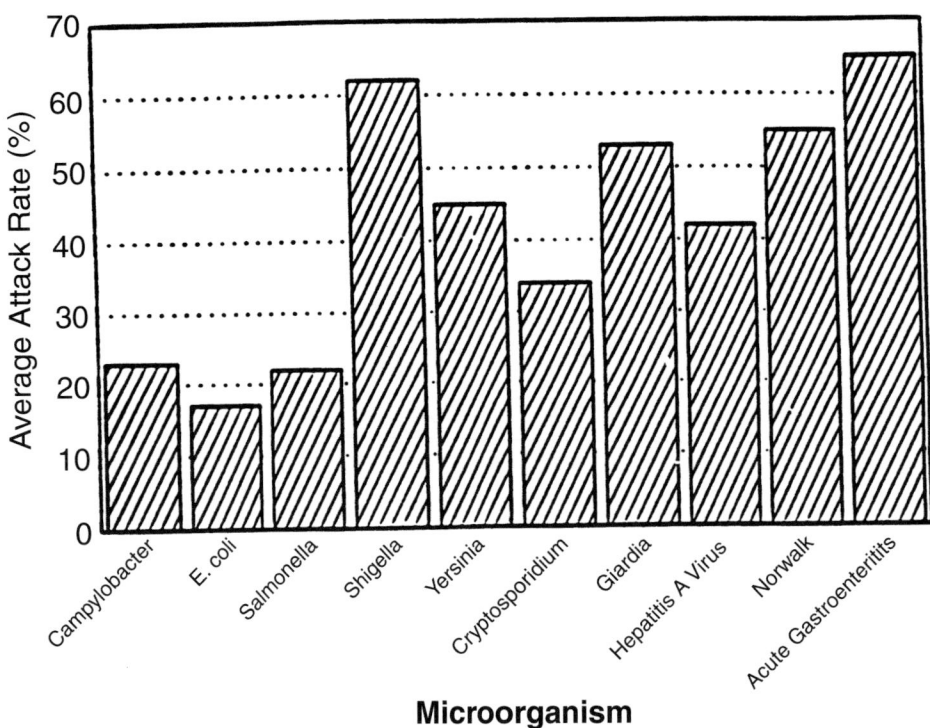

FIGURE 11 Average attack rates by microorganism during waterborne outbreaks. (Source: Haas et al. 1999.)

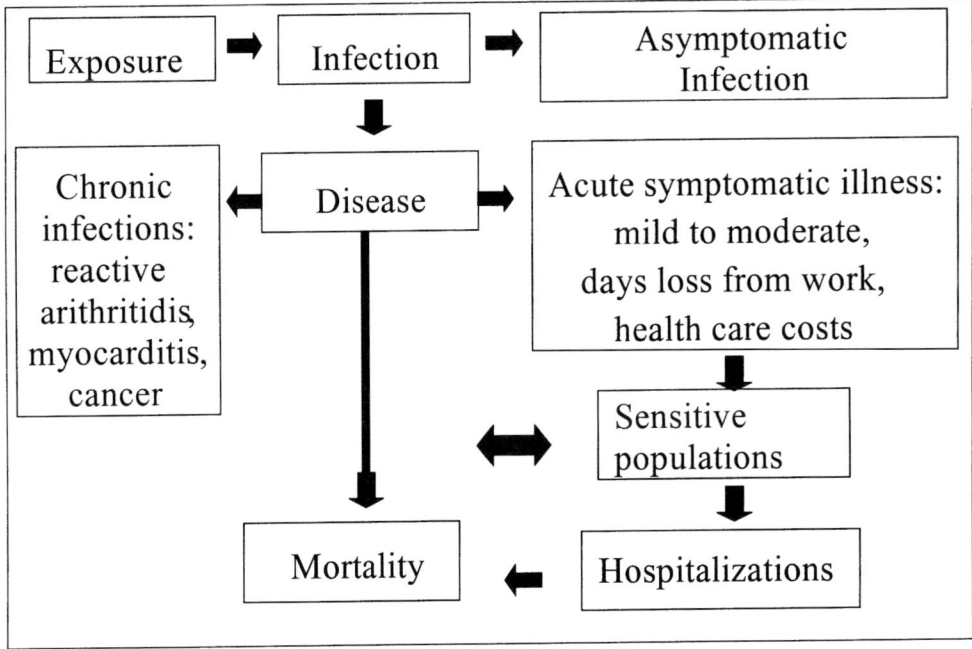

FIGURE 12 Outcomes of the infection process for quantification. (Source: Haas et al. 1999.)

Figure 12 demonstrates the various outcomes that need to be assessed during exposure and infections. It has been difficult to predict, based on the current health databases, the quantitative probability of each possible outcome because it might be microorganism-specific, even isolate-specific, and can depend on the host's status. The goal of hazard identification, however, is to define these outcomes to the extent possible. Each outcome can be described as a ratio or percentage, but the numerator and denominator need to be adequately defined, as well as the populations that are associated with the data.

Health Outcome Databases Associated With Biological Weapons and Terrorist Attacks

Figures 13 and 14 demonstrate the outcomes of the *Salmonella* and *Shigella* outbreaks associated with the tainted food sources during suspected terrorist acts (Torok et al. 1997; Kolavic et al. 1997). During the *Salmonella* event, lettuce was contaminated at several restaurants. Employees and customers were exposed. For employees, infection was determined by clinical diagnosis based on excretion of the bacteria in the feces for those with no symptoms, or mild symptoms, and by self-reporting at least three (reporting symptoms of fever, chills, headache, nausea, abdominal pain, vomiting, or bloody stools), for those with case-definition symptoms. Based on this, a 53% attack rate was established and could be used to estimate the impact of the contamination (692 cases/0.53 = 1,306). With 53% and 32% being the illness rate and infection rate, respectively, the estimate of the total number affected would be ~ 4,081 (1,306/0.32). There was no estimate of the number of individuals exposed. Severity was shown to be 6.5%, based on hospitalizations (45/692). There were no deaths. Although chronic outcomes were not followed, secondary transmission was estimated at 1%. In contrast, the *Shigella* event involved very high levels of contamination of muffins that were consumed by 12 individuals (although 45 people had access to the muffins), all of whom became ill (100% attack rate). The illness was more severe with 42% and 30% visiting the emergency room and being hospitalized, respectively. No deaths occurred and no chronic outcomes were evaluated.

Figures 15 and 16 show the dose-response models for the two bacteria. *Shigella* (N_{50} = 1,120; hospitalization 30%) has a greater infectivity and severity than *Salmonella* (N_{50} = 23,600; hospitalization 6.5%). However, the magnitude of the *Salmonella* outbreak is greater (45 hospitalized compared with 4 in the *Shigella* outbreak) due to the amount and nature of the exposure (more people, multiple days, and multiple restaurants). The dose-response models could determine the average dose from the outbreak data, by setting the attack rate (4,081 infected/total exposed) equal to P_i and then solving for N. These types of quantitative assessments allow the building of exposure scenarios whereby thresholds associated with ineffectiveness in the troops in a given time frame can be determined for specific agents.

Table 13 shows some of the other data that would be required in determining health outcomes.

Assessment of Exposure

Critical to the risk-assessment processes is the ability to quantify exposure to pathogens. Methods used in environmental applications are available to isolate and identify bacteria, fungi, protozoa, and viruses, as well as microbiological toxins (Hurst 1997). Standard methods have and continue to be used, such as those published in *Standard Methods for the Analysis of Water and Wastewater* (APHA 1998). However, newer methods using immuno-magnetic capture systems and molecular techniques are now being applied to foods for detection of *E. coli* 0157:H7 in hamburger.

Much of the past microbial occurrence data are nonquantitative, reported as presence or absence, and developed with very different protocols and monitoring approaches. Thus, often the issue is not the

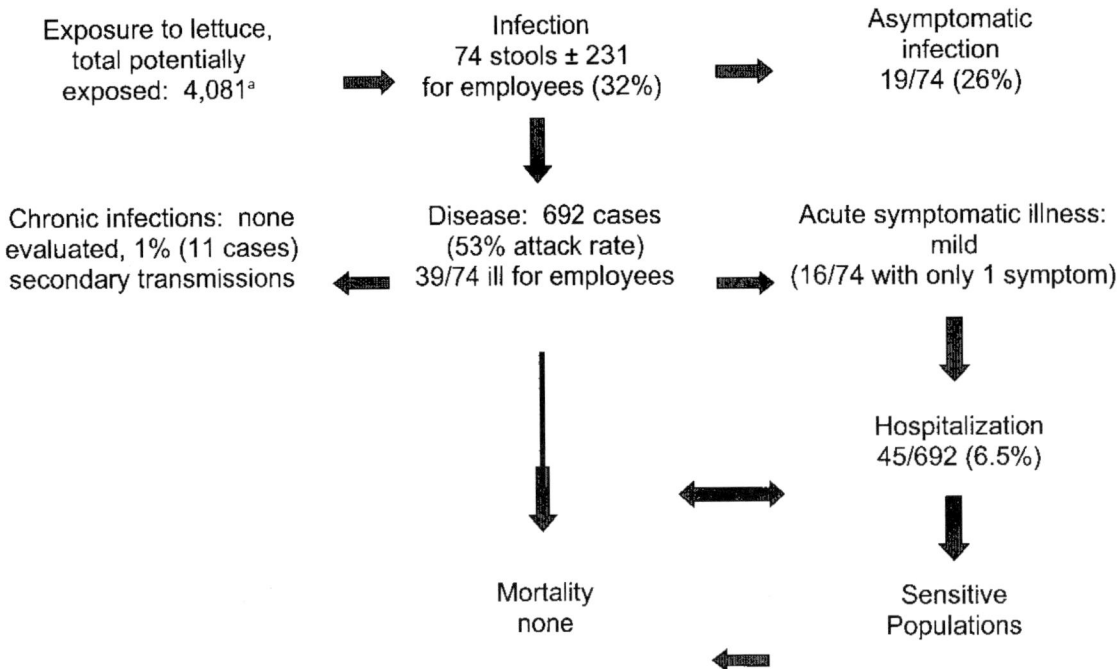

ᵃEstimated; exact total unknown.

FIGURE 13 Outcomes associated with an intentional contamination of *Salmonella* leading to an outbreak. (Source: Torok et al. 1997.)

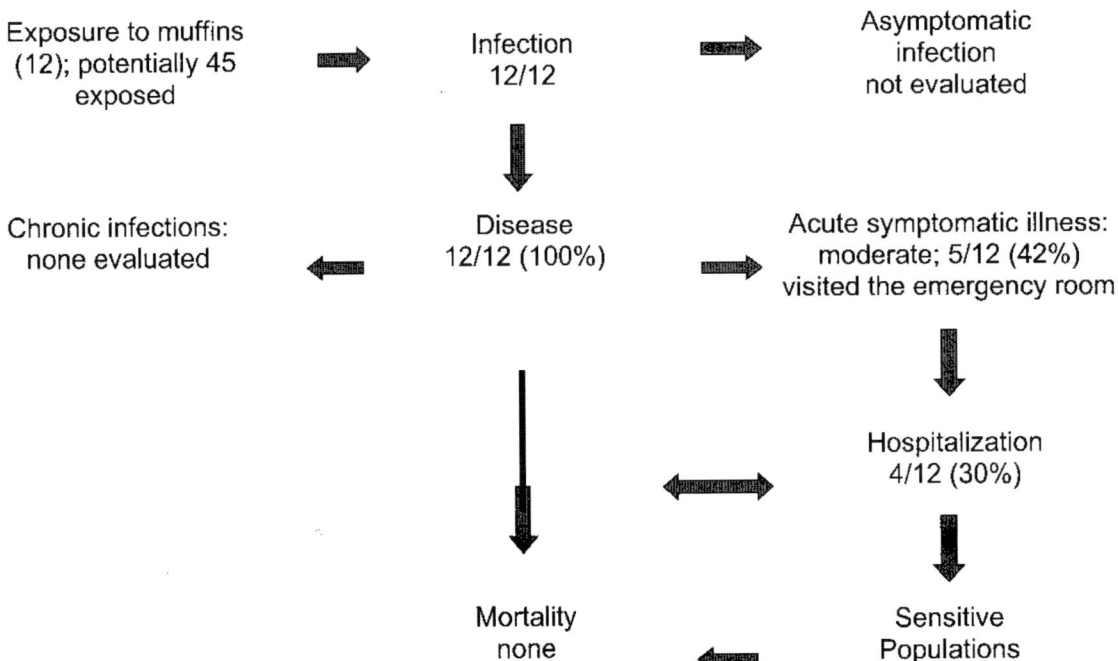

FIGURE 14 Outcomes associated with an intentional contamination of *Shigella* leading to an outbreak. (Source: Kolavic et al. 1997.)

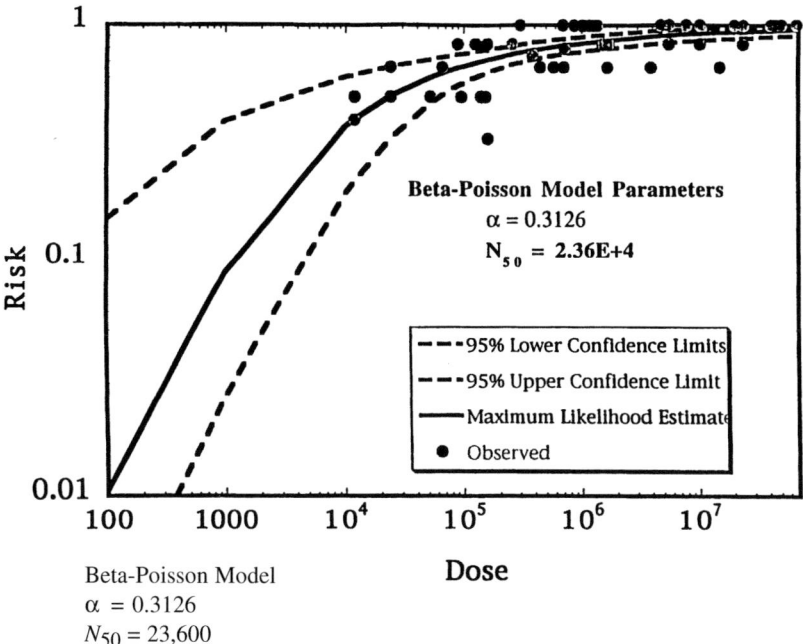

FIGURE 15 Dose-response model for *Salmonella*. (Source: Haas et al. 1999.)

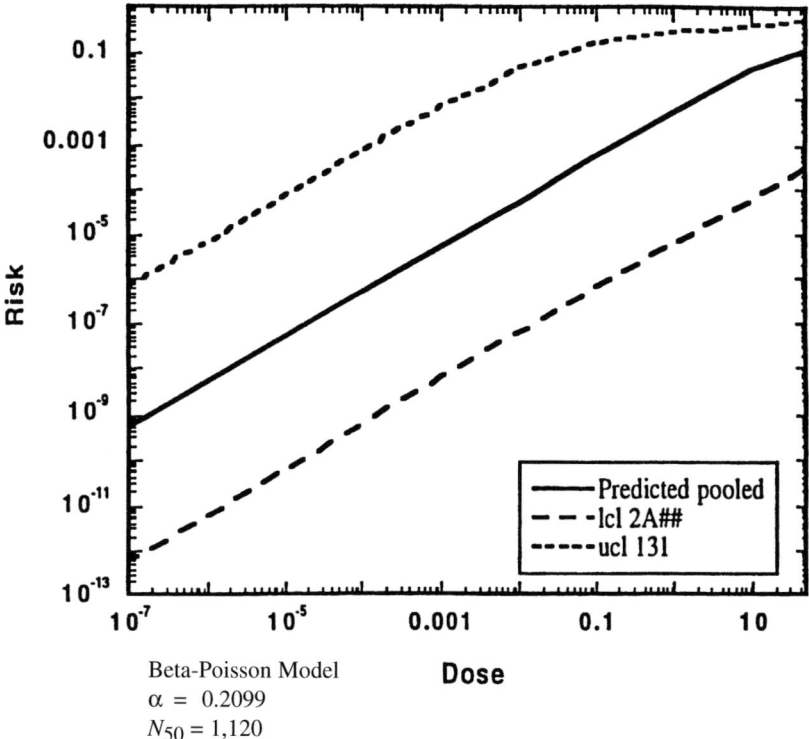

FIGURE 16 Dose-response model for *Shigella*. (Source: Crockett et al. 1996.)

TABLE 13 Assessment of Health Outcome[a]

Health Effects	Data Needs
Evaluation of outbreaks	Magnitude of community impact, attack rates, hospitalization and mortality, demographics, sensitive populations, level of contamination, duration, medical costs, community costs. Course of immune response and secondary transmission. Follow-up long-term outcomes.
Evaluation of endemic disease	Incidence, prevalence, geographic distribution, temporal distribution, percentage associated with various transmission routes (e.g., water versus food), demographics, sensitive populations, hospitalization, individual medical costs. Antibody prevalence, infection rates and illness rates.
Immune status	Protection versus issues for depression of the immune system.
Description of microbial pathogens	Mechanism of pathogenicity (how does it cause disease), virulence factors, virulence genes, antibiotic resistance.
Disease description	Types of diseases, duration, severity, medical treatment and costs, days lost, chronic sequelae, contributing risks (i.e., pregnancy, nutritional status, lifestyle [i.e., smoking and *Legionella*], immune status).
Methods for diagnosis	Available, routinely in use, require special requests, ease in use, cost, time.

[a]Clinical diagnostic tests must be available before other databases can be adequately established.
Source: Haas et al. 1999.

detection method per se but the sampling protocols and schemes and the interpretation of the data. These data have limited application for quantitative risk assessment. It is now recognized that quantitative, statistically evaluated databases must be developed because lack of exposure databases is often the major data gap for adequate risk assessments. These databases must be combined with models for prediction of transport and fate of microorganisms through the environment and through water and food treatment processes. By doing so, the field of predictive microbiology is a rapidly developing area that will be able to fill some of the data gaps on exposure assessment.

Exposure assessment could be defined as monitoring the source of the exposure over time, up to contact, that is, the final food product prior to consumption, the glass of water from the tap, or the aerosol that is inhaled. This is a difficult and impossible task in most cases. Microorganisms, unlike chemicals, act as particles, and their concentrations in water, soil, air, food, and on surfaces are not normally or homogeneously distributed. Microorganisms can change concentrations through die-off or growth over time. The sources of the microorganisms (e.g., animal wastes or sewage) are also diverse in concentrations over time (e.g., seasonal and climatic influences). Finally, many controls have already been implemented (disinfection) to reduce the concentrations and the exposure. Therefore, other strategies have been developed for assessing exposure and developing occurrence databases for microorganisms. These include the monitoring of indicators and pathogens for

- assessing the sources of microorganisms,
- assessing the transport and fate of microorganisms, and
- assessing the reduction through the use of treatment and process controls of microorganisms.

These approaches include field data and laboratory-based data and the use of models for evaluating transport (e.g., subsurface migration) and fate (e.g., inactivation rates). Ecosystem studies are necessary for evaluating most microorganism transport and fate (e.g., *Legionella* in biofilms and release during

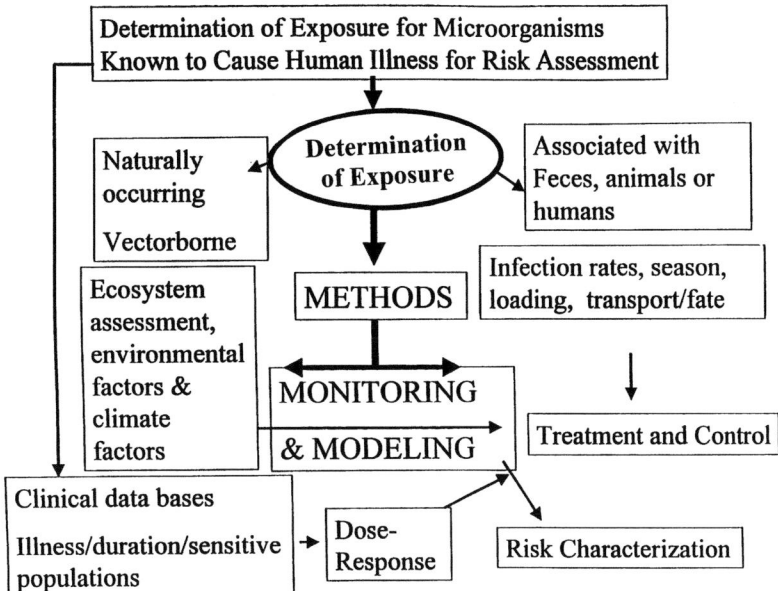

FIGURE 17 Framework for determination of exposure.

aerosolization), and more ecosystem modeling is needed. In the area of food safety, the concept of farm-to-table is being used to follow the microbial contaminants from their source on the farm through harvest and production to the final packing of the food product. For drinking water, a similar system based on watershed assessment, drinking-water treatment efficacy, and distribution-system integrity is being promoted. In some of these cases, an understanding of infections in the animal or human populations, waste disposal practices, and the transport patterns, survival, and growth of the microorganisms must be gained and monitoring data must be developed to support the likelihood of exposure through the various pathways. Therefore, the evaluation of exposure will require the extensive development of a variety of databases and models.

Figure 17 shows an example of how the exposure determination is tied to the risk assessment.

Assessment of Dose-Response and Disease Modeling

There have been over 40 dose-response data sets analyzed to date (Haas et al. 1999). Tables 14 and 15 show a summary of some of these data and Figure 18 shows a comparison of the models.

The development of a quantitative dose-response relationship is a primary step in performing a risk analysis. In QMRA microbial risk assessment, the dose-response relationship enables estimates to be made of the likelihood of an infection occurring, that is, the ability of the microorganism to colonize the body, specifically in the intestinal tract or the respiratory tract, for example. In the environment, exposures to microorganisms are usually at doses that are too low to measure via direct dose-response experiments. The exceptions to this are with BWs and bacterial growth in foods. In addition, microbial toxins may be modeled more as a chemical dose response than a microbial but very little data on toxins have been modeled to date.

TABLE 14 Best-Fit Values for Some Fecal-Oral Microorganisms

| | | Best-Fit Model Values | | |
| | | Exponential | Beta-Poisson[a] | |
Microorganism	Subject (doses)	k	α	N_{50} (β)
E. coli	Human (19)	na	0.1748	2.55×10^6
Campylobacter	Human (6)	na	0.145	896
Salmonella nontyphoid	Human	na	0.3126	2.36×10^4
Shigella	Human (13)	na	0.2099	1.12×10^3
Cryptosporidium	Human (8)	238	na	
Giardia	Human (9)	50.2296	na	
Coxsackie B viruses	Mice (4)	129	na	
Rotavirus	Human (8)	na	0.265	5.597

[a] Using a modified Beta-Poisson model: $P_i = 1 - [1 + N/\beta]^{-\alpha}$.
Source: Haas et al. 1999.

TABLE 15 Best-Fit Parameters for Additional Microorganisms

| | | Best-Fit Model Values | | |
| | | Exponential | Beta-Poisson | |
Organism	Subject (doses)	k	α	N_{50}
Adenovirus	pigs (3)	3375.3500	n/a	n/a
Adenovirus type 4	pigs (3)	267.0500	n/a	n/a
Astrovirus	humans (3)	16.5×10^5	n/a	n/a
Conjunctivitis[a]	humans (6)	38.5×10^1	n/a	n/a
Conjunctivitis[b]	humans (4)	8.3700	n/a	n/a
Conjunctivitis[c]	humans (12)	n/a	.4041	1.11
Cyanobacteria	mice (8)	23.7×10^1	n/a	n/a
Echovirus	humans (3)	78.3×10^1	n/a	n/a
Endamoeba coli	humans (5)	n/a	.1008	34.1×10^2
Influenza type 2	humans (5)	77.9×10^5	n/a	n/a
Influenza type 3	hamsters (9)	4.8301	n/a	n/a
Porcine enterovirus[d]	pigs (3)	3375.3500	n/a	n/a
Porcine enterovirus[e]	pigs (3)	267.0500	n/a	n/a
Rhinovirus type 14	humans (6)	n/a	.2011	9.22
Rhinovirus type 39	humans (5)	n/a	.2245	3.29
RSV[f]	humans (3)	15.0×10^4	n/a	n/a
RSV	humans (7)	n/a	.1639	41.9×10^4
RSV	primates (6)	n/a	.1136	86.8×10^4
Rubella	humans (2)	94.6000	n/a	n/a

[a] IC Cal strain.
[b] IC Cal 8 YS10 strain.
[c] IC Cal 8 YS10 and IC Cal 8 strain.
[d] PE3-ECOPO-6 strain.
[e] PE7-O51 strain.
[f] Respiratory Syncytial Virus.
Source: Haas et al. 1999.

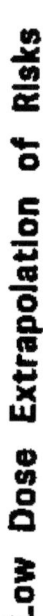

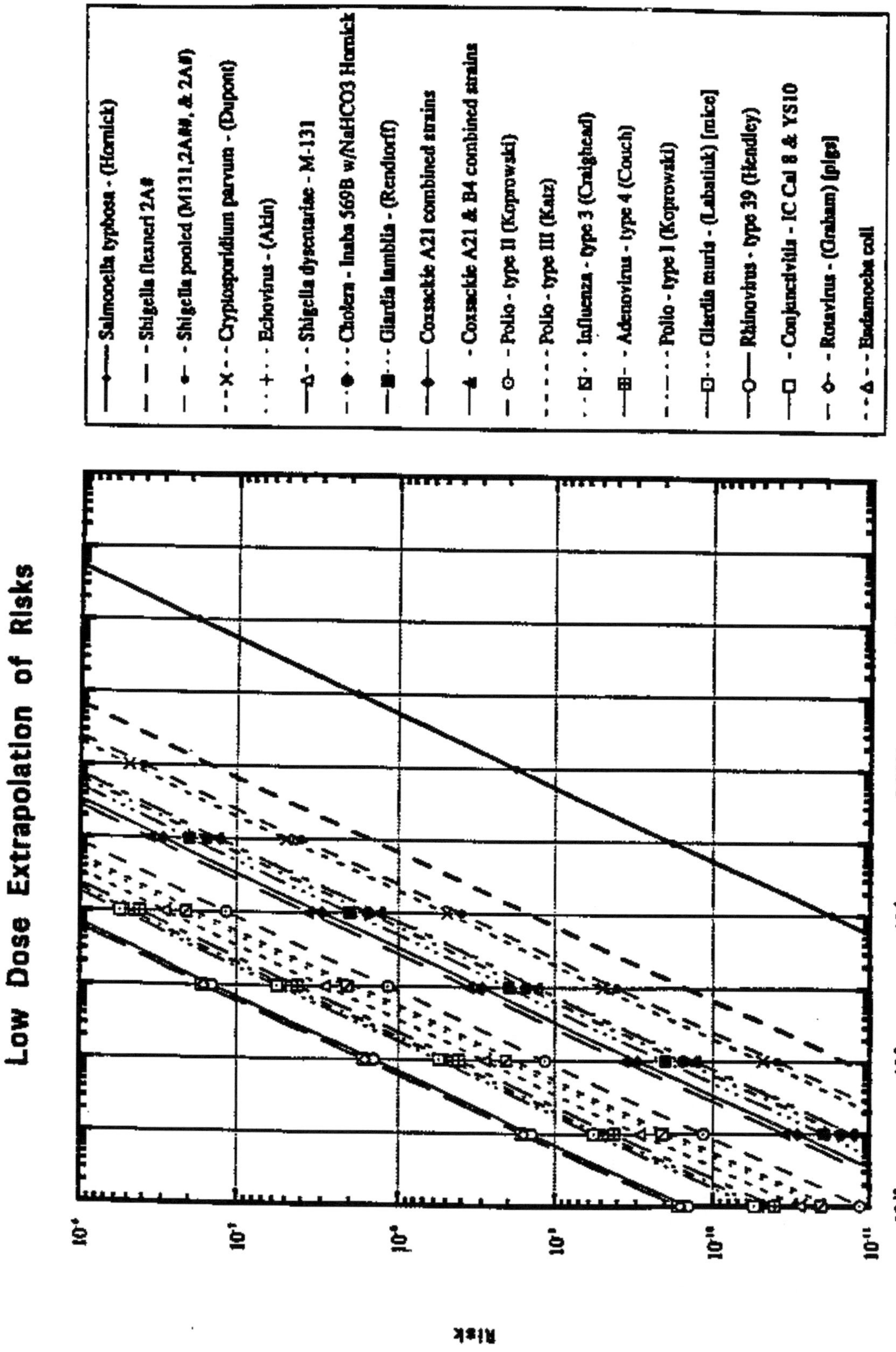

FIGURE 18 Comparative dose-response models at low-level exposure. (Source: Haas et al. 1999.)

Methodological Issues and Types of Data Sets

Obtaining data from a study designed to test the dose-response relationship of a specific organism on a human host is the ideal situation. However, it will be necessary at times to use data from studies designed for animals. Besides extrapolation from animals to humans, other issues identified in building databases include:

- How the dose was administered. This includes information about the type of system that was used to measure and administer the dose.
- Identification of the criteria used for a positive response. In most cases colonization was the criterion used, referred to as infection (clinical diagnosis or antibody response [serology]).
- The number of exposures.
- High-dose experiments without low doses tested.

Data can be pooled from many studies, as was the case for the *Shigella* and *Salmonella* models, or there might be a single study that would lead to the model. With either approach, upper and lower confidence limits can be determined for the models.

Both infection and the development of symptomatic disease can be measured, but in many experimental data sets not all the pertinent information is reported. However, there are several studies that do measure both, and in these situations a morbidity analysis can be performed (dosages required for infection to result in illness). In some cases, the illness was independent of the dose (such was the case for *Cryptosporidium*, Haas et al. 1996).

The data demonstrate that once infection had occurred the microorganism had some inherent virulence, that is, for example, 50% of those who became infected became ill.

As an example of infectivity, one might examine the data on the Hanta virus (Haas, C.N., Drexel University, Philadelphia, Penn., personal communication, 1999). The Hanta virus is transmitted through the aerosolization of the virus from urine from infected rodents. (As one of the types of viruses that cause hemorrhagic fever, it has also been placed on the list of BWs.) The infectivity of this virus can be modeled based on data reported by Nuzum et al. (1988). Mice were the host used and the dose was given in a single exposure by nasal aerosolization. Seroconversion (antibody response) was used as the measure of infectivity. The beta-Poisson model is shown in Figure 19. The data demonstrate that this virus is highly infectious. Interestingly, the inability to fully characterize the dose based on current methodologies was shown, because less than 1 PFU (plaque forming unit, the culturable unit for measuring viruses) could initiate the infection and the serological conversion. Morbidity, severity, mortality, and the other outcomes previously discussed would need to be further assessed.

Vectorborne Disease Modeling

Climatic issues have spurred the development of models for predicting disease outcomes associated with vectorborne transmission and changes in temperature and precipitation, particularly for malaria and dengue (Martens et al. 1994; Patz et al. 1998). These models combine elements of population epidemiological modeling as the outcome assessment associated with exposure to the infected vector (Figure 20). The density of the vectors, their age, their infectivity, and biting frequency can be predicted based on environmental conditions associated with precipitation and temperature. Thus, although not traditional

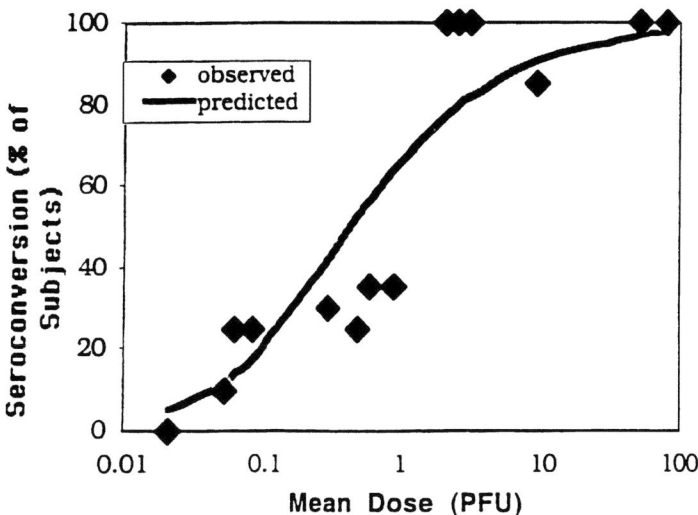

FIGURE 19 The beta-Poisson dose-response model for Hanta virus. (Source: based on the data of Nuzum et al. 1988.)

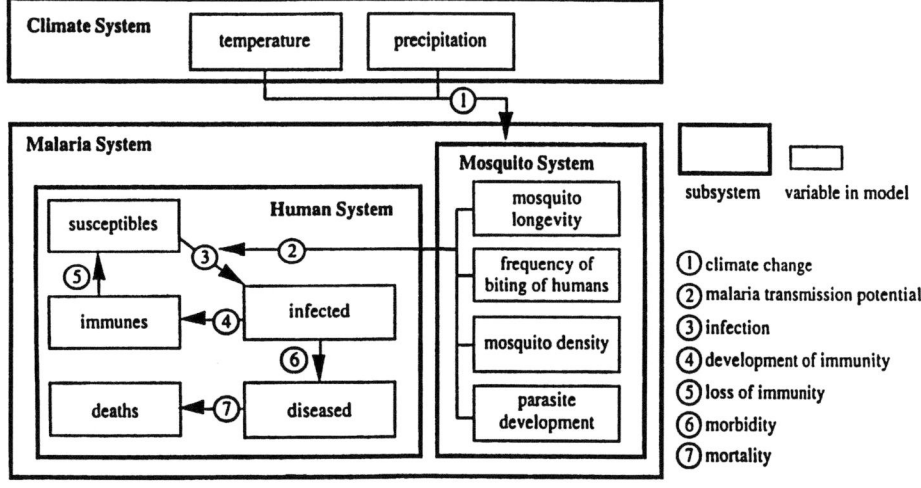

FIGURE 20 Disease model for malaria. (Source: Martens et al. 1994.)

dose-response models, these climatic models are extremely useful for comparing risks to various populations and could be used to examine the risks to deployed troops. Data should be gathered on geographic and climatic conditions, along with knowledge on the distribution and density of the vector and the level of infection of the parasite in the vector. Rapid methods (using molecular techniques) for assessing the level of virus or protozoan present in the vector population could be used in modeling the potential risk redeployment.

DOD INFECTIOUS DISEASE RESEARCH LABORATORIES

Summary of the Laboratories' History and Missions

There are nine DOD infectious disease research laboratories, three in the Washington, DC, area in the United States and one in each of the following countries, Peru, Brazil, Kenya, Egypt, Indonesia, and Thailand. Table 16 is a brief summary of the laboratories.

Early in the history of the United States, it was clearly recognized that conflicts, wars, and deployment of troops carried with them special medical needs in regards to infectious disease. No doubt the high morbidity and mortality associated with early conflicts such as the Civil War led to the realization of the importance of disease in these situations. In the late 1800s and early 1900s, great strides were being made in science and medicine. Methods were being developed for diagnosing diseases and characterizing microorganisms. There was a greater understanding of the disease process and transmission, and vaccines were being developed. In 1893, the Army Medical School was established to train physicians in the art and science of military medicine. Now known as the Walter Reed Army Institute of Research (WRAIR), this is the oldest and largest facility.

The current mission of the WRAIR is "biomedical research focused on soldier health and readiness." Early in its history, the development of a vaccine for typhoid fever and the study of yellow fever by Major Walter Reed in Cuba during the Spanish-American War were major accomplishments that led to a recognition of the benefits from such an organization. Since that time WRAIR has been involved in addressing the key plagues of the troops (such as malaria, hepatitis, dysentary, dengue) from WWI through the Bosnian conflict. Vaccine development, treatments, diagnostics, surveillance, assistance with deployments, and education have remained key components of the facility. Infectious diseases, combat casualty care, army operational medicine and medical chemical and biological defense are the four areas where research is conducted.

Although WRAIR is the largest laboratory within the U.S. Army Medical Research and Materiel Command, three other units were established outside of the United States. The largest of the three, the Armed Forces Research Institute of Medical Sciences (AFRIMS), functions as a Special Foreign Activity of the WRAIR. Established in 1959 in Bangkok, Thailand, the original mission was to research the cholera epidemic as was a part of the Southeast Asia Treaty Organization Cholera Research Laboratory. Command is with the Royal Thai Army and joint research on tropical diseases has included studies on Japanese encephalitis, hepatitis A and E, dengue, diarrhea, malaria, and drug-resistant scrubtyphus. The scientists have also been responsible for field-testing new drugs and vaccines. Epidemiological investigation, surveillance, rapid diagnostics, and advice on tropical diseases are part of the primary objectives of the laboratory.

TABLE 16 Rate of Infection and Clinical Cryptosporidiosis

Dose of oocysts	Exposed	Infected	Ill
30	5	1	0
100	8	3	3
300	3	2	0
500	6	5	2
>1000	7	7	2

Source: DuPont et al. 1995

Two smaller laboratories, known as U.S. Army Medical Research Units (USAMRU) were established, Unit K in Nairobi, Kenya, in 1969 and Unit B in Brazil (Rio De Janeiro and several other satellite locations) in 1973. U.S. personnel are limited at these facilities and they house host-country scientists and medical personnel. USAMRU B collaborates with PAHO, Institute of Biology of the Brazilian Army, University of Espirtu Santu, Vitoria and Instituto de Medicina Tropical do Amazonas to study emerging infectious disease agents in the Brazilian Amazon. The USAMRU K is affiliated with the Kenya Medical Research Institute and works out of two main facilities, a central laboratory in Nairobi and a field laboratory in Kisumu/Kisian in western Kenya. There are many joint collaborations with other organization including the U.S. Centers for Disease Control (CDC) and the Japanese International Cooperative Agency. The research has focused on drug resistance and vectorborne disease (tryptosomiasis, leishmaniasis, arboviruses). Molecular techniques such as PCR are used for microbial detection and characterizations and the facility houses a rearing laboratory for sand flies and mosquitoes.

Originally established in 1956 and officially named in 1969, the U.S. Army Medical Research Institute of Infectious Diseases (USAMRIID) was established in Ft. Detrick, Maryland. This is the second largest Army facility with approximately 450 scientists and other personnel. Their mission is to "conduct research to develop strategies, products, information, procedures and training programs for medical defense against biological warfare threats and infectious diseases." The research here is focused on deployment, and special scientific teams are developed and dispatched to assist in various types of investigations. The facility has one of the few biological level (BL)-4 containment laboratories to work on highly infectious and deadly diseases. The research is focused on biological weapons in addition to other areas including vaccine and drug development. The Navy Medical Research Institute (NMRI) was established in 1942 and is located in Washington, D.C. During the war NMRI's mission was focused on immediate operational problems and in particular was commissioned to study the atomic bomb survivors and develop methods for treatment of radiation exposure. The facility housed the first tissue bank in the world and pioneered studies on freeze-drying techniques used in preservation of human tissues for grafting and use of hypothermia for open-heart surgery. Among the recent accomplishments, scientists have also developed handheld assays for identification of BWs, and a PCR-based diagnosis system for *Campylobacter*. The NMRI and the WRIAR work as co-tenants (as a combined Army-Navy medical research program) and will soon be housed in a new facility in Forest Glen, Maryland.

In 1940 and 1942, Naval Medical Research Units (NAMRU) 2 and 3 were established in Guam (relocated to Taipei, Thailand) and Cairo, Egypt, respectively. Unit 2 is focusing on significant diseases in Asia, and is a WHO-collaborating center for emerging infectious diseases. Because it houses an animal facility, research on hemorragic fevers is of interest. Unit 3 has historically studied rickettsial disease, cholera, smallpox and meningitis, but has begun examining drug-resistant malaria, enterotoxogenic *E. coli, Campylobacter, Shigella,* and emerging viruses. This unit is also a WHO-collaborating facility for the study of the new strains of cholera and also has an animal facility.

Finally, in 1983, the Naval Medical Research Institute Detachment (NMRID) was established in Lima, Peru (10 years after USAMRU B in Brazil). Antibiotic resistance and drug-resistance in malaria were of interest and the research moved to address the dengue virus using PCR. This laboratory also contains an animal facility.

DOD Global Emerging Infectious Surveillance and Response System

The formal expansion of DOD's mission on emerging infectious diseases in June 1996 by Presidential Decision Directive NSTC-7 now includes global surveillance, training, research, and response. A 5-year strategic plan has been developed in parallel with CDC. Four goals have been articulated and are described in Table 17.

TABLE 17 DOD Infectious Disease Laboratories

Lab	Date Established/Location	Approximate Personnel Level	Focus and Special Activities
Naval Medical Research Institute Detachment (NAMRID	1983; Lima, Peru	8 Americans	Animal laboratory facility Antibiotic resistance Malaria drug resistance PCR: dengue
Naval Medical Research Unit 2 (NAMRU2)	1940; Guam then relocated to Taipei, Thailand (Indonesia)	21 Americans 120 Indonesians	Infectious disease Military significance in Asia WHO collaborating Center for Emerging Diseases of S.E. Asia
U.S. Army Medical Research Unit B (USAMRUB)	1973; Rio de Janeiro, Brazil and satellite locations limited	15 Brazilians U.S. personnel	Animal laboratory PAHO U.S. Collaborating
Naval Medical Research Unit 3 (NAMRU3)	1942; Cairo, Egypt	19 Americans 165 Egyptians	Rickettsia Cholera Smallpox Meningitis Emerging viruses Drug-resistant malaria Enterotoxogenic *E. coli*/*Campylobacter*/*Shigella* Animal facility WHO collaborating (19 personnel) CDC-Cholera OB9
U.S. Army Medical Research Unit K (USAMRUK)	1969; Nairobi, Kenya	8 Americans Kenyan personnel of the Medical Research Institute	Drug-resistant malaria Tryptosomiasis Leishmaniasis Arboviruses Viral infections CDC/Japan International Cooperative Agency PCR (insect facilities)

Institute	Founded; Location	Personnel	Research Areas
Armed Forces Research Institute of Medical Science (AFRIMS)	1959; Bangkok, Thailand	Numbers not given (largest of the USAMRU)	Cyclospora Diseases Scrubtyphus Malaria Hepatitis Diarrhea Dengue Japanese encephalitis Risk assessment New drugs/vaccines/diagnostics PCR Flow cytometry Animal facility
U.S. Army Medical Research Institute of Infectious Diseases (USAMRIID)	Ft. Detrick, MD	450 Americans	Deploy teams for investigation Vaccines/drugs BW Biological lab Level 4 (BL 4) Lab
Naval Medical Research Institute (NMRI)	1942; Washington, D.C.	Numbers unavailable	Navy tissue bank Operational problems Radiation study Handheld devices for BW PCR
Walter Reed Army Institute of Research (WRAIR)	1893; Washington, D.C.	700 Americans	Biomedical research Vaccine development Treatments, diagnostics, surveillance Assistance with deployments Infectious diseases Combat casualty care Army operational medicine Medical chemical and biological defense

One of the major assets in implementing this new directive is the overseas research laboratory system that is currently in place. All of the laboratories are undertaking various aspects related to all four goals. Clearly, although geographic locale is of some interest for some of the diseases, there is widespread global distribution of many of the microbial hazards. New resources will likely be needed to enhance not only the laboratory infrastructure and equipment but also to address personnel gaps. The evaluation and assessment of each laboratory is needed. Although specific activities matched to each laboratory's capabilities have been identified under each of the goals, there is no formal process for identifying and setting priorities for the various hazards, the specific activities, and the resources distribution. The use of risk-assessment methodologies offers an opportunity to use a scientific-based process for identifying and setting priorities for the most efficient and productive allocation of resources to the overseas laboratories.

Opportunities for Research Using a Risk-Assessment Method

It is proposed that a risk-assessment framework be used to develop criteria documents or briefs on the various microbial hazards, dose-response models, exposure assessments, and risk characterization, followed by a risk-management strategy. These documents can be used to fill data gaps and then be matched to the capabilities of the various laboratories. Clearly, laboratories with animal facilities could begin to fill gaps on dose-response and mixtures data. Laboratories with insect facilities can further evaluate the vectorborne models that have been developed. The overseas laboratories involved in treatment and vaccine development will fall into a category associated with risk-management research. However, one of the greatest needs will be to adapt the available tools to quantitate the hazards and, in particular, the exposure assessment in a prospective manner.

Environmental health programs focusing on exposure assessment using modeling and monitoring data will need to be developed. Data on the quality of food, water, air, and environment (surfaces) and health surveillance of the people will be needed. This will spur the development of better methods for environmental monitoring and lead to evaluation of the current tools. At a minimum, each laboratory staff should be trained in risk-assessment methods, should have PCR capabilities, and be trained in the use of the Geographical Information Systems (GIS) for maintaining and analyzing the database.

LESSONS LEARNED AND RECOMMENDATIONS

Lessons Learned from Deployments and Disease Surveillance

1. Intestinal illness and upper respiratory infection remain one of the greatest threats to deployed troops. These are largely of an unknown etiology and the hazards have not been properly identified. The illnesses are also time-dependent, with the greatest risk associated with early deployment.

2. There is seasonality and geographic variation in the diseases, although the factors associated with these trends are often not known.

3. Indigenous foods, fruits and vegetables, and bottled waters are associated with gastrointestinal risks.

4. The indoor environment is associated with upper respiratory illness.

5. Despite vaccination programs, with evolution will come new strains of pathogens that will continue to emerge (e.g., influenza) causing illness in troops. Assessment of these episodes will provide insight into the spread of disease globally.

6. Although vectorborne disease remains a concern, predeployment assessment of risk and preven-

tion has been shown to be successful; however, diligence is needed because exposures as low as a few hours can result in serious illness.

7. Although much is known about types of biological weapons that could be used, concerns regarding availability of vaccines has emerged, as well as the ability to detect and respond to an attack.

8. Some emerging infectious diseases are being studied and assessed in troops; however, the data are limited. Of concern are the emergence of antibiotic-resistant bacteria, resistant forms of parasites, and the lack of vaccines for many of these diseases. These factors have led to a limitation in treatment options, and better prevention strategies are needed.

Some Recommendations

Emerging Hazards

- Coxsackieviruses can exhibit chronic outcomes and these infections should be followed with serology.
- The use of urinary antigen could be used to screen for prevalence for *Legionella* as a cause of indoor respiratory disease.
- All Hanta virus and rodent distributions should be mapped.
- Streptococci skin infections and associated upper respiratory disease should be of interest.

Risk Assessment

- Health surveillance databases need to include asymptomatic infections and quantitative outcomes.
- Dose-response databases should be developed.
- Geographic, climatic, seasonal, dose-response, and exposure scenarios can be used to develop tools for setting priorities for assessment of predeployment risks.
- Risk models can be evaluated for plausibility during outbreak investigations or disease surveillance operations. Exposure and health outcomes must be better assessed.
- The use of quantitative assessments allows one to begin to build exposure scenarios in which thresholds associated with ineffectiveness in the troops in a given time frame can be determined for specific agents.

Biological Weapons

- Dose-response models should be developed.
- Time and concentration exposure and consequence scenarios should be built and evaluated.

Mixtures and Multiple Stressors

- Microbial hazards should be added to animal research studies to test for mixtures effects (e.g., vaccination followed by coxsackieviruses, metals and viruses effects, and nutrition and infection). Special focus should be given to those microorganisms with possible immunological and neurological outcomes.

DOD Infectious Disease Research Laboratories

• One of the major assets in implementing DOD's expand mission on emerging infectious diseases is the overseas research laboratory system that is currently in place. At a minimum, each laboratory staff should be trained in risk-assessment methods, should have PCR capabilities, and be trained in the use of GIS for maintaining and analyzing the databases.

REFERENCES

Abbaszadegan, M., P. Stewart, and M. LeChevallier. 1999. A strategy for detection of viruses in groundwater by PCR. Appl. Environ. Microbiol. 65(2):444-449.

American Public Health Association, American Water Works Association and Water Environmental Federation. 1998. Standard Methods for the Examination of Water and Wastewater, Supplement, 18th Ed. American Public Health Association, Washington, D.C.

Ashford, R.W. 1979. Occurrence of an undescribed coccidian in man in Papua New Guinea. Ann. Trop. Med. Parasitol. 73:497-500.

Axon, A.T.R. 1995. Review article: is Helicobacter pylori transmitted by the gastro-oral route. Ailment. Pharmacol. Ther. 9:585-588.

Bendinelli, M. and H. Friedman. 1988. Coxsackieviruses: A General Update. New York, NY: Plenum Press.

Benenson, M.W., E.T. Takafuji, S.M. Lemon, R.L. Greenup, and A.J. Sulzer. 1982. Oocyst-transmitted toxoplasmosis associated with ingestion of contaminated water. N. Engl. J. Med. 307:666-669.

Beneson, A. 1995. Dengue Fever. Pp. 128-130. In: Control of Communicable Diseases Manual. 16th Ed. Washington, D.C: American Public Health Association.

Beck, M., P.C. Kolbeck, Q. Shi, L.H. Rohr, V.C. Morris, and O.A. Levander. 1994. Increased virulence of a human enterovirus (Coxsackievirus B3) in seleniu-deficient mice. J. Infect. Dis. 170:351-7.

Bryan, R.T. 1995. Microsporidiosis as an AIDS-related opportunistic infection. Clin. Infect. Dis. 21(Suppl. 1):S 62-65.

Buck, A.C. and E.M. Cooke. 1969. The fate of ingested Pseudomonas aeruginosa in normal persons. J. Med. Microbiol. 2:521-525.

Buzby, J.C., T. Roberts, and B.M. Allos. 1997. Estimated Annual Costs of Campylobacter-Associated GBS. Econ. Res. Serv., USDA. (July).

Canadian Water Works Association. 1995. Special report: Victoria toxoplasmosis outbreak traced to water supply. CWWA Bulletin (October):3-4.

Cascio, A., M. Bosco, E. Vizzi, A. Giammanco, D. Ferraro, and S. Artista. 1996. Identification of picobirnavirus from faeces of Italian children suffering from acute diarrhea. Eur. J. Epidemiol. 12(5):545-7.

CDC (Centers for Disease Control and Prevention). 1997. Emerging Infectious Diseases. 3(4) (Oct. - Dec.)

Chandra, R. 1997. Picobirnavirus, a novel group of undescribed viruses of mammals and birds: a minireview. Acta Virol. 41(1):59-62.

Chant, K., R.Chan, M.Smith, D.E. Dwyer, and P. Kirkland. 1998. Probable human infection with a newly described virus in the family Paramyxoviridae. Emerg. Infect. Dis. 4(2):273-5.

Cooper, R.C., A.W. Olivieri, R.E. Danielson, P.G. Badger, R.C. Spear, and S. Selvin. 1986. Evaluation of Military Field-Water Quality, Vol. 5. Infectious Organisms of Military Concern Associated With Consumption: Assessment of Health Risks, and Recommendation for Establishing Related Standards. Lawrence Livermore National Laboratory UCRL-21008. U.S. Army Medical Research and Development Command, Fort Detrick, Frederick, MD.

Craun, G.F. 1996. Water Quality in Latin America:Balancing the Microbial and Chemical Risk in Water Disinfection. Washington, D.C.: International Life Science Institute Press.

Crockett, C., C.N. Haas, A. Fazil, J.B. Rose, and C.P. Gerba. 1996. Prevalence of shigellosis in the U.S.: Consistency with dose-response information. Int. J. Food Microbiol. 30(1-2):87-99.

Dev, V.J., M. Main, and I. Gould. 1991. Waterborne outbreak of Escherichia coli O157. [letter]. Lancet. 337:1412.

Dowd, S.E., C.P. Gerba, and I.L. Pepper. 1998. Confirmation of the human-pathogenic microsporidia Enterocytozoon bieneusi, Encephalitozoon intestinalis, and Vittaforma corneae in water. Appl. Environ. Microbiol. 64(9):3332-5.

Dubey, J.P., C.A. Speer, and R. Fayer. 1990. Cryptosporidiosis of man and animals. Boca Raton, Fla.: CRC Press.

DuPont, H.L., C.L. Chappell, C.R. Sterling, P.C. Okhuysen, J.B. Rose, and W. Jakubowski. 1995. The infectivity of Cryptosporidium parvum in healthy volunteers. N. Engl. J. Med. 322:855-859.

EPA (United States Environmental Protection Agency). 1989. National Primary Drinking Water Regulations; Filtration and Disinfection; Turbidity; Giardia Lamblia, Viruses, Legionella, and Heterotrophic Bacteria. Fed. Regist. 54(124): 27486-27541.

Eurogast Study Group. 1993. An international association between Helicobacter pylori infection and gastric cancer. Lancet. 341:1359-1362.

Fauci, A.S. 1998. New and reemerging diseases: the importance of biomedical research. Emerg. Infect. Dis. 4(3):374-378.

Ferrieri, P., A.S. Dajani, L.W. Wannamaker, and S.S. Chapman. 1972. Natural history of impetigo. I. Site sequence of acquisition and familial patterns of spread of cutaneous streptococci. J. Clinical Inv. 51:2851-2862.

Fitzen, E., J. Paulin, T. Cleslak, G. Christopher, and R. Culpepper. 1998. Medical Management of Biological Casualties. U.S. Army Medical Research Institute of Infectious Disease. Ft. Detrick, MD.

Franz, D.R., P.B. Jahrling, A.M. Friedlander, D.J. McClain, D.L. Hoover, W.R. Bryne, J.A. Pavlin, G.W. Christopher, and E.M. Eitzen, Jr. 1997. Clinical recognition and management of patients exposed to biological warfare agents. JAMA 278 (5):399-411.

Gajdusek, D. 1962. Virus hemorrhagic fevers. J. Oediatr. 60:841-57.

Gale, P. 1998. Quantitative BSE risk assessment: relating exposures to risk. Lett. Appl. Microbiol. 27(5):239-42.

Gale, P., C. Young, G. Stanfield ,and D. Oakes. 1998. Development of a risk assessment for BSE in the aquatic environment. J. Appl. Microbiol. 84(4): 467-77.

Gallimore, C.I., H. Appleton, D. Lewis, J. Green, and D.W. Brow. 1995. Detection and characterization of bisegmented double-stranded RNA viruses (picobirnaviruses) in human faecal specimens. J. Med. Virol. 45(2):135-40.

Geldreich, E.E., K.R. Fox, J.A. Goodrich, E.W. Rice, R.M. Clark, and D.L. Swerdlow, 1992. Searching for a water supply connection in the Cabool, Missouri disease outbreak of Escherichia coli O157:H7. Water Res. 26:1127-1137.

Gerba, C.P. and C.N. Haas. 1988. Assessment of risks associated with enteric viruses in contaminated drinking water. ASTM Special Technical Publication 976:489-494.

Gerba, C.P. and J.B. Rose. 1990. Viruses in source and drinking water. Pp. 380-396. In: Drinking Water Microbiology. G.A. McFeters, ed. New York, NY: Springer-Verlag.

Glynn, A.W., Y. Lind, E. Funseth, and N.G. Ilback. 1998. The intestinal absorption of cadmium increases during a common viral infection (coxsackie virus B3) in mice. Chem. Biol. Interact. 113:79-89.

Goodgame, R.W. 1996. Understanding intestinal spore-forming protozoa: cryptosporidia, microsporidia, isospora and cyclospora. Ann. Intern. Med. 124:429-441.

Grabow, W.O., M.O. Favorov, N.S. Khudyakova, M.B. Taylor, and H.A. Fields. 1994. Hepatitis E seroprevalence in selected individuals in South Africa. J. Med. Virol. 44:384-388.

Gubler, D.J., and G.G. Clark. 1995. Dengue/dengue hemorrhagic fever: the emergence of a global health problem. Emerg. Infect. Dis. 1(2):55-7.

Gust I.D. and R.H. Purcell. 1987. Report of a workshop: waterborne non-A, non-B hepatitis. J. Infect. Dis. 156(4):630-5.

Haas, C.N. 1983. Estimation of risk due to low doses of microorganisms: A comparison of alternative methodologies. Am. J. Epidemiol. 118:573-582.

Haas, C.N, J.B. Rose, C. Gerba, and S. Regli. 1993. Risk assessment of virus in drinking water. Risk Anal. 13:545-552.

Haas C.N., C.S. Crockett, J.B. Rose, C.P. Gerba, and A.M Fazil. 1996. Assessing the risk posed by oocysts in drinking water. J. Am. Water Works Assoc. 88:131-136.

Haas, C.N, J.B. Rose, and C.P. Gerba. 1999. Quantitative Microbial Risk Assessment, New York, NY:John Wiley and Sons.

Halstead, S.B. 1988. Pathogenesis of dengue: challenges to molecular biology. Science 239(4839):476-81.

Hancock, C.M., J.B. Rose, and M. Callahan. 1998. Crypto and giardia in US groundwater. J. Am. Water Works Assoc. 90(3):58-61.

Hentges, D.J., A.J. Stein, S.W. Casey, and J.U. Que. 1985. Protective role of intestinal flora against infection with Pseudomonas aeruginosa in mice: Influence of antibiotics on colonization resistance. Infect. Immun. 47:118-122.

Hepatitis Control Report. 1998. Using an epidemic approach, El Paso takes aim at endemic hepatitis A. 3(2):1-8.

Hurst, C.J. 1997. Detection of viruses in environmental waters, sewage, and sewage sludge. Pp. 168-175. In: Manual of Environmental Microbiology, C.J. Hurst, G. R. Knudsen, M.J. McInerney, L.D. Stetzenbach, and M.V. Walter, eds. Washington, D.C.: ASM Press.

Hyams, K., F.S. Wignall, and R. Roswell. 1996. War syndromes and their evaluation: from the U.S. Civil War to the Persian Gulf War. Ann. Inter. Med. 125:398-405.

Hyams, K.C., K. Hanson, F.S. Wignall, J. Escamilla, and E.C. Oldfield 3rd. 1995. The impact of infectious diseases on the health of U.S. troops deployed to the Persian Gulf during operations Desert Shield and Desert Storm. Clin. Infect. Dis. 20:1497-1504.

ILSI (International Life Sciences Institute). 1996. A conceptual framework to assess the risks of human disease following exposure to pathogens. Risk Anal. 16:841-848.

Joseph, C.A., T.G. Harrison, D. Ilijic-Car, and C.L. Bartlett. 1998. Legionnaires' disease in residents of England and Wales: 1997. Commun. Dis. Pub. Health 1(4):252-258.

JSC (Joint Chiefs of Staff). 1998. Memorandum: Deployment Health Surveillance and Readiness. MCM-251-98. Office of the Chairman, Washington, D.C. (dated December 4, 1998.)

Klein, P.D., D.Y. Graham, A. Gaillour, A.R. Opekun, and E.O. Smith. 1991. Water source as risk factor for Helicobacter pylori infection in peruvian children. Lancet 337:1503-1506.

Kiode, H., Y. Kitaura, H. Deguchi, A. Ukimura, K. Kawamura, and A. Hirai. 1992. Genomic detection of enteroviruses in the myocardium—studies on animal hearts with coxsackievirus B3 myocarditis and endomyocardial biopsies from patients with myocarditis and dilated cardiomyopathy Jpn. Circ. J. 56:1081-1093.

Klingel, K, C. Hohenadl, A. Canu, M. Albrecht, M. Seemann, G. Mall, and R. Kandolf. 1992. Ongoing enterovirus-induced myocarditis is associated with persistent heart muscle infection: quantitative analysis of virus replication, tissue damage and inflammation. Proc. Natl. Acad. Sci. U.S.A. 89:314-318.

Kolavic, S.A., A. Kimura, S.L. Simons, L. Slutsker, S. Barth, and C.E. Haley. 1997. An outbreak of Shigella dysenteriae type 2 among laboratory workers due to intentional food contamination. JAMA. 278(5):396-398.

Lee, S.H., S.T. Lai, J.Y. Lai, and N.K. Leung. 1996. Resurgence of cholera in Hong Kong. Epidemiol. Infect. 117(1) 43-49.

Lederberg, J. 1997. Infectious disease as an evolutionary paradigm. Emerg. Infect. Dis. 3(4):417-423.

Lisle, J.T. and J.B. Rose. 1995. Cryptosporidium contamination of water in the USA and UK: a mini review. Aqua 44(3):103.

Llback, N.G., J. Fohlman, and G. Friman. 1994. Changed distribution and immune effects of nickel augmented viral-induced inflammatory heart lesions in mice. Toxicology 91:203-219.

MacKenzie, W.R., N.J. Hoxie, M.E. Proctor, S. Gradus, K.A. Blair, D.E. Peterson, J.J. Kazmierczak, K. Fox, D.G. Addiss, J.B. Rose, and J.P. Davis. 1994. A massive outbreak in Milwaukee of cryptosporidium Infection transmitted through the public water supply. N. Engl. J. Med. 331(3):161-167.

Martens, W.J.M., J. Rotmans, and L.W. Niessen. 1994. Pp 37. In: Climate change and malaria risk: an integrated modeling approach. GLOBO. Report 3. No. 461502003.

Martin, S., J. Gamble, J. Jackson, N. Aronson, R. Gupta, E. Rowton, M. Perich, P. McEvoy, J. Berman, A. Magill, and C. Hoke. 1998. Leishmaniasis in the United States Military. Milit. Med. 163:801-807.

Mas, P., J.L. Pelegrino, M.G. Guzman, M.M. Comellas, S. Resik, M. Alvarez, R. Rodriguez, M. Mune, V. Capo, A. Balmaseda, L. Rodriguez, M.P. Rodriguez, J. Handy, G. Kouri, and A. Llop. 1997. Viral isolation from cases of epidemic nueropathy in Cuba. Arch. Pathol. Lab. Med. 121:825-833.

Meng, J. and M.P. Doyle. 1998. Emerging and evolving microbial foodborne pathogens. Bull. Inst. Pasteur. 96:151-164.

MSMR (Medical Surveillance Monthly Report). 1995. Guillain-Barre Syndrome Following Influenza Immunization, Fort Sam Houston, Texas. Vol.1. No. 9. p. 9. Available: http://www.amsa.army.mil. U.S. Army Center for Health Promotion and Preventative Medicine (ACHPPM), Fort Detrick, Maryland.

MSMR (Medical Surveillance Monthly Report) (MSMR). 1996a. Project Gargle: U.S. Air Force Influenza Surveillance Program Summary, 1995-1996. Vol. 2, No. 10, p. 8. Available: http://www.amsa.army.mil. U.S. Army Center for Health Promotion and Preventative Medicine (ACHPPM), Fort Detrick, Maryland.

MSMR (Medical Surveillance Monthly Report). 1996b. Leptospirosis, Tripler Army Medical Center. Vol. 2, No. 7, p. 7. Available: http://www.amsa.army.mil. U.S. Army Center for Health Promotion and Preventative Medicine (ACHPPM), Fort Detrick, Maryland.

MSMR (Medical Surveillance Monthly Report). 1997a. Reportable Conditions Reported Through Medical Surveillance System, Jan.-Dec. 1996. Vol. 3, No. 3. Available: http://www.amsa.army.mil. U.S. Army Center for Health Promotion and Preventative Medicine (ACHPPM), Fort Detrick, Maryland.

MSMR (Medical Surveillance Monthly Report). 1997b. Adult Respiratory Distress Syndrome (ARDS), Fort Lewis, Washington. Vol. 3, No. 5, p. 9. Available: http://www.amsa.army.mil. U.S. Army Center for Health Promotion and Preventative Medicine (ACHPPM), Fort Detrick, Maryland.

MSMR (Medical Surveillance Monthly Report). 1997c. Hospitalizations, Operation Joint Endeavor, Bosnia Part II. Hospitalization Experience in Diagnostic Subcategories. Vol. 3, No. 6, p. 12. Available: http://www.amsa.army.mil. U.S. Army Center for Health Promotion and Preventative Medicine (ACHPPM), Fort Detrick, Maryland.

MSMR (Medical Surveillance Monthly Report). 1997d. Ross River Virus Disease ("Epidemic Polyarthritis"), Exercise Tandem Trust 97, Queensland, Australia, Vol. 3, No. 7, p. 13. Available: http://www.amsa.army.mil. U.S. Army Center for Health Promotion and Preventative Medicine (ACHPPM), Fort Detrick, Maryland.

MSMR (Medical Surveillance Monthly Report). 1997e. Late Presentations of Vivax Malaria of Korean Origin, Multiple Geographic Sites. Vol. 3, No. 5, p. 3. Available: http://www.amsa.army.mil. U.S. Army Center for Health Promotion and Preventative Medicine (ACHPPM), Fort Detrick, Maryland.

MSMR (Medical Surveillance Monthly Report). 1998a. Reportable Conditions Reported Thorough Medical Surveillance System, Jan.-Dec. 1997. Vol. 4, No. 1. Available: http://www.amsa.army.mil. U.S. Army Center for Health Promotion and Preventative Medicine (ACHPPM), Fort Detrick, Maryland.

MSMR (Medical Surveillance Monthly Report). 1998b. Active Duty Hospitalizations, United States Army, 1997. Vol. 4, No. 3, p. 18. Available: http://www.amsa.army.mil. U.S. Army Center for Health Promotion and Preventative Medicine (ACHPPM), Fort Detrick, Maryland.

MSMR (Medical Surveillance Monthly Report). 1998c. Influenza Among Immunized Members of Aviation Squadron, U.S. Navy, Hawaii. Vol. 4, No. 2, p. 12-13. Available: http://www.amsa.army.mil. U.S. Army Center for Health Promotion and Preventative Medicine (ACHPPM), Fort Detrick, Maryland.

MSMR (Medical Surveillance Monthly Report). 1998d. Hospitalizations Among Active Duty Soldiers for "Fevers of Unknown Origin." Vol. 4, No. 1, p. 2. Available: http://www.amsa.army.mil. U.S. Army Center for Health Promotion and Preventative Medicine (ACHPPM), Fort Detrick, Maryland.

MSMR (Medical Surveillance Monthly Report). 1998e. Morbidity Surveillance During a Joint Multinational Field Training Exercise (OPERATION GOLD COBRA 98), Thailand. Vol. 4, No. 6, p. 2. Available: http://www.amsa.army.mil. U.S. Army Center for Health Promotion and Preventative Medicine (ACHPPM), Fort Detrick, Maryland.

MSMR (Medical Surveillance Monthly Report). 1998f. Visceral Leishmaniasis among Children of Active Duty U.S. Navy Members, Signolla, Italy. Vol. 4, No. 1, p. 9. Available: http://www.amsa.army.mil. U.S. Army Center for Health Promotion and Preventative Medicine (ACHPPM), Fort Detrick, Maryland.

MSMR (Medical Surveillance Monthly Report). 1998g. Leptospirosis in the Pacific: Tripler Army Medical Center. Vol. 4, No. 3, p. 12. Available: http://www.amsa.army.mil. U.S. Army Center for Health Promotion and Preventative Medicine (ACHPPM), Fort Detrick, Maryland.

Nchinda, T. 1998. Malaria: a reemerging disease in Africa. Emerg. Infect. Dis. 4(3): 398-403.

Notermans, S. and G.C. Mead. 1996. Incorporation of elements of quantitative risk analysis in the HACCP system. Int. J. Food Microbiol. 30:157-173.

NRC (National Research Council). 1994. Science and Judgment in Risk Assessment. Washington, D.C.: National Academy Press.

Nuzum, R.O., C.A. Rossi, E.H. Stephenson, and J.W. LeDuc. 1988. Aerosol transmission of Hantaan and related viruses to laboratory rats. Am. J. Trop. Med. Hyg. 38(3):636-40.

Ortega, Y.R., C.R. Sterling, R.H. Gilman, M.A. Cama, and F. Diaz. 1993. Cyclospora species—a new protozoan pathogen of humans. N. Engl. J. Med. 328:1308-1312.

Patz, J.A., J.M. Martens, D.A. Flocks, and T.H. Jetten. 1998. Dengue fever epidemic potential as projected by general circulation models of global climate change. Environ. Health. Perspect. 106(3):147-153.

Philbey, A.W., P.D. Kirkland, A.D. Ross, R.J. Davis, A.B. Gleeson, R.J. Love, P.W. Daniels, A.R. Gould, and A.D. Hyatt. 1998. An apparently new virus (family Paramyxovirdae) infectious for pigs, humans, and fruit bats. Emerg. Inf. Dis. 4(2):269-71.

Regli, S., J.B. Rose, C.N. Haas, and C.P. Gerba. 1991. Modeling the risk from *Giardia* and viruses in drinking water. Am. Water Works Assoc. 83:76-84.

Rose, J.B. and C.P. Gerba. 1991. Use of risk assessment for development of microbial standards. Water Sci. Technol. 24:29-34.

Rose, J.B. and T.R. Slifko. 1999. Giardia, Cryptosporidium and Cyclospora and their impact on foods—a review. J. Food Prot. 62(9):1059-1070.

Rose, J., C.N. Haas, and S. Regli. 1991. Risk assessment and control of waterborne giardiasis. Am. J. Pub. Health. 1:709-713.

Rubin, L.G. 1987. Bacterial colonization and infection resulting from multiplication of a single organism. Rev. Infect. Dis. 9(3):488-493.

Schmaljohn, C. and B. Hjelle. 1997. Hantaviruses: a global disease problem. Emerg. Infect. Dis. 3(2):95-104.

Shadduck, J.A. 1989. Human microsporidiosis and AIDS. Rev. Infect. Dis. 11:203-207.

Shadduck, J.A. and M.B. Polley. 1978. Some factors influencing the in vitro infectivity and replication of Encephalitozoon cuniculi. J. Protozool. 25:491-496.

Soave, R. and W.D. Johnson, Jr. 1995. Cyclospora: conquest of an emerging pathogen. Lancet 345:667-668.

Swerdlow, D.L. B.A. Woodruff, R.C. Brady, P.M. Griffin, S. Tippen, H.D. Donnel, E.E. Geldreich, B.J. Payne, A. Meyer, J.G. Wells, K.D. Greene, M. Bright, N.H. Bean, and P.A. Blake. 1992. A waterborne outbreak in Missouri of Escherichia coli O157:H7 associated with bloody diarrhea and death. Annals Int. Med. 117:812-819.

Taylor, D.N. and M.J. Blaser. 1991. The epidemiology of Helicobacter pylori infection. Epidemiol. Rev. 13:42-58.

Thomas, J.E., G.R. Gibson, M.K. Darboe, A. Dale, and L.T. Weaver. 1992. Isolation of Helicobacter pylori from human faeces. Lancet 340:1194-1195.

Torok, T.J., R.V. Tauxe, R.P. Wise, J.P. Livengood, R. Sokolow, S. Mauvais, K.A. Birkness, M.R. Skeels, J.M. Horan, and L.R. Foster. 1997. A large community outbreak of salmonellosis caused by intentional contamination of restaurant salad bars. JAMA 278(5):389-95.

Wagenknecht, L.E., J.M. Roseman, and W.H. Herman. 1991. Increased incidence of insulin-dependent diabetes mellitus following an epidemic of coxsackievirus B5. Am. J. Epidemiol. 133:1024-1031.

Waller, T. 1979. Sensitivity of Encephalitozoon cuniculi to various temperatures, disinfectants and drugs. Lab Anim. 13:227-230.

WRAIR (Walter Reed Army Institute of Research). 1998. DOD-Global Emerging Infections Surveillance and Response System. Addressing emerging infectious disease threats, a strategic plan for the Department of Defense. Presidential decision Directive NSTC-7. Emerg. Infect. Dis. 4(3). (July - Sept.).

Yates, M.V. and S.R. Yates. 1988. Modeling microbial fate in the subsurface environment. Crit. Rev. Environ. Control 17:307-344.

Approaches for Using Toxicokinetic Information in Assessing Risk to Deployed U.S. Forces

by Karl K. Rozman[1]

ABSTRACT

If there is no exposure, there is no toxicity. If there is exposure, toxicity might ensue when exposure exceeds a certain dose or time, a topic discussed under toxicokinetics and toxicodynamics. Analysis of the fundamental equation of toxicity yields the recognition of three independent time scales. One is the dynamic time scale, which is an intrinsic property of a given compound (what does a chemical do to an organism). The second is the kinetic time scale, which is an intrinsic property of a specific organism (what does an organism do to a chemical). The frequency of exposure denotes the third time scale, which is independent of dose and of the dynamic and kinetic time scales. Frequency of exposure depends on the experimental design or nature, but not on the organism or substance. A liminal condition occurs when the frequency becomes infinite, which corresponds to continuous exposure. Continuous exposure forces the dynamic and kinetic time scales to become synchronized, thereby reducing complexity to three variables: dose, effect, and one time scale. Keeping one of those variables constant allows one to study the other two variables reproducibly under isoeffective, isodosic, or isotemporal conditions. However, any departure from continuous exposure will introduce the full complexity of four independent variables (dose, and the kinetic, dynamic, and frequency time scales) impacting on the effect (dependent variable) at the same time. The examples discussed in this paper demonstrate how nature in the form of long half-lives provides liminal conditions when either kinetic or dynamic half-lives force synchronization of all three time scales.

The original charge for this paper was to conceptualize the role of toxicokinetics in the risk assessment of deployed forces exposed to chemicals. Most toxicologists familiar with current trends in toxicology are aware of the tremendous proliferation of publications combining physiologically based pharmacokinetic (PBPK) models with various dose-response extrapolation models, usually with the linearized multistage (LMS) model, or more recently with the benchmark (BM) curve-fitting approach.

---

[1]Department of Pharmacology, Toxicology and Therapeutics, University of Kansas Medical Center, Kansas City, KS, 66160 and Section of Environmental Toxicology, GSF-Institut für Toxikologie, Neuherberg, 85758 Germany.

This author has used both PBPK and classical pharmacokinetics in many experiments. Although both are conceptually sound, there is one fundamental difference: classical pharmacokinetics uses time as an explicit function, whereas PBPK deals with time mostly as a variable, to be predicted based on physiological and physicochemical parameters. Therefore, the concepts of classical pharmacokinetics were helpful in the development of the initial core of a theory of toxicology, as presented in this document, whereas the concepts of PBPK were not as useful. This is not to say that combining PBPK with a theoretically sound biological model will not provide appropriate answers in some instances. However, as long as PBPK is used in conjunction with biologically implausible models (LMS, BM), it will lead (not surprisingly) to insignificant improvements. Central to the development of the concepts presented here was the notion that time is a variable equivalent to dose in toxicology. This idea has been around among toxicologists for almost exactly 100 years. Nevertheless, claims of exceptions to this idea as embodied in Haber's Rule prevented the development of time as a variable of toxicity. Even today toxicologists tend to focus on the so-called "exceptions" when effects are overwhelmingly dose— but not time—dependent. They do not realize that they are studying extreme parts of a spectrum under liminal conditions (e.g., a highly reversible effect on a short time scale), and they use experimental models with insufficient time resolution. When time resolution is satisfactory (such as pungency on a scale of seconds), clear summation effects emerge.

Recognition of the limits of the current risk-assessment paradigm made a paradox clear: none of the current risk projections include time as a variable even though any and all such risk predictions are by definition made in time. From this recognition it was concluded that something that is basically flawed cannot be fixed. Therefore, a new risk-assessment paradigm that includes time as a variable of toxicity, is being suggested. It is clear that although dose is a simple function (number of molecules), time is a complex variable, which runs on many different scales, at least three of which are interacting with dose to provide the complexity that seems to have bewildered generations of toxicologists. The three time scales are the toxicokinetic and toxicodynamic half-lives and the frequency of exposure. Thus, there are three liminal conditions:

1. When the toxicokinetic half-life is very long, it keeps the frequency of exposure essentially infinite (continuous exposure), and the toxicodynamic half-life by definition will be the same as the toxicokinetic one. Under these liminal conditions, $c \times t = k$ for isoeffective experiments, because there is only dose-dependence and one time-dependence.

2. When the toxicodynamic half-life is very long, it requires no additional injury to occur to keep injury constant nor the continuous presence of the noxious agent to result under isoeffective conditions in $c \times t = k$, because there is only dose-dependence and one time-dependence.

3. When the toxicokinetic/toxicodynamic half-lives become very short, they will blur the distinction between the kinetic and dynamic time scales and both will become less important, because in that case the frequency of exposure dominates the time-dependence. Under liminal (continuous exposure = infinite frequency) and isoeffective conditions, this will also lead to $c \times t = k$.

When experiments are conducted under isodosic or isotemporal conditions, then the relationship will obey the equation $c \times t = k \times Effect$. The vast majority of exposure scenarios are of course far from these liminal situations (ideal conditions) and will, therefore, yield $c \times t^x = k$. There are clear suggestions in this paper for the type of experiments that need to be done to determine x with exactitude. In the meantime, practical suggestions are included, which illustrate how to use a decision tree or available databases to conduct risk assessments for deployment situations that are less arbitrary by using both dose and time as variables of toxicity.

The decision tree approach uses a top-to-bottom analysis of identifying rate-determining or rate-

limiting steps in the toxic action of a given compound for a specific effect. The advantage of this approach is its flexibility of determining at what level to contemplate modeling (risk assessment) of toxicity without having to rely on default assumptions. As recognized by other scientific disciplines, understanding of complexity is always advanced at three levels of investigations: experimental, computational, and theoretical. For the most part, toxicologists were and are engaged in experimental and computational studies with very little, if any, progress having been made in developing a comprehensive theory of toxicology. The combined theory and decision-tree analysis presented here should allow rapid progress in improving predictions of toxicity, if experimental design, computational goal, and theory come into equilibrium in terms of checks and balances. Instead of claiming exceptions, the three questions to be asked should be:

1. Why do some experimental results deviate from $c \times t = k$ (isoeffective) or $c \times t = k \times Effect$ (isodosic, isotemporal)?

2. What kind of computational (modeling) approach, and what level of integration, is needed to transform $c \times t^x = k$ or $c \times t^x = k \times Effect$ back to $c \times t = k$ or $c \times t = k \times Effect$?

3. How does exploration of Questions 1 and 2 improve the theory of toxicology, specifically the understanding of k?

It must be recognized that eventually experiments will be conducted under ideal conditions ($c \times t = k$ or $c \times t = k \times Effect$). Once it is known how to transform $c \times t^x = k$ or $c \times t^x = k \times Effect$ (real-life situations) back to the ideal conditions, then any projection will also be possible in the opposite direction. Thus, it can be expected that the vast majority of experiments conducted under less-than-ideal conditions will then become interpretable by using a related study, which has been conducted under ideal conditions.

TOXICITY

Introduction

Toxicity (T) is a function of exposure (E) and E is a function of dose (c) and time (t) ($T = f[E(c,t)]$). Toxicity is the manifestation of an interaction between molecules constituting some form of life and molecules of exogenous chemicals or forms of life affected by physical insults. Consequences of molecular interactions or physical insults might propagate, through causality chains, all the way to the organismic level. There are two fundamental ways to view this interaction: (1) what does an organism do to a chemical, and (2) what does a chemical do to an organism? Dealing with the first question led to the development of the discipline of pharmacokinetics, which was later incorporated into some toxicity studies; in that context it would be more appropriately called toxicokinetics (K). The other question was addressed by the discipline of pharmacology in the form of pharmacodynamic experiments, which again in the context of toxicity, would be more properly termed toxicodynamics (D). Thus, toxicity (T) might be defined as a function of E, K, and D.

$$T = f(E,K,D)$$

A definition of toxicity according to Rozman and Doull (1998) runs as follows "[toxicity] is the accumulation of injury over short or long periods of time, which renders an organism incapable of functioning within the limits of adaptation." This definition implies that toxicity is a function of time in addition to the dose. The latter was already recognized by Paracelsus 500 years ago. A closer scrutiny of the earlier definition of toxicity indicates that the relationship between toxicity, dose (c)

and time (t) is a complex one because toxicokinetics itself is dose- and time-dependent [$K = f(c,t)$] as is toxicodynamics [$D = f(c,t)$]. It is noteworthy that the various time-dependencies seldom run on the same time scale.

Conceptually, K might also be viewed as a function of the dynamic change between absorption (*Abs*) and elimination (*El*),

$$K = f(Abs, El)$$

because it is the ratio between entry rate (absorption) and exit rate (elimination) that determines the time course of a compound in an organism. In the simplest case of an iv bolus injection (instantaneous absorption), the time course is determined by the rate of elimination alone for a compound obeying a one-compartment model. Usually absorption is faster than elimination-making processes related to elimination (distribution, biotransformation, excretion) rate-determining or rate-limiting in most instances.

By analogy, D might be viewed as a function of the dynamic change between injury (I) and recovery (R),

$$D = f(I, R)$$

because it is the ratio of injury to recovery that determines the time course of an adverse effect in an organism. The simplest case for such an injury would be when an organism would recover from an acute injury in accordance with a one-compartment toxicodynamic model. Again, processes related to recovery are usually slower than the rate of injury. Therefore, recovery (adaptation, repair, reversibility) will more often be rate-determining or rate-limiting.

Most often compounds do not behave in an organism according to a one-compartment model. The reason for this is that elimination from the systemic circulation itself can be a function of excretion (*Ex*), distribution (*Dist*), and biotransformation (*Bio*).

$$El = f(Ex, Dist, Bio)$$

When any or all of these processes become rate-limiting, two- or multi-compartmental models are needed.

Again, by analogy to K, recovery (R) in a D model might not be a simple function of, for example, reversibility (*Rv*), but could also require repair (*Rp*). In addition, adaptation (*Adp*) might also be occurring.

$$R = f(Adp, Rp, Rv)$$

In such instances, two- or multi-compartment toxicodynamic analyses are needed to describe the toxicity of a compound that affects any or all of these processes. Absorption and injury can be thought of as being analogous manifestations of K and D. Absorption is a function of site (S) and mechanism (M) as is injury.

$$Abs = f(S, M)$$
$$I = f(S, M)$$

This analysis can be continued all the way to the molecular level. It is clear that any rate-determining or rate-limiting steps, originating at the level of molecular interactions, will then propagate through causality chain(s) to the levels depicted in Figure 1, which represents a schematic illustration of this concept.

Each of these processes might be dose- and time-dependent, although past experiments often failed to demonstrate this because they were conducted with preponderant emphasis on one or the other variable; for example, D was mainly studied as a function of dose and K mainly as a function of time.

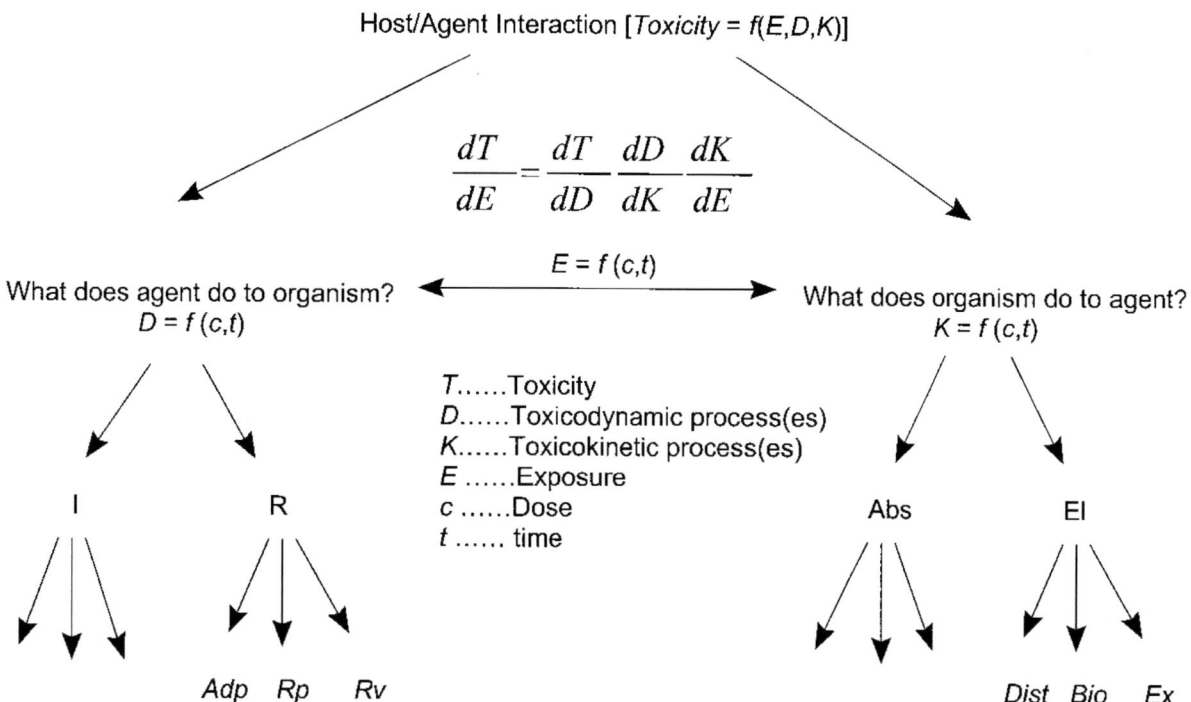

FIGURE 1 Schematic presentation of the decision-tree concept and a mathematical description of toxicity as a function of exposure, kinetics, and dynamics using the chain expansion.

History

Time has always been an important factor in designing toxicological experiments, yet time as an explicit variable of toxicity has been afforded very little attention. It is even more interesting that after Warren (1900) was severely criticized by Ostwald and Dernoscheck (1910) for his analogy of $c \times t = k$ to $P \times V = k$ of ideal gases, the entire issue was forgotten. Even though $c \times t = k$ kept surfacing repeatedly (e.g., Flury and Wirth 1934; Druckrey and Küpfmüller 1948; Littlefield et al. 1980; Peto et al. 1991), an analogy to thermodynamics was not contemplated again, at least not to this author's knowledge! With the "rediscovery" of the $c \times t = k$ concept in still another context (delayed acute oral toxicity), some reevaluation regarding the role of time in toxicology in a historical context is required.

Ostwald and Dernoscheck's (1910) analogy of toxicity to an adsorption isotherm is problematic, because adsorption entails processes far from ideal conditions. Much more reasonable is Warren's (1900) analogy to $P \times V = k$ for ideal gases as a comparison to ideal conditions in toxicology. Reducing the volume of a gas chamber containing a given number of molecules or atoms of an ideal gas will decrease the time for any given molecules or atoms to collide with the wall of the chamber and will lead to increased pressure, which is simply an attribute of the increased number of molecules per unit volume, which is concentration. Thus, $c \times t = k$ and $P \times V = k$ are compatible with each other if looked at mechanistically. Of course, Ostwald and Dernoscheck's comparison of toxicity to an adsorption isotherm is much closer to the real-life situation of toxicology where the most frequent finding is that of $c \times t^x = k$.

These thought experiments and some discussions led to the recognition that toxicologists did everything the opposite of what thermodynamicists did. Instead of starting out with the simplest model (ideal gas in thermodynamics corresponds to ideal conditions in toxicological experiments) and building into it step by step the increasing complexity of the real world, toxicologists tried to predict from one complex situation to another complex situation. In addition, time was largely ignored, although it is one of two fundamental variables of toxicity (Rozman 1998). It is unlikely that a better understanding of biological processes at the molecular level alone will lead to improved risk predictions in toxicology, as long as the experimental designs of toxicological studies provide the wrong reference points for departure from ideal to real conditions. For example, the standard inhalation toxicity protocols (6 h/d for 5 d/wk) cannot yield $c \times t = k$ because after 6 h intoxication, there are up to 18 h of recovery, and on weekends there are up to 66 h of recovery, at least for compounds of short half-life. This would require at least two additional functions to correct for departure from steady state. The real-life situation is even more complex when departures from the ideal condition (steady state) are highly irregular. Nevertheless, it is reasonable to expect that risk predictions will be possible for even the most irregular exposure scenarios once the reference points are established as dose- and time-responses under ideal conditions (toxicodynamic or toxicokinetic/toxicodynamic steady state) and then departures of increasing complexity are defined.

In 25 years of studying the toxicity of tetrachlorodibenzodioxin (TCDD) and related compounds, the concept of $c \times t = k$ did not emerge in any other experimental context except in the two recent subchronic and chronic toxicity studies, which were conducted under conditions of toxicokinetic steady state (Rozman et al. 1996; Viluksela et al. 1997, 1998). Nevertheless, a general interest in the role of time in toxicology pervaded the line of thinking presented here for many years (Rozman et al. 1993; Rozman et al. 1996; Rozman and Doull 1998; Rozman 1998). Most toxicologists are familiar with Haber's Rule of inhalation toxicology and its applicability to war gases and some solvents. Much less reference has been made to Druckrey's work (Druckrey and Küpfmüller 1948, Druckrey et al. 1963, 1964, 1967), which extended the $c \times t$ concept to lifetime cancer studies by oral rather than inhalation exposure. And finally, there is very little cross-referencing of the $c \times t = k$ data, which were generated by entomologists (e.g., Peters and Ganter 1935; Busvine 1938; Bliss 1940) and those established by toxicologists. History demonstrates that a fundamental relationship in science keeps reappearing in different contexts, as is the case with $c \times t = k$. During this period many apparent exceptions seem to be occurring with no satisfactory explanation. Attempts at generalization usually fail until a commonality is detected among all experiments, as is the case among those that yielded $c \times t = k$. This commonality is toxicokinetic steady state or irreversibility of an effect, which of course can be interrelated. Anesthesia, like intravenous infusion, leads to rapid and sustained steady state for compounds of short half-life. Most anesthetics and solvents do have short half-lives and many obey Haber's Rule, except when measurements are taken while an adaptive process is under way, that is, induction of a protein. Druckrey and the ED_{01}-Study used feeding as a route of exposure, which yields a better steady state for compounds of intermediate half-life than, for example, gavage. However, the exponent x in the term of Druckrey's general formula increases above one rapidly as the half-life of compounds becomes shorter, because there is intermittent recovery between bouts of feeding. Most of the entomology studies were related to fumigation, which often but not always resulted in fairly rapid steady state. And finally 1,2,3,4,5,6,7,8-heptachlorodibenzo-p-dioxin (HpCDD), which has a half-life of 314 days (Viluksela et al. 1997) in female rats yields virtual steady state for a 70-d observation period after any route of administration but not TCDD with a half-life of 20 d. However, when TCDD's toxicity was studied under steady-state conditions, its subchronic and chronic toxicity also occurred according to $c \times t = k$ (Rozman et al. 1993).

DOSE AND TIME AS VARIABLES OF TOXICITY

Definition of Dose and Time

Before analyzing dose and time relationships further, it is useful to come up with clear definitions of these fundamental variables of toxicity. Due to historical developments, neither dose nor time has been defined with clarity as variables of both toxicokinetics and toxicodynamics. It is customary to use the term acute dose and acute effect as if the two were interchangeable. In fact, an acute dose can lead to chronic effects (Druckrey et al. 1964) and multiple doses can trigger a fulminant episode of toxicity (Garrettson 1983). In risk (safety) assessment it is always the total dose delivered that is of concern, although in therapeutics the daily dose is often referred to simply as the dose. Therefore, a useful definition of dose in toxicology, would be:

$$Dose = \sum_{n=1}^{n} Dose\ Rates$$

According to this definition a single acute dose would represent the liminal case when the dose rate equals the dose. This definition would be valid for any kind of irregularity in the dosing regimens and is analogous to the definition of dose in radiation biology.

Ever since the dawn of human consciousness, humanity has struggled with the notion of time. It is not possible to predict what influence the concept of toxicological time will have on our perception of time. Suffice it to say at this junction, it is not possible to think of toxicty without the implicit presence of time as a variable, although in toxicological studies, time received only semiquantitative designations (acute, subacute, subchronic, chronic). In fact, one could view organisms as instruments exquisitely sensitive to time. Important for toxicology is that the time course of a toxicant in an organism (kinetics) is very often different than the time course of toxicity (dynamics). Underlying biological processes (absorption, distribution, elimination, injury, adaptation, recovery) have their own time scales, depending on the molecular events behind each process (e.g., enzyme induction, receptor regulation either directly or via gene expression). Thus, in toxicology the dose is a pure variable, but there are many different processes occurring on different time scales yielding different $\int cdt$ integrals leading to complex interactions, which can be described as $c \times t^x$. In spite of this complexity, science can deal with it in a traditional, analytical fashion. Because only knowledge of rate-limiting steps is required to accurately describe toxicity, this will often reduce complexity to manageable proportions.

Dose and Time Relationships

Consequences of interactions between a toxic agent and an organism at the molecular level propagate through toxicodynamic or toxicokinetic/toxicodynamic causality chains all the way to the manifestation of toxicity at the organismic level (Figure 1). If the recovery (adaptation, repair, and reversibility) half-life of an organism is longer than the half-life of the causative agent in the organism, then toxicodynamics become rate-determining (one-compartment model) or rate-limiting (multi-compartment model). If the toxicokinetic half-life of the compound is longer than the recovery half-life, then toxicokinetics will be rate-determining (rate-limiting), in which case the toxicokinetic area under the curve (AUC) will be identical to the toxicodynamic AUC. There are three liminal conditions for $c \times t = k$ that emerge when the causality chain propagates through either toxicodynamic or toxicokinetic/toxicodynamic processes:

Toxicodynamics

1. In case of no recovery (no reversibility, no repair, no adaptation) linear accumulation of injury will occur according to a triangular geometry ($c \times t/2 = k$) following repeated doses or according to a rectangular geometry after a single dose ($c \times t = k$), provided that the $c \times t$ lifetime threshold has been exceeded, which occurs when $c_{threshold} \times t_{lifespan} = k$.

2. After recovery (reversibility, repair, adaptation) steady state has been reached, injury will occur according to a rectangular geometry ($c \times t = k$), after exceeding the $c \times t$ lifetime threshold.

Toxicokinetics

1. No elimination will lead to linear accumulation of a compound and, as a consequence, to accumulation of injury according to a triangular geometry ($c \times t/2 = k$) after repeated doses or according to rectangular geometry after a single dose ($c \times t = k$) above the $c \times t$ lifetime threshold.

2. After toxicokinetic (and as a consequence toxicodynamic) steady state has been reached, injury will occur above the $c \times t$ lifetime threshold according to a rectangular geometry ($c \times t = k$).

Exposure Frequency

As the toxicokinetic and toxicodynamic half-lives become shorter and shorter, the distinction between elimination and recovery half-lives becomes less important, because another time-dependence, that of the frequency of exposure, starts dominating the time-dependence.

1. Compounds having very short toxicokinetic/toxicodynamic half-lives will reach steady state rapidly and yield $c \times t = k$ upon continuous exposure according to a rectangular geometry, provided that adaptation and repair are also at steady state.

2. Other types of geometries certainly can be created by elaborate, but regular, dosing regimens. These scenarios are less likely to play a practical role in toxicology, although they might be of theoretical interest.

It should be kept in mind that the mathematics of first-order processes, when appropriate, are valid for bi-molecular reactions (e.g., receptor binding), which result in the propagation of the causality chain to the level of modeling (Figure 1). Therefore, 90% of toxicodynamic steady state will not be reached until 3.32 recovery half-lives have elapsed. Thus, Haber's Rule will be obeyed only if the observation period is outside of about 4 recovery half-lives or if recovery is a zero order process.

Thus, the various ($c \times t = k$) scenarios represent liminal conditions. The magnitude of the $c \times t$ product is a function of the potency of the compound, of the susceptibility of the organism, and of the deviation from the ideal conditions and will yield $c \times t^x = k$ for nonliminal conditions. (Large $c \times t^x$ product indicates either low potency, lack of susceptibility, or low exposure frequency.) It must be recognized that the dose (c) does not have exponential properties, but time (t) does have such properties, because under nonideal conditions toxicity is a function of at least two independent time scales. One independent time scale is the half-life of the rate-determining step (toxicodynamic or toxicodynamic/toxicokinetic) of the intoxication (intrinsic property of compound or organism), the other one is the frequency and duration of exposure, which is independent of both the compound and the organism.

In conclusion, these data and considerations of a significant body of evidence accumulated over the last 100 years suggest that $c \times t = k$ is a fundamental law of toxicology, and possibly of biology in general, that can be seen only under ideal conditions. If confirmed using other classes of compounds and the ideal conditions described here, then Paracelsus' famous statement might have to be supplemented to read *Dosis et tempus fiunt (faciunt) venenum* (Dose and time together make the poison). Implications for risk assessment are that the margin of exposure (MOE) must be defined in terms of both dose and time. This can be done by relating the real-life exposure scenario to that of the ideal exposure condition:

$$MOE = \frac{c \times t^x}{c \times t}$$

Above the $c \times t$ lifetime threshold, this will yield the margin of safety and its reciprocal, the margin of risk.

Figure 1 might also be viewed as a decision tree to identify critical steps needed for modeling to predict toxicity. It is important to note that a high degree of irreversibility and toxicokinetic steady state are rare phenomena in toxicology, although both can be seen any time when the observation period is much shorter than the recovery or the elimination half-life. In the real-life situation, there are usually at least two or three rate-limiting steps in toxicokinetics and likely as many in toxicodynamics. It must be emphasized though, that multiple toxicokinetic compartmental models do not necessarily require multiple toxicodynamic models, and vice versa. However, if there are three different rate-limiting processes occurring on different time scales in toxicokinetics and three different rate-limiting processes taking place on three different time scales in toxicodynamics, such a scenario would represent a formidable computational task for a theoretical treatise. Therefore, a practical approach would be to conduct experiments at toxicodynamic steady state (which of course would require a preexisting toxicokinetic steady state in many instances) as a point of reference clearly defined by $c \times t = k$. Then, experiments need to be carried out for different compounds with different half-lives to establish model parameters, which describe departures from toxicokinetic/toxicodynamic steady state of increasing frequency and irregularity.

In summary, $c \times t = k$ represents the most efficient (a kind of worst-case) exposure scenario for producing an effect, namely continuous exposure until manifestation of an effect. Experimentally, this condition is often met by continuous inhalation exposure (e.g., Gardner et al. 1977), or daily oral administration of compounds that have toxicodynamic/toxicokinetic half-lives of a few days or longer or effects that are essentially irreversible. It must be emphasized that any departure from the worst-case scenario will result in a change of $c \times t = k$ into $c \times t^x = k$. Departures are represented by regular or irregular interruptions of exposure or intermittent recovery from injury. The larger the departure, the larger will be x, and with that k. It is somewhat counterintuitive, but increasing x and k are equivalent to decreasing toxicity. This is entirely logical, however, when it is recognized that increasing interruptions of exposure or injury will result in longer and longer periods of time needed to cause equivalent toxicity to that of continuous exposure, because of increasing intermittent recovery. A liminal condition for first-order processes will be reached when exposure occurs outside of 6.6 toxicokinetic/toxicodynamic half-lives, because at that time 99% elimination or recovery will have occurred. Under such conditions (which are closest to the real-life situation for most compounds), toxicity will be less dose-dependent and toxicokinetic/toxicodynamic time-dependent, and mainly the frequency of exposure will determine x. If x is then determined experimentally, for example, for 1, 2, 4, 8, 16, and 32 days for a compound with a toxicokinetic/toxicodynamic half-life < 3.6 h after continuous versus intermittent exposure under isoeffective conditions, then plotting the data will allow extrapolation to any exposure scenario outside of 6.64 half-lives (which corresponds to 1 day). Most dietary constituents fall in this category. For zero-order processes, 2 half-lives are needed for elimination or recovery. It should be kept in mind that the half-life of zero-order processes (unlike that of first-order processes) is dependent on concentration.

Analogy to Thermodynamics

In physics, Boyle's Law of ideal gases, gave rise to thermodynamics, and molecular and mechanistic considerations led to a theory of gas reactions. The former is based on the idea of finding the minimum number of fundamental variables that can describe the simplest possible dynamic system ($P \times V = k$ for ideal gases). The latter required a great deal of knowledge about the mechanism of chemical reactions, such as wall reaction and activation energy. Both of these approaches have been attempted in toxicology with, as yet, limited success, as shown in subsequent discussions in this paper. The reason for the lack of advance in theoretical toxicology is probably due to the fact that, unlike thermodynamicists, toxicologists did not start out with defining the simplest possible toxicological conditions with a minimum number of variables as a point of departure toward more complexity. Coincidentally, experiments were conducted under such ideal conditions and in every such instance Haber's Rule proved to be applicable (Gardner et al. 1977), even though researchers might have failed to notice it (Sivam et al. 1984).

The lack of conceptualization of the three variables of toxicity resulted in arbitrary study designs, which further eroded the predictability from one experiment to another. It is this author's opinion that analogous thinking to thermodynamics might help to optimize study design and eventually to build a theory of toxicology. Thermodynamics, like toxicology, has three fundamental variables ($P, V,$ and T versus $c, t,$ and W). (W [German for Wirkung]) will be used for effect, because of the many Es ([exposure, elimination, effect, excretion] in English.) Before the development of a comprehensive theory of thermodynamics, it was clear to scientists that to study an independent and a dependent variable, a third or other variables had to be kept constant. This has not been done in toxicology, although most dose-response studies have been conducted at constant time (isotemporal). However, to study the relationship between time and effect, the dose needs to be kept constant (isodosic). Moreover, to examine the relationship between dose and time, the effect must be kept constant (isoeffective). The $c \times t$ product will not emerge from the equation of ergodynamics (Figure 2) until after elucidation of the relationship between specific effect at constant time and specific effect at constant dose. In other words, more must be learned about k before significant theoretical advance is possible. As mentioned before, most experiments have been conducted isotemporally in the past (14 d, 90 d, 104 wk), which is appropriate for dose-response studies. The arbitrary choice of these time points and the inexactitude of diagnosis (stuff them and count them) led to a great deal of confusion in the 14-day studies, because different dose responses with different mechanisms were often lumped together. Experiments in toxicology have frequently been conducted under isoeffective conditions, mainly with the endpoint being 100% of an effect (mortality, cancer). However, systematic investigation of $c \times t = k$ has not been done, for example, at 20 or 80% of an effect. Finally, there have been very few experiments conducted under isodosic conditions, because this requires that the concentration be kept constant at the site of action. The only experiment-driven condition when this is often the case is inhalation exposure. Gardner et al. (1977) have reported such data after continuous exposure of experimental animals to benzene and SO_2 when the endpoint in question was measured immediately after termination of exposure (chronaxy, leukopenia). However, when the endpoint of measurement was not immediately done (streptococcal infection-related mortality) after cessation of NO_2 exposure, the time response started flattening out (Gardner et al. 1979). A systematic investigation of these issues has been done recently for HpCDD after oral administration with as yet only one endpoint of toxicity (delayed acute toxicity), although preliminary analysis indicates that there are other valid endpoints such as anemia and lung cancer (Rozman 1999). These data provide support for the suggestion of Rozman et al. (1996) that the dose-time-response be viewed as a 3-dimensional surface area similar to, but conceptually distinctly different from, the model of Hartung (1987) (Figure 3). Experiments conducted under isoeffective conditions

ERGODYNAMICS

$$dW = \left(\frac{\partial W}{\partial c}\right)_t dc + \left(\frac{\partial W}{\partial t}\right)_c dt$$

$$-\left(\frac{\partial W}{\partial c}\right)_t dc = \left(\frac{\partial W}{\partial t}\right)_c dt$$

$dW = 0$ isoeffective

$$dW = \left(\frac{\partial W}{\partial c}\right)_t dc$$

$$dW = \left(\frac{\partial W}{\partial t}\right)_c dt$$

$dt = 0$ isotemporal

$dc = 0$ isodosic

FIGURE 2 Definition of toxicity in analogy to thermodynamics.

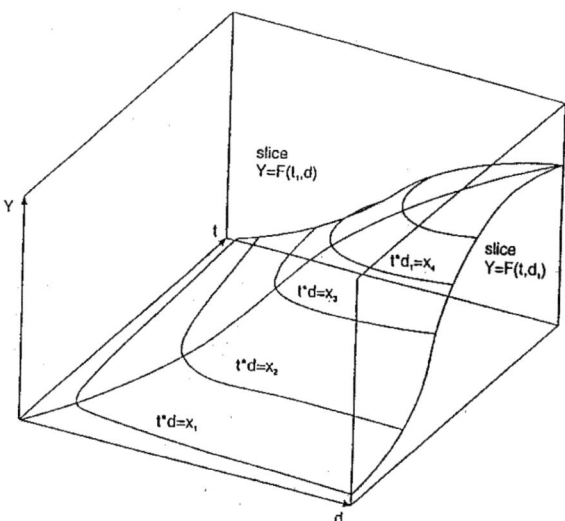

FIGURE 3 Schematic presentation of the dose-time-response surface area showing slices for isoeffective (hyperbolas), isodosic (S-shaped time response), and isochronic (S-shaped dose response) responses.

(slices parallel to the dose-time plane) correspond to Haber's Rule of $c \times t = k$ represented by hyperbolas. Studies carried out under isotemporal conditions (slices parallel to the time-effect plane) yield S-shaped dose-response curves along which $c \times t = k \times W$ whereas isodosic investigations (slices parallel to the dose-effect plane) produce S-shaped time-response curves along which $c \times t = k \times W$ also. Indeed, plotting the $c \times t$ product against effect (W) for HpCDD for doses causing about 10 to 90% wasting/hemorrhage, yielded a straight line of high correlation ($r^2 = 0.96$) (Figure 4). This is the beginning core of a theory of toxicology, which is analogous to $P \times V = k$ for isotherms, and $P \times V = k \times T$ for isobars or isochors. Of course, thermodynamicists know that $k = n \times R$ (n = number of moles; R = gas constant), but toxicology is not yet there. What is clear already at this junction is that the dimension of $P \times V$ is energy, whereas the dimension of $c \times t$ is energy × time, which is action and is called effect in toxicology (Figure 5).

DECISION TREE

A recent series of articles explored how other disciplines deal with complex systems (Goldenfeld and Kandanoff 1999; Whitesides and Ismagilov 1999; Weng et al. 1999; Koch and Laurent 1999). Goldenfeld and Kandanoff (1999) made some important observations, that are relevant for toxicology. Simple laws of physics give rise to enormous complexity when the number of actors is very large. The same paradox exists in toxicology in that the $c \times t$ concept is very simple, but the "real world" of the manifestation of toxicity is very complicated. Their other observation is equally relevant; "Use the right

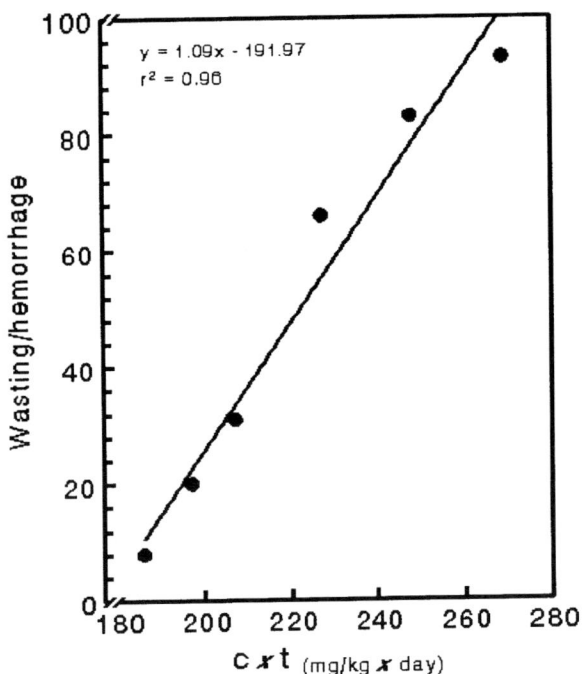

FIGURE 4 A $c \times t$ wasting/hemorrhage plot in HpCDD-treated rats. Data were taken from Rozman (1999) and the second lowest dose added.

Ergodynamics:

$c \times t = k \times W$

W..........Effect (Wirkung)
c...........dose
t........... time

Thermodynamics:

$P \times V = n \times R \times T$

$dW = \left(\frac{\partial W}{\partial c}\right)_t dc + \left(\frac{\partial W}{\partial t}\right)_c dt$

Physics:

Action = Energy x Time

Toxicology:

W = Dose x Time

Dose is a form of energy.

FIGURE 5 Additional analogies between thermodynamics and ergodynamics.

level of description to catch the phenomena of interest. Don't model bulldozers with quarks." The decision tree (Figure 1) was developed to aid toxicologists and modelers to identify both the appropriate phenomena and the right level of modeling. Toxicologists can avoid much unnecessary experimentation by using this top to bottom approach rather than the currently fashionable bottom to top approach.

Toxicokinetics [$K = f(Abs, El)$]

This discipline deals with the mathematical modeling of the question, "What does an organism do to a chemical?" Pharmacokinetics is, and was, dominated by investigations of the time course of drugs and other chemicals in humans and in animals. Dose-dependence was seldom studied, except when a saturation phenomenon resulted in some unexpected data. This is understandable, because the therapeutic range is in the (hormetic) dose region of adaptation or improved repair and not in the toxic range. However, toxicity (such as body weight loss or renal or liver damage) is certain to alter the kinetics of the toxicant or of other toxicants, as has been demonstrated repeatedly (e.g., Weber et al. 1993; Roth et al. 1994; El-Masri et al. 1996). Procedurally, toxicokinetics needs to be determined at a nontoxic and a highly toxic dose. It would be advisable to do the kinetics right after a toxicological dose-range finding. Ideally, the kinetics should also be determined in humans at a nontoxic dose. Early determination of toxicokinetics is very important, because the design of toxicodynamic experiments might be critically dependent on the half-life of a compound and on other kinetic information (Figure 1).

For analytical purposes, toxicokinetics can be divided into separate considerations of absorption and elimination (biotransformation, distribution, and excretion). Although they are overlapping, each of these processes has its own dose- and time-dependence. The notion of AUC, which is the integration of dose over time, is well recognized in K.

Absorption [$Abs = f(S,M)$]

There are three main entries for chemicals into the body: oral, inhalation, and dermal. There are a number of minor portals of entry, such as the eyes and the nasal mucosa, as well as artificially created ones like intramuscular, subcutaneous, intravenous, and intraperitoneal. Oral absorption is by far the most common route of exposure to chemicals. It should be kept in mind that this route of exposure is well controlled by the food supply of highly developed countries, but not so in less developed nations. Inhalation and dermal exposure to chemicals is usually an involuntary process with varying contributions to total exposure. In general, absorption is much less likely to be a rate-determining or rate-limiting step than elimination is.

Oral Absorption

This process is dose- and time-dependent. Dose-dependence is usually due to saturation phenomena (active transport, facilitated diffusion, limited solubility). Time-dependence of absorption is linked to the dynamism of the gut (passage of ingested material). Determination of the time course of absorption is standard practice in pharmacokinetic studies of drugs. In toxicological studies, measurement of oral absorption is, unfortunately, not standard practice. But, it is not fundamentally different from the absorption of drugs, and it has been done often enough to arrive at generalizations (Aungst and Shen 1986; Rozman and Klaassen 1996). The time course of oral absorption is limited by the dynamism of the gastrointestinal (GI) tract and the physicochemical properties of the chemicals being absorbed. Absorption of amphophilic chemicals is quite efficient from the hydrophilic contents of the gut. Highly hydrophilic chemicals, such as metal ions, penetrate the GI tract to a very limited extent because their large hydration shells prevent movement with bulk flow of water through aqueous pores. Often there are active transport processes to carry such molecules across membranes, but transporters are usually saturated at low concentrations. Highly lipophilic chemicals are absorbed in the context of lipid digestion (e.g., micelles and chilomicrons) via the lymphatics. The residency time of the GI contents sets a limit for absorption. Contents move rapidly through the duodenum and jejunoileum, traversing about half of the small intestine in about 20 min after leaving the stomach. They reach the ileocecal valve after about 1 h. Contents remain for up to 36 h in the large intestine, being churned there by peristalsis and antiperistalsis, but absorption of chemicals other than water is limited in this part of the GI tract. Oral absorption entails chemicals entering the systemic circulation after being transported to the liver by the portal vein. Most compounds will be detoxified, in the liver, to more readily excretable metabolites. Metabolic activation and subsequent hepatotoxicity must be considered, although this is the exception. Allometric species differences must be taken into account when animal data are interpreted for humans.

This discussion illustrates that oral absorption of chemicals can be well managed during other than customary circumstances of short- or long-term exposure. The critical factor is control of the food and drinking water supplies, which determine the dose-dependence (source, size of meals and drinks) and time-dependence (frequency of meals, duration of exposure) of oral absorption. Ingestion of particulate matter (dust, sand, and aerosol) is of low concern, because exposure by inhalation will be the major route of their uptake. The best way to protect deployed forces from potential oral exposure to toxicants is to provision them with food and water from the home country by meals ready to eat (MRE), until the safety of local resources has been ascertained.

Inhalation

Due to the enormous surface area of the lungs, absorption here can be much more efficient than in the GI tract, particularly for volatile compounds. There are no special transport processes for ions or lipids in the lungs, with corresponding consequences for their absorption by inhalation. For a more detailed discussion of absorption by inhalation, see Casarett and Doull's Toxicology (Rozman and Klaassen 1996). For purposes of this paper, it is important to consider at what point absorption by inhalation will represent a rate-determining or rate-limiting step on the decision tree (Figure 1). Absorption by inhalation is either ventilation (high solubility in blood) or blood-flow-limited (low solubility in blood). In either case, absorption in the lungs is almost as rapid as intravenous infusion, which means that it is rarely, if ever, rate-determining. Nevertheless, it should be kept in mind that, as with iv infusion, 99% of steady state will be reached by inhalation after about 7 elimination half-lives.

Protection of deployed forces from exposure to toxicants by inhalation is the most difficult task. Defense against war gases utilizes a combination of a prophylactic antidote administration and gas masks. However, this is not a topic here, although interesting kinetic considerations are also applicable in that context. Inhalation exposure will become rate-determining only for compounds with low lung clearance such as silica, asbestos, dusts of various kinds, and soot. Due to their low clearance, they tend to accumulate in the lungs and cause mechanical injury or sustained immunoresponse. Exposure to these agents is often unavoidable, because it is part of the deployment conditions. According to considerations depicted in Figure 1, the toxicity of such substances will be determined by toxicokinetics and, hence, by the toxicokinetic/toxicodynamic AUC generated, which implies that it will occur according to $c \times t = k$ above the lifetime threshold. A deviation from 1 as exponent on t will depend on the low lung clearance, although such deviation is expected to be minor. A practical way to determine the risk (safety) of such substances for various lengths of deployment is to identify appropriate standards of the Occupational Safety and Health Administration (OSHA), the American Council of Governmental Industrial Hygienists (ACGIH), or the Environmental Protection Agency (EPA) and calculate a $c \times t$ for a particular deployment situation. For example, ACGIH recommends a no-observed-adverse-effect level (NOAEL) of 0.1 fiber/cm^3 of asbestos for a 45-yr working life, at 8-h/d, 5 d/wk.

> Amount of air inhaled in 8 h: 10 m^3
> Amount of fibers inhaled in 45 yr: 0.1×10^6 fibers/m^3 (cm$^3 \rightarrow$ m^3) $\times$ 10 m^3 (air inhaled) $\times$ 5 d/wk $\times$ 52 wk $\times$ 45 yrs = 1.17×10^{10} fibers
> Amount that might be inhaled in 14 d: 1.17×10^{10} fibers
> In one day: $1.17 \times 10^{10}/14 = 8.357 \times 10^8$ fibers/d
> Amount of air inhaled in 24 h: 20 m^3
> $8.357 \times 10^8/20$ m^3 = 4.178×10^7 fibers/m^3, or $4.178 \times 10^7/1 \times 10^6$ cm^3 = 41.8 fibers/cm^3
> 14-day deployment exposure limit (DEL): 41.8 fibers/cm^3

It is a risk-management decision how much reserve capacity needs to be retained for the remaining life expectancy. This example illustrates that a simple calculation, by using the $c \times t$ concept when appropriate, will yield a safe level of exposure for any length of deployment.

Dermal Absorption

The skin is an effective barrier separating higher organisms from their environment. The rate-determining process in dermal absorption is the stratum corneum, which is a dead keratinized cell layer, composed mainly of ceramides. Physicochemical properties of molecules determine whether or not a particular compound will or will not (and to what extent) penetrate this barrier. Highly water-soluble and highly lipid-soluble compounds have the poorest penetration rates, whereas compounds most similar to ceramides have the highest penetration rates. For more detail, see Cassarett and Doull's Toxicology (Rozman and Klaassen 1996). For conceptual purposes, unlike the GI-tract and the lungs, dermal penetration can be rate-limiting in the toxicokinetics of compounds, because elimination of substances by biotransformantion (often a first-order process) and excretion are often more rapid than the rate of dermal absorption (often a zero-order process). For these reasons, systemic effects after dermal exposure are not as frequent as generally believed. The most frequent toxicodynamic sequel of dermal exposure is local irritation or allergic reaction, for which exposure itself is rate-determining. For systemic considerations, dermal absorption will be critical only if it results in accumulation of injury, as in the case of soman, or if a large surface area is exposed to a small, rapidly penetrating molecule like chloroacetic acid.

Considering that deployed forces will be wearing uniforms most of the time when dermal exposure to toxicants might be occurring, the only sites of exposure will be the hands and facial area. Although penetration rates of chemicals are variable, they are seldom faster than a few $\mu g/cm^2$. Therefore, dermal exposure under usual deployment conditions will have few or no toxicological consequences for the vast majority of toxicants, with the notable exceptions of irritants and allergens.

Elimination [$El = f(Ex, Dist, Bio)$]

Elimination terminates the interaction between molecules of an organism and molecules that invaded it. It is most often the rate-determining step in the dynamic equilibrium between absorption and elimination. Therefore, in instances when toxicokinetics determines the toxicodynamic process or processes, this is the step that requires modeling. Elimination means removal of a compound from the systemic circulation. This can be due to distribution, sequestration in non-target tissues, biotransformation, or excretion.

Excretion

This process ends the presence of a chemical in an organism. In the simplest case of an iv bolus injection of a toxicant, if the compound is excreted mainly by urinary excretion, one would obtain a straight line (one-compartment model), on a log C_p versus time plot. For chemicals that are very rapidly cleared, excretion will not be rate-determining, because biotransformation is usually a slower process, and hence it will dominate the overall time course of elimination.

Renal Excretion. This is most often the main route of excretion. It is well understood, including the consequences of its impairment in the pharmacokinetics of drugs (Gibaldi and Perrier 1975). It will seldom represent the rate-determining or rate-limiting step in the toxicodynamic action of chemicals, because of its rapidity. Modeling of urinary excretion of toxicants will be useful only if there is no other rate-limiting step in the disposition of a compound.

Fecal Excretion. Bile and direct transfer across the intestinal mucosa are the two major sources of toxicants in feces. Both processes are reasonably well understood (Gregus and Klaassen 1986; Rozman 1986). After hepatic biotransformation, biliary excretion is usually fast and conjugates will be rehydrolyzed in the GI tract, leading to reabsorption and often followed by urinary excretion. A small fraction might escape hydrolysis and be excreted in feces. The half-life of a compound excreted with bile with or without enterohepatic circulation can be, nevertheless, quite short. The major route of excretion of chemicals that are resistant to biotransformation is also fecal excretion. Important for risk assessment is when fecal excretion represents the slowest step in the disposition of toxicants and, at the same time, toxicokinetics represents the rate-determining step in the toxicodynamic action of a compound. This is the case for the infamous class of compounds generically called "dioxins." Half-lives of chemicals become very long when biotransformation is highly inefficient and excretion occurs primarily by nonbiliary intestinal processes, such as desquamation of intestinal epithelium or direct diffusion from the capillary bed into the GI contents. Both are slow processes, exfoliation being limited by the proliferation of the intestinal mucosa and intestinal excretion being limited by the small volume of distribution of the GI contents and their slow flow rate. Interestingly, in spite of their supposed unimportance, these processes can dominate the toxicodynamics of certain classes of chemicals, whereas urinary excretion as the major route of elimination much less frequently determines toxicodynamics.

Biotransformation

This is perhaps the most extensively studied part of the elimination process of chemicals (e.g., Hodgson et al. 1991; Parkinson 1996). Rightly so, because it probably represents, most frequently, the rate-limiting step in the elimination of chemicals from the body. Therefore, in instances when toxicokinetics is responsible for a given toxicodynamic AUC, biotransformation requires careful evaluation. It is not the purpose of this paper to review any part of the vast literature on Phase I and Phase II biotransformations. Rather, the aim is to outline under what conditions biotransformation becomes rate-determining or rate-limiting. Most often, biotransformation is a process of recovery from a toxic insult, because both Phase I and more so, Phase II metabolism leads to more water-soluble, and hence more readily excretable, metabolites. Sometimes, however, biotransformation leads to metabolic activation, that is, to more toxic derivatives. If toxicodynamics rather than toxicokinetics is rate-determining then metabolic activation is of no consequence, because the dynamics of recovery from the lesion will dominate the time course of the effect. For example, an enormous amount of effort has gone into understanding the mechanism of toxicity of benzene in terms of metabolic activation. However, the half-life of benzene is about 8 h in humans and not much different in animals (Brugnone et al. 1992; ATSDR 1997), whereas the hematopoietic system replenishes erythrocytes on a time scale of about 120 days (e.g., Winthrobe and Lee 1974). In equilibrium, this must be the rate of maturation of erythrocytes from stem cells. The propagation of any lesion at any step of this process will be subject to this time scale. Therefore, the dynamics of benzene toxicity will be dominated by the dynamics of the lesion and not by kinetics. Consequently, risk assessment of benzene exposure should be driven by the frequency of exposure above the lifetime threshold and not by some low-level continuous environmental exposure. According to these considerations, once a month exposure to very high concentrations of benzene would result in accumulation of residual damage (according to $c \times t$ after reaching steady state), until the individual's aplastic anemia (or leukemia on still another time scale) threshold has been exceeded. Therefore, preventive measures regarding benzene toxicity should focus on reducing peak concentrations and the frequency of exposure (ideally peak-exposure frequency should be reduced to less than once in 100 days). If safety considerations were to be based erroneously on toxicokinetics, the conclusion would be that continuous exposure to lower levels of benzene would be more dangerous (larger AUC) than intermittent exposures to high-peak concentrations. In any event, understanding of the mechanism of action of a chemical helps to identify the rate-determining or rate-limiting step (or steps), because the dose- and time-responses ($c \times t = k$) of a causally related precursor event must be parallel to that of the effect itself. It must be remembered that biotransformation leading to usually less toxic, more easily excretable metabolites is most often the rate-determining step in the elimination of chemicals because processes related to excretion occur on a faster time scale. Thus, the toxicodynamic consequence of biotransformation is that the AUC of elimination will be identical to the AUC of recovery. A very important exception is when a more toxic chemical is produced by an organism than the invading compound itself (metabolic activation). In this case, production of the more reactive metabolite will determine the rate of injury and hence the rate-determining step changes from elimination to the time scale of recovery from the injury. Similar considerations need to be made for the interaction between Phase I and Phase II metabolism regarding detoxification and toxification.

Distribution. This is the process when a compound is transferred from the systemic circulation into tissues. With regard to tissues, this amounts to absorption into them. Distribution can be rate-limiting, but seldom rate-determining. Almost all chemicals eventually get eliminated, which sometimes represents the slowest, and hence rate-determining, process (e.g., biotransformation). Therefore, chronic effects (when driven by K) will occur according to laws ruled by the terminal half-life of chemicals. However, in instances when the effect occurs during the distribution phase of a chemical, its dynamics will be determined by the distribution half-life rather than its terminal half-life. An example is chloroacetic acid-induced coma and death.

Toxicodynamics $[D = f(I,R,)]$

Toxicodynamics deals with the quantitative description of the answer to the question "What does a particular chemical do to an organism?" Although K has been dominated by studies of its time-dependence, D has been overwhelmingly dominated by dose-response studies, which have ignored time whenever possible. This was probably the reason for a lack of conceptualization of time as a variable of toxicodynamics. D might be viewed as the dynamic (therefore time-dependent) equilibrium between the occurrence of injury and recovery from it. At steady state, the rate of injury equals the rate of recovery. Whichever is the rate-determining step will rule the dynamics of this equilibrium similar to toxicokinetics, where elimination most often represents the rate-determining step. In toxicodynamics, recovery is most frequently found to be rate-determining. It is not common practice to use the concept of AUC in D, although often the toxicodynamic AUC will be the only rate-determining process in the manifestation of toxicity. This is perhaps the most neglected area of toxicology, as shown by the scarcity of data on recovery from injury. The reason for this is probably that toxicologists focused mainly on the process of injury, including its time course, although injury is much less often rate-determining than recovery because the time course of injury is usually (much) faster than that of recovery.

Injury $[I = f(S,M)]$

Understandably, but also regrettably, injury is the most widely studied part of toxicity, because much, if not most, of the time, the process of setting an injury is very rapid and hence not rate-determining. Recovery is usually slower, making it most often the rate-determining step. The definition of toxicity as the accumulation of injury (occurring usually, but not always, according to the dynamic time scale of recovery) to the point when it becomes incompatible with life indicates that death is the ultimate endpoint of all toxic effects. The important question is whether or not a particular toxic insult will or will not be rate-determining in the incapacitation and ultimate demise of an organism. There are extremely rapid rates of accumulation of injury, particularly when the process of recovery is very inefficient (hydrogen cyanide). There are also exceedingly slow rates of accumulation of injury, as in the formation of precursor lesions to cancer, when a particular form of recovery (repair) is very efficient.

Cancer caused by initiators might be viewed as being driven by dynamics because the rate of producing viable mutated cells is much slower than the repair of the DNA damage, which is often very efficient. It takes considerable time to accumulate a critical number of viable mutated cells to have a finite probability that some stimulatory or inhibitory signal will trigger sustained proliferation of such cells. In contrast, promoters do not act by a dynamic, but rather a kinetic, rate-determining step. They do not bind to DNA, but due to their long half-life (dioxins) or continuous exposure (phorbol esters), they alter for a prolonged period of time hormonal constellations or signal transduction pathways, which increase the probability of triggering proliferation of fewer initiated cells (background initiation). Thus, dynamically acting chemicals (initiators) increase the number of initiated cells, whereas kinetically acting compounds (promoters) provide a more favorable environment for cell proliferation.

Injury can theoretically accumulate linearly when there is no recovery. However, this is very seldom the case, because it only happens when the organism dies, before any recovery could occur. For example, the recovery half-life from arsine-induced hemolysis will be identical to the production half-life of erythrocytes. At very high doses, when time to death will be shorter than a fraction of the recovery half-life, injury will accumulate linearly (zero-order process). However, at lower doses, when animals do not die, hemolysis will reach steady state between injury and recovery, and if the dosing interval is within 100 days, chronic consequences might ensue.

Death

One of the major problems in dealing with toxicity is that death of an individual usually does not occur under conditions of a toxicodynamic or a toxicokinetically determined toxicodynamic steady state, but at any place along ascending or descending exponential functions of injury or recovery. This makes it essentially impossible to recognize any patterns other than under ideal conditions, when $c \times t$ becomes constant.

Death is the ultimate end-point of toxicity, because the question is always if an insult to the organism contributes to reducing the natural life-span of that individual. The answer is only if the insult becomes rate-determining or rate-limiting. But, it must be emphasized that one, or many, exposure episodes will remain inconsequential if $c_{threshold} \times t^x_{lifespan} = k$ is not exceeded.

Incapacitation

This is a precursor condition to death, best exemplified by the parallel dose-responses for the various stages of anesthesia (Storm and Rozman 1998). However, all toxic insults lead to incapacitation before death occurs. Recovery from incapacitation can occur without adverse residual effects according to the rate-determining steps of processes involved in recovery. However, in the worst case scenario, irreversible damage can occur, which then will become the rate-determining step.

Residual damage

A great deal is known about residual damage. For conceptual purposes it is important to consider residual damage that relates to toxicity and residual damage that is coincidental. For example, organophosphates deplete acetylcholinesterase (AChE) in the brain and in erythrocytes. Erythrocytes cannot synthesize AChE and, therefore, residual damage will persist according to the dynamics of erythrocyte production. Thus, organophosphate exposure to toxic levels can be seen for up to 60 days, and possibly longer, after exposure when determining AChE in erythrocytes (Sidell 1974). Therefore, if soldiers are deployed for 30 to 90 days, exposure to organophosphates could be quantitated, if pre- and post-deployment blood samples were available, even though this effect has no toxicological relevance other than as marker of exposure. One major advantage of drawing pre- and post-deployment blood samples from the same individual would be an elimination of the considerable interindividual variability in terms of AChE. Some toxicities of organophosphates are due to depletion of AChE at neuronal or neuromuscular junctions, where release subsequent to synthesis of AChE is only a matter of time. Therefore, toxicity will depend on whether the rate of deactivation (covalent binding) or synthesis of new enzymes represents a rate-determining step. Usually, degradation of enzymes is slower than synthesis of new enzymes. However, binding of reactive organophosphates, such as soman to serine residues, occurs on a time scale of minutes as compared with normal degradation of enzymes, which proceed on a time scale of longer than a day. Thus, in such instances, synthesis of new enzymes, rather than their degradation, becomes rate-determining for recovery.

However, it should be kept in mind that soman-induced seizure is thought to occur in animals with rapid accumulation of acetylcholine (ACh) in the synaptic junctions. But, this is only possible if inactivation of AChE is still faster. Nevertheless, the rate-determining step in this case will become irreversible injury of the central nervous system (CNS) due to hypoxia during seizure, and not depletion of AChE. On the other hand, respiratory failure is thought to be (mainly) due to inhibition of AChE in the respiratory center. In this case, recovery (synthesis of new enzymes) will become rate-determining. Individuals survive on artificial respiration with no residual damage. Many phenomena of adaptation are related to this interplay between injury and recovery, particularly to the switch in which one, or the other, is becoming rate-determining.

Residual damage can be due to toxicokinetics, but most frequently it is related to a lack of complete recovery or the lack of any recovery. In any event, the recovery half-lives of causally related effects must be the same. Thus, if the recovery half-life from soman intoxication is 12 to 24 h (estimated from Sterri et al. 1980) and the recovery half-life of brain AChE is more than a week (Tripathi and Dewey 1989), then the two are not directly related, although, theoretically, a small amount of newly synthesized enzyme could initiate recovery.

Recovery [$R = f(Adp, Rp, Rv)$]

Most unfortunately, recovery is not a well studied part of the toxicity of chemicals. Pharmacologists routinely examine the reversibility of receptor binding, although its time-dependence is usually "hidden" in affinity constants. This author has seen very few studies in which the time course of recovery from an injury was systematically studied. Of course, there are standard protocols to study recovery (most often called reversibility) after subchronic exposure. Usually one single time point is chosen after cessation of exposure, which does not permit any kind of quantitative analysis of the dynamics of recovery. It is also clear that there are formidable experimental difficulties in investigating recovery in all or none type effects, because of aging and the limits imposed by life-span in chronic studies. No matter how much the injury caused by a chemical is studied, if its recovery half-life is much longer than the injury half-life, then the latter will dominate the dynamics of the overall process of toxicity. Another important question is whether toxicokinetics or toxicodynamics will play a rate-determining role in the recovery process. If it is toxicokinetics, the recovery process will be determined by the elimination of the compound from the organism. This is the case with dioxins and, indeed, all their effects occur according to $c \times t$ even after acute oral exposure. However, if recovery is slower than the kinetic half-life of a compound, then the recovery process will dominate toxicity. For example, clearance of aniline from blood of rats is very rapid after cessation of inhalation exposure. In agreement with this, Kim and Carlson (1986) found no accumulation of aniline in blood of rats after 8- or 12-h inhalation shifts for 5 and 4 days, respectively. However, methemoglobinemia accumulated to steady state after 12-h shifts, but not after 8-h shifts. This is compatible with the slower recovery half-life of methemoglobinemia (about 3 h). After 12-h shifts, 4 recovery half-lives elapse between exposures (about 90% clearance), whereas after 8-h shifts, 5.3 recovery half-lives pass by before the next exposure (about 97% clearance), which explains why the accumulation is measurable after 12-h, but not after 8-h, shifts of exposure. This demonstrates that accumulation of damage (methemoglobinemia) to a steady state occurs according to the recovery half-life of methemoglobinemia and not according the half-life of aniline (Kim and Carlson 1986).

Adaptation

Adaptation is a well-known phenomenon, but also controversial, probably because it has not been studied nearly as thoroughly as injury. There are strong indications that adaptation might be the rate-determining effect in radiation hormesis (e.g., Caratero et al. 1998; Hoel and Li 1998). When adaptation is not rate-determining, but rate-limiting, its investigation is more difficult. The only way that appears feasible is to study recovery very carefully and to plot the recovery data to determine whether or not the process of recovery is monophasic or multiphasic (biphasic). Curve-stripping would then yield a slope for adaptation. This author is not aware of any studies having performed such analysis.

Repair

Repair is a similarly neglected field, although much more information is available on repair than on adaptation. It is not the purpose of this analysis to do an exhaustive search of the literature for papers dealing with tissue repair, but to illustrate that whenever repair is the rate-determining (slowest) process, then repair rather than injury needs to be studied. This has been done extensively for DNA repair (Pitot and Dragan 1996). A semiquantitative relationship between the half-life of adducts and carcinogenic potency has been recognized. Unfortunately, the time-course studies were less than ideally designed from the point of view of dynamics. Nevertheless, some of the better studies provide support for the concepts presented here (Swenberg et al. 1985). The significance of tissue repair or the lack thereof in the manifestation of toxicity has been recognized (Mehendele 1995), but few people study this important phenomenon other than Mehendele's group.

Reversibility

When an effect is reversed, it ends the action of a chemical in an organism. This can occur simultaneously with the elimination of a compound or with a lag period (equal to the toxicodynamic half-life), which is a measure of the reversibility or irreversibility of an effect. Considering how central reversibility is to toxicology, it is a neglected field that has been paid much less attention than the process of injury itself. Perhaps due to the fact that the majority of effects is mediated by receptors, reversibility is reasonably well understood in pharmacology (Lauffenburger and Linderman 1993). However, reversibility is much more difficult and sometimes impossible (when organisms die) to study in toxicology. This is no excuse for the relative paucity of quantitative data in terms of reversibility half-lives of effects. Even when such data are available (Swenberg et al. 1985), the experiments have not been ideally designed; this entails defining the reversibility plot for about 7 reversibility half-lives to obtain the terminal slope (if reversibility is bi- or multiphasic). The lack of quantitative information on reversibility is very disturbing, because this will most frequently be the rate-determining step when compounds act by toxicodynamic mechanisms.

CONCLUSIONS

If there is no exposure, there is no toxicity. If there is exposure, toxicity might ensue above a certain dose and time, a topic discussed under toxicokinetics and toxicodynamics. Analysis of the fundamental equation of toxicity (Figure 1) yielded the recognition of three independent time scales. One is the dynamic time scale which is an intrinsic property of a given compound (what does a chemical do to an organism), and the other is the kinetic time scale which is an intrinsic property of a specific organism (what does an organism do to a chemical). The frequency of exposure denotes a third time scale, which is independent of dose and of the dynamic and kinetic time scales. Frequency of exposure depends on the experimentalist or nature, but not on an organism or substance. A liminal condition occurs when the frequency becomes infinite, which corresponds to continuous exposure. Continuous exposure forces the dynamic and kinetic time scales to become synchronized, thereby reducing complexity to three variables: dose, effect, and one time scale. Keeping one of those variables constant allows one to study the other variables reproducibly under isoeffective, isodosic, or isotemporal conditions. However, any departure from continuous exposure will introduce the full complexity of four independent variables (dose and the kinetic, dynamic, and frequency time scales) impacting on the effect (dependent variable) at the same time. The examples discussed here demonstrate how nature in the form of long half-lives provides liminal conditions when either kinetic or dynamic half-lives force synchronization of all three time scales.

The original charge for this paper was to conceptualize the role of toxicokinetics in the risk assessment of deployed forces exposed to chemicals. Most toxicologists familiar with current trends in toxicology are aware of the tremendous proliferation of publications combining physiologically based pharmacokinetic (PBPK) models with various dose-response extrapolation models, usually with the linearized multistage (LMS) model or more recently with the benchmark (BM) curve-fitting model. This author has used both PBPK and classical pharmacokinetics to model numerous experiments (Scheufler and Rozman 1984; Roth et al. 1994; Roth et al. 1995). Although both are conceptually sound, there is one fundamental difference: classical pharmacokinetics uses time as an explicit function, whereas PBPK deals with time as a predicted variable based on partition coefficients, tissue volumina, and blood flow rates. Therefore, concepts of classical pharmacokinetics were helpful in the development of the initial core of a theory of toxicology, as presented in this document, whereas the concepts of PBPK were not as useful. This is not to say that combining PBPK with a theoretically sound biological model will not provide appropriate answers in some instances. However, as long as PBPK is used in conjunction with biologically implausible models (LMS, BM), it will lead (not surprisingly) to insignificant improvements (Storm and Rozman, 1997; Storm and Rozman 1998). Central to the development of the concepts presented here was the notion that time is a variable equivalent to dose in toxicology. This idea has been around among toxicologists for almost exactly 100 years (Warren 1900). Nevertheless, claims of exceptions to this idea as embodied in Haber's Rule prevented the development of time as a variable in toxicology. Even today toxicologists tend to focus on the so-called "exceptions" when effects are overwhelmingly dose—but not time—dependent. They do not realize that they are studying extreme parts of a spectrum under liminal conditions (e.g., a highly reversible effect on a short time scale), and they use experimental models with insufficient time resolution. When time resolution is satisfactory (such as pungency on a scale of seconds), clear summation effects emerge (Cometto-Muñiz and Cain 1984).

Thinking about how to fix current risk assessments made a paradox clear: risk projections using elaborate mathematical models do not include time as a variable even though any and all risk predictions are by definition made in time. From this recognition it was concluded that something that is basically flawed cannot be fixed. Therefore, a new risk-assessment paradigm that includes time as a variable of toxicity is being suggested. It is clear that although dose is a simple function (number of molecules), time is a complex variable, which runs on many different scales, at least three of which are interacting with dose to provide the enormous complexity that seemed to have bewildered generations of toxicologists. The three time scales are the toxicokinetic and toxicodynamic half lives and the frequency of exposure. Thus, there are three liminal conditions:

1. When the toxicokinetic half-life is very long, it keeps the frequency of exposure constant (continuous exposure), and the toxicodynamic half-life by definition will be the same as the toxicokinetic one. Under these liminal conditions $c \times t = k$ for isoeffective experiments, because there is only dose-dependence and one time-dependence.

2. When the toxicodynamic half-life is very long, it requires no additional injury to occur to keep injury constant nor the continuous presence of the noxious agent to result under isoeffective conditions in $c \times t = k$, because there is only dose-dependence and one time-dependence.

3. When the toxicokinetic/toxicodynamic half-lives become very short, they will blur the distinction between the kinetic and dynamic time scales and both will become less important, because in that case the frequency of exposure dominates the time-dependence. Under liminal (continuous exposure = infinite frequency) and isoeffective conditions, this will also lead to $c \times t = k$.

When experiments are conducted under isodosic or isotemporal conditions then the relationship will obey the equation $c \times t = k \times \mathit{Effect}$ (Figure 4). The vast majority of exposure scenarios are of course far from these liminal situations (ideal conditions) and will, therefore, yield $c \times t^x = k$. There are clear suggestions in this paper for the type of experiments that need to be done to determine x with exactitude. In the meantime, practical suggestions illustrate how to use a decision tree or available databases to conduct less arbitrary risk assessments than currently done for any conceivable deployment situation by using the new risk paradigm, which includes both dose and time as variables of toxicity.

To Summarize:

1. The charge was to conceptualize the role of kinetics in risk assessment. The current trend is to use PBPK rather than classical kinetics. The author prefers classical kinetics, because time is an explicit variable there.

2. Adding time to dose as an independent variable in toxicology allows a new risk assessment paradigm, which does not depend on defaults and uncertainties associated with current methodology (reference dose, linear multistage extrapolation, etc.) in which the only independent variable is dose.

3. A decision-tree approach is outlined in Appendix 1 in which the first step is the identification of the target species and chemical and the specific adverse effect to be applied to the deployment scenario. The second step involves the use of the kinetic and dynamic information relative to this scenario to define the rate-limiting or rate-determining steps. The final step is to use the kinetic or dynamic half-life, together with the anticipated schedules, to predict exposure thresholds for the deployed forces.

4. Examples are provided to illustrate various liminal conditions where $c \times t = k$ (very long kinetic or dynamic half-lives versus very short kinetic or dynamic half-lives where exposure frequency becomes the limiting condition). Examples are also provided for the more common exposure situation where $c \times t^x = k$ as well as the methodology for risk predictions.

5. A somewhat simplified approach using occupational exposure limits as the starting point is described in Appendix 2, together with examples of how this approach could be used to protect deployed forces.

APPENDIX 1

Examples to Illustrate the Use of the Decision Tree Concept in Risk Analysis

Dioxin (TCDD)

Toxicodynamics

    half-life unknown, but unlikely to be rate-determining

Injury
    Death: wasting, hemorrhage, anemia, cancer
    Incapacitation: little
    Residual damage: chloracne (human)
                      multiple (animals)

Recovery
    Adaptation
        Pretreatment: induction of enzymes (ineffective)
        Exercise: unlikely
        Stress: unlikely
        Temperature: unlikely
    Repair
        DNA repair: no DNA damage
        Apoptosis: some
        Cell replication: yes
    Reversibility
        Receptor binding: strong
        Chemical bonding: no
        Hydrogen bonding: no
        Ion-Ion interaction: no

Toxicokinetics (Figure 6)

    half-life 7 years (humans)
    half-life 20 days (rats)
    This will be the rate-determining process.

Absorption
    Oral: 90%
    Inhalation: negligible
    Dermal: negligible
    Other: negligible

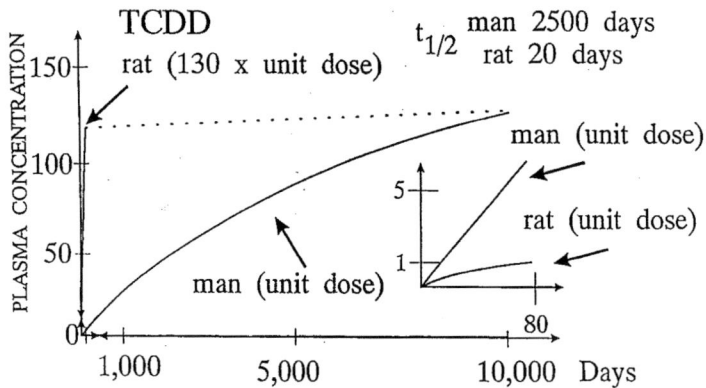

FIGURE 6 Schematic illustration of the effect of different half-lives of TCDD on steady-state concentrations in humans and rats given the same daily dose rates.

Elimination
    Distribution
        Adipose tissue: sequestration
        Liver protein: sequestration
        Bone matrix: negligible
    Biotransformation
        Phase I: rapid, very little
        Phase II: rapid, but not much
        Polymorphism: unimportant because of lack of biotransformation
    Excretion
        Renal: negligible
        Fecal: slow (rate-determining)
        Biliary/enterohepatic circulation: very little
Minor routes: negligible

Risk Assessment for Dioxin

It takes 6.64 half-lives (46.5 years) to eliminate 99% of a single dose of TCDD. TCDD will accumulate and reach 99% of steady state after 6.64 half-lives (46.5 years) following repeated exposure.

Thus, x, of the $c \times t^x$ term, will be very close to unity for this compound, implying very little margin of safety above the $c \times t$ lifetime threshold. This, combined with the lack of possibility for toxicokinetic intervention (which is the rate-determining step), makes it mandatory that the source of exposure must be controlled, which is the food.

Because toxicokinetics is the rate-determining step in the toxicity of dioxins, interpretation of animal data has to take into account the large difference in half-lives between humans (half-life = 7 years) and laboratory animals (half-life = 20 days). If $c \times t$ estimates are derived from rat data, they have to be divided by 128 to ascertain that the AUC will not be larger in humans in 46.5 years than in rats after 133 days (Figure 6).

These types of compounds will be detectable in exposed people for the rest of their lives. Moreover, the magnitude of their exposure can be extrapolated back in time with just a few assumptions about exposure scenarios. The accuracy of these projections is very high.

During 1- to 30-day deployments, it will not matter much in terms of risk assessment if exposure will be due to a single hostile act or to insidious repeated exposures.

It can be derived from the $c \times t = k$ relationship (Table 1) that the lifetime lowest-observed-adverse-effect level (LOAEL) for HpCDD-induced lung cancer in female rats with a life expectancy of 1,000 days would be a dose of 1,180 µg/kg. Because the difference between LD_{100} and LD_0 is a factor of 2, virtually all female rats will be protected from lung cancer by a dose of 590 µg/kg of HpCDD. In terms of daily dose rate, this corresponds to 0.59 µg/kg/day. Due to the long half-life of HpCDD (314 days in female rats), exposure would be continuous and therefore $x = 1$ (approximately) for all biological endpoints. Thus, any dose of HpCDD that would not cause minimum enzyme induction (ethoxyresorufin-o-deethylase [erod]) would represent a margin of safety (MS) that would correspond to a 59-fold margin of safety or a 1.7×10^{-2} margin of risk.

$$MS = \frac{c \times t_{lungcancer}}{c \times t_{erod}}$$

Conversion of these margins for humans would require an adjustment for the longer life expectancy of humans (25,550 days versus 1,000 days) under an assumption of equal sensitivity, resulting in a 2.3-fold margin of safety or a 4×10^{-1} margin of risk for humans at this dose. It is a risk management decision to reduce these numbers by arbitrary safety factors. However, because exposure has been reduced to subthreshold levels, no additional safety will be gained by the application of large safety factors. As the relative potency of dioxins to cause cancer (Rozman et al. 1993) is the same as that to cause other effects, these calculations can also be applied to other dioxins to calculate the margins of safety and risk. For tetra-dioxin (toxic equivalent factor [TEF] of TCDD [1] versus HpCDD [0.007]), this calculation yields a daily lifetime dose rate of 4.1 ng/kg. Assuming that risk is linearly decreasing, also below the threshold, this calculation would yield a risk of 0.4×10^{-6} for a daily exposure to 4.1 ng/kg of TCDD. According to the $c \times t$ concept, lung cancer could occur in a sensitive human being after 10,250,000 days, or 28,082 years, of exposure to TCDD at this daily dose rate.

Soman

Toxicokinetics

half-life $\cong$ 10 to 100 min in animals (Benschop and De Jong, 1991)
half-life unknown in humans (unlikely to be much different from animals)
↓
not rate-determining

Toxicodynamics

half-life $\cong$ 12 h (animals)
half-life unknown (humans) (unlikely to be much different from animals)

Injury: very rapid (not rate-determining)
    Death: cholinergic crisis/hypoxia

Incapacitation: cholinergic crisis
Residual damage: CNS/hypoxia
Recovery: slow (rate-determining)
    half-life $\cong$ 12 h (Sterri et al. 1980)
    Synthesis of new enzyme at critical sites (CNS)
Adaptation: limited
    Pretreatment:
        Pretreatment with soman does not change its toxicity
        Pretreatment with agents, which bind to the same site reversibly provides possibility for therapeutic intervention
    Exercise:
    Increases rate of respiration and therefore will lead to higher systemic exposure
    Stress:
        Same as for exercise
    Temperature:
        There is a temperature effect
Repair
    DNA repair: not critical
    Apoptosis: not critical
    Cell proliferation: coincidental impact
    Synthesis of new biological entity: slow (rate-determining)

Cell Proliferation:

This is not a critical step in the assessment of soman toxicity. However, it is important in the assessment of exposure to soman. Soman binds promiscuously to all sites capable of nucleophilic displacement of flouride (Fl^-), which includes erythrocytes. Although this in itself does not have toxic consequences, it produces a rate-determining step (production of new erythrocytes) that allows an exposure assessment much longer than the rate-determining step of toxicity (synthesis of new acetylcholinesterase [AChE] in CNS). If both pre- and post-deployment blood samples were available, significant exposure to anticholinesterase compounds could be demonstrated for up to 90 days after an acute, subchronic, or chronic intoxication situation. This method would be somewhat nonspecific and time-dependent because all acetylcholinesterase inhibitors, including organophosphate and carbamate pesticide, would also temporarily inhibit AChE.

Synthesis of a biochemical entity:

It appears from the literature that the rate-determining step in soman intoxications is recovery in the form of synthesis of new AChE in the CNS, specifically in the respiratory center (Lintern et al. 1998). Injury (binding to AChE) is very rapid and hence not rate-determining. The estimated half-life of recovery is about 12 h (Sterri et al. 1980), which is in good agreement with the half-life of synthesis of some enzymes. This represents a reversal of the normal situation when degradation of a protein is the rate-determining step in maintaining a steady-state concentration of an enzyme. This is the therapeutic window when reversibly binding agents can protect newly synthesized AChE from irreversible reaction with soman before natural degradation becomes rate-limiting again. As useful as these mechanistic considerations might be for the development of therapeutic intervention, knowledge of the mechanism of toxicity is not needed for risk assessment. What is essential though, is identification of the rate-determining step and its modeling to obtain a half-life of that process.

Risk Assessment for Soman

Single dose, subcutaneous exposure:
　　$c \times t$ = 17,858 µg/kg/min (Sivam et al. 1984)
　　17,858 / (24 × 60) = 12.4 µg/kg/day
This is valid if exposure is continuous and effect entirely irreversible.

Primates are about 10 times more sensitive, because of the lower levels of the nonspecific esterases (as a detoxification sink) (Anzueto et al. 1986; 1990)
　　12.4/10 = 1.24 µg/kg/day
Primates are very similar to each other, including humans (Talbot et al. 1988)
The dose response for soman is extremely steep, at most a factor of 2
　　1.24/2 = 0.62 µg/kg/day (Aas et al. 1985)
Recovery half-life from soman intoxication is estimated at 12 h (Sterri et al. 1980; Lintern et al. 1998)
Therefore, if exposure occurs outside of 6.64 recovery half-lives, there will be no accumulation of injury.

If exposure occurs within 6.64 recovery half-lives, there will be accumulation of injury to steady state after 6.64 half-lives.

As a first approximation, the daily reference dose needs to be divided further by the number of days exposure occurred.

Oral
　　1-day deployment exposure limit (DEL) by ingestion: 0.62 µg/kg/day
　　14-day DEL by ingestion: 0.04 µg/kg/day
　　30-day DEL by ingestion: 0.02 µg/kg/day
These are probably very conservative estimates because organophosphates have strong hepatic first-pass effect and these numbers were derived from subcutaneous injection, which is kinetically closer to inhalation than ingestion. This notion is supported by the similarity of the $c \times t$ product after inhalation and subcutaneous injection.

Inhalation (Aas et al. 1985)
　　$c \times t$ = 520 mg/m^3/min at a concentration of 21 mg/m^3
　　t = 24.8 min
　　Rats (~150 to 200) inhale about 500-600 ml air/min (Druckrey et al. 1967)
According to calculations using metabolic body size and caloric utilization (Kleiber, 1975; Kleiber, 1975), rats of this size should have a breathing rate of 481 ml/min, which is close to Druckrey's estimate.

Converting inhalation to oral dose:
　　500 ml/min air inhaled for 24.8 min → 12,400 ml → 12.41 → 0.0124 m^3
　　at 21 mg/m^3 → 0.2604 mg/rat for a 260 g rat → 1.002 mg/kg = 1,002 g/kg
　　$c \times t$ = 24,848 g/kg/min
This is very similar to the subcutaneous $c \times t$ (17,858 µg/kg/min).
　　$c \times t$ = 520 mg/m^3/min
Primates 10 times more sensitive than rats (Anzueto et al. 1990)
　　$c \times t$ = 52 mg/m^3 /min
Steep dose response of factor 2
　　$c \times t$ = 26 mg/m^3/min (LOEL)
　　$c \times t$ = 433 µg/m^3/h
　　$c \times t$ = 18.0 µg/m^3/day

Breathing-rate conversion of rat to human's ~ 3.7

$c \times t = 66.6$ µg/m³/day

Because this represents an estimated lowest-observable-effect level (LOEL), risk managers might divide it by a safety factor of 10 to ascertain that no one will be exposed to near toxic concentrations of soman.

1-day deployment exposure limit (DEL): 7 µg/m³
14-day DEL: 0.5 µg/m³
30-day DEL: 0.2 µg/m³

These values are DELs for continuous exposure. If exposure is intermittent, the following rule will provide protection: If exposure occurs outside of 6.62 recovery half-lives (3.3 days at a half-life of ~ 12 h) the 1-day DEL will provide protection for all scenarios, because there will be no accumulation of injury.

The 1-day DEL should not be exceeded if exposure occurs for shorter durations (e.g., 1 h or 10 min), because in 24 h there will be only 75% recovery and injury will proceed to steady state, and after 3.32 half-lives it will be accumulating according to $c \times t = k$.

APPENDIX 2

Strategies for Developing Exposure Guidelines of Deployed Forces

Development of exposure guidelines from existing databases (ACGIH, NIOSH, OSHA):

(1) Identify if compound exerts its rate-determining step(s) by toxicodynamic or toxicokinetic means (Figure 1).

(2) Narrow down critical step(s) to injury/absorption or elimination/recovery or further to adaptation/distribution, repair/biotransformation, and reversibility/excretion.

(3) Estimate half-life of critical step(s).

This is a very important step. Failure to identify the proper process and its half-life can lead to erroneous conclusions. This can be illustrated with a pharmacological example to indicate the universality of this approach.

Omperazole is a H^+-ion pump inhibitor. The binding half-life to its receptor is 24 h. Its biological half-life is about 1 h. If the therapeutic dose would be based on the biological half-life of the compound, the conclusion would be that after 6.64 half-lives (6.64 h) 99% of the drug would be eliminated. Therefore, a dosing regiment entailing the administration of the drug every 6 h still would yield a very poor steady state and, with that, moderate to low therapeutic efficacy. Omperazole in fact is given daily once or every other day in accordance with its pharmacodynamic half-life of 24 h. It has been reported that it takes 3 days for maximum effect (clinically indistinguishable from 3.32 half-lives) and 3 to 5 days for cessation of effect, which is clinically also indistinguishable from 3.32 reversibility half-lives. The action of this drug is entirely dominated by D and any opinion, based on K, would be in error.

(4) Because threshold limit values (TLVs), short-term exposure limits (STELs) and ceilings (ACGIH), permissible exposure limit (PELs) (OSHA), and recommended exposure levels (RELs) (NIOSH) represent NOAELs, one could use these values and convert them to any given deployment situation by considering duration and frequency of exposure along with the half-life of the critical step, which could be designated as exposure kinetics (see equation in Figure 1). A twofold critical question is: When are time-weighted averages (TWAs) and when are peak concentrations important for converting these standards into standards for various deployment situations?

Derivation of DEL When Toxicokinetics Is Rate-Determining

Very long toxicokinetic half-lives

Compounds having half-lives of years or longer (e.g., mirex, dioxins, cadmium, asbestos) are the simplest to deal with. (It is amazing that regulatory agencies have been struggling with this for decades.)

For such compounds, any $c \times t$ conversion will be fairly accurate without regard to route and frequency of exposure. A single high dose exposure will not be much different from exposure to proportionally smaller daily dose rates. Thus, for these types of compounds, there is little difference between TWA and peak exposure.

Example: *cadmium* half-life $\cong$ 30 years (in humans)

Inhalation
TLV (ACGIH): 0.01 mg/m^3, 8-h TWA for 5 days/week for 45 years at 10 m^3/8 h
    Total dose: 1,170 mg/70 kg person
      16.7 mg/kg
1-day limit by inhalation: 1,170 mg/20 m^3 = 58.5 mg/m^3 at 20 m^3 (air inhaled/24 h)
Similar to radiation, this is a ceiling value for total exposure, which might not be exceeded. Persons must be protected from further exposure. It is a risk management decision to reduce this number, e.g., by dividing it by 10.
 1-day deployment exposure limit (DEL) by inhalation: 5.9 mg/m^3
 14-day DEL by inhalation: 0.4 mg/m^3
 3-month DEL by inhalation: 0.2 mg/m^3

Oral
Conversion of inhalation to oral dose:
20 m^3 × 5.9 mg/m^3 ÷ 70 kg = 1.69 mg/kg
Absorption of cadmium salts in the GI tract is very limited at 5 to 8% of dose (Goyer 1996), which provides additional safety.
1-day DEL by ingestion: 1.69 mg/kg
14-day DEL by ingestion: 0.12 mg/kg/day
3-month DEL by ingestion: 0.06 mg/kg/day

It is a risk management decision to reduce these numbers to leave room for reserve capacity, although the safety factor does not have to be large, because of low fractional absorption, which reduces systemic exposure by nearly a factor of a 100.

Dermal
Dermal penetration of cadmium salts and of highly lipophilic compounds of very long half-life is very inefficient.

Intermediate toxicokinetic half-lives

For compounds having a half-life 3.6 h or longer, but shorter than months or years, elimination will not be complete within 24 h after a single dose. This is important, because, as a consequence, recovery from injury will also not be complete. Recovery from injury by chemicals having intermediate half-lives will be probably as often rate-determining (rate-limiting) as the biological half-life. Therefore, a discussion of these types of chemicals will be also found in the toxicodynamic section as well. For such compounds, peak exposures as well as TWA concentrations will be of consequence. Therefore, particular attention must be paid to the ratio between the biological half-life and various exposure scenarios when setting DELs for such chemicals. It is worthwhile to consider that the half-life of 3.6 h represents among this class of compounds the best case scenario, because the longer the half-life, the higher the accumulation will be by the time a steady state is reached.

Example: *monochloroacetic acid (MCA)*
    half-life $\cong$ 4 h (rats)

The half-life is probably very similar in humans because the mechanism of toxicity is the same and the rat's LD_{50} = 75 mg/kg is similar to the human's lethal dose $\cong$ 220 mg/kg.

Inhalation
    TLV recommendation: 2 mg/m^3, 8-h TWA for 5 days/week for 45 years at 10 m^3/8 h
    Total dose: 234,000 mg/70 kg person
                      3,343 mg/kg
    1-day DEL by inhalation: 1 mg/m^3 at 20 m^3/24 h
    14-day DEL by inhalation: 0.07 mg/m^3
    3-month DEL by inhalation: 0.03 mg/m^3

This is the most conservative conversion, assuming continuous exposure. A comparison of the 1-day total DEL (20 mg) with the total occupational exposure limit (OEL) in 45 years (234,000 mg) indicates how sensitive these type of compounds are to the frequency of exposure.

After 6.64 half-lives, 99% of steady state will be reached. The half-life of MCA is about 4 h, and steady-state concentration will be reached after about 1 day. Thereafter, the AUC will increase according to $c \times t$ (above the lifetime threshold) if exposure is uninterrupted.

However, if exposure is intermittent, say for 1 h every day, then higher levels might be tolerated without adverse effect, because complete (99%) elimination/recovery will occur between any two episodes of exposure.

1-hour DEL by inhalation: 16 mg/m^3 at 1.25 m^3/h air inhaled

Oral
    Assuming six (three eating and drinking and three additional drinking) intake episodes per day with a half-life of 4 h, almost 99% of steady state will be reached after 1 day. Continuous exposure for 14 or 30 days will be occurring with smaller or larger fluctuations between $C_{\text{maximum serum contration}}$ and $C_{\text{minimum serum concentration}}$ if eating/drinking are not equally paced, which will not effect the average AUC. Therefore, safe levels can be calculated for oral exposure according to $c \times t = k$ also for this compound.

Conversion of inhalation dose to oral dose:
    1 mg/m^3 × 20 m^3 (air inhaled/ 24 h) = 20 mg/70 kg person = 0.3 mg/kg

The same (cumulative) dose can be ingested safely during 14 or 30 days of deployment according to the most conservative conversion, which assumes repeated exposures every day.

    1-day DEL by ingestion: 0.3 mg/kg
    14-day DEL by ingestion: 0.02 mg/kg/day
    30-day DEL by ingestion: 0.01 mg/kg/day

Again 1-h ingestion (single daily exposure) might be higher since there will be 99% elimination/recovery within 24 h.

1-hour DEL by ingestion: 7.1 mg/kg if no further exposure occurs on that day.

Dermal

Dermal toxicity of MCA is similar to its oral toxicity as dermal penetration of MCA is extremely efficient, particularly at higher temperatures. Therefore, the same numbers are recommended for dermal exposure as for oral exposure.

As the half-life of compounds becomes longer than about 4 h, accumulation to steady state will take correspondingly longer. Nevertheless, $c \times t$ conversions will remain conservative (but not extremely conservative and not arbitrary) estimations of safe levels of exposure, because the increase of AUC during the ascending phase of the exposure curve will be smaller than at steady state. With increasing half lives, deviations from $c \times t = k$ will become less dependent on the frequency and duration of exposure.

Very short toxicokinetic half lives

If half-lives are shorter than 3.6 h then more than 99% of the compound will be eliminated within 24 h of exposure. With such compounds, the frequency of exposure will become more and more important as the half-life decreases further, because of increasing periods of recovery between exposure episodes.

Example: *Methylene chloride (MCl)*
    half-life $\cong$ 5 to 40 min (humans), indicating an average of 22.5 min

Inhalation

TLV: 174 mg/m^3, 8-h TWA for 5 days/week for 45 years at 10 m^3/8 h

For compounds of very short half-life, it is not meaningful to use the $c \times t$ conversion unless exposure is continuous, because of rapid elimination/recovery after cessation of exposure. Rapid elimination/recovery in turn reduces time-dependence of toxicity. Compounds having very short half-lives will be mainly concentration-dependent, particularly when considering short time scales such as 1 day, 14 days, or 30 days. In fact, toxicity of such compounds depends primarily on the time scale of frequency and duration of exposure in addition to the dose (concentration). For these reasons, an OEL of 25 to 50 parts per million (ppm) (86.8 to 174 mg/m^3) was derived for MCl from impaired flicker fusion reflex data (4-h exposure) in humans (Storm and Rozman 1998). Although this behavioral effect is highly reversible, it impairs optimum performance. Therefore, in a deployment situation these values could be used as ceilings not to be exceeded. Because these values were derived with continuous exposure, the 1-hour DEL (continuous exposure) could be set based on $c \times t$ yielding 100 to 200 ppm (348 to 696 mg/m^3). However, longer-term intermittent exposures should use the ceiling approach:

    1-day DEL by inhalation: 174 mg/m^3
    14-day DEL by inhalation: 174 mg/m^3
    30-day DEL by inhalation: 174 mg/m^3
    1-hour DEL by inhalation: 696 mg/m^3

Oral

Because of significant first-pass biotransformation, oral DELs require additional considerations, but they would be higher than those obtained for inhalation.

Derivation of DEL When Toxicodynamics is Rate-Determining

Compounds having very long recovery half-lives

There are few examples for recovery taking place on a time scale of years or longer. Damage to neurons (e.g., lead encephalopathy) is the closest example that comes to mind. Because of the enormous reserve capacity and plasticity of the nervous system, it is difficult to conduct conclusive studies in this area. Unlike compounds with very long toxicokinetic half-lives (which amounts to continuous exposure), both the frequency and duration and the kinetics of compounds are important when dynamics of the effects are rate-determining. When the toxicokinetic half-life of a compound is long (lead), a TWA approach ($c \times t = k$) will be the best way to protect deployed forces, whereas in the case of short half-life compounds (methanol), the ceiling approach must be applied to prevent the beginning of accumulation of injury.

Example: *lead*
    half-life $\cong$ 20 years

Inhalation
    TLV: 0.05 mg/m^3, 8-hr TWA for 5 days/week for 45 years at 10 m^3/8h
    Total dose: 5,850 mg
    5,850 mg/20 m^3 = 293 mg/m^3
    It might be advisable to reduce these numbers by a safety factor of 10.
    1-day DEL: 29.3 mg/m^3
    14-day DEL: 2.1 mg/m^3
    30-day DEL: 1.0 mg/m^3
    1-hour DEL should not significantly exceed the TWA, even if exposure remains infrequent.

Oral
Conversion of inhalation to oral dose:
    20 m^3 × 29.3 mg/m^3/70 kg = 8.4 mg/kg
Adults absorb 5 to15% of ingested lead, which provides enough margin of safety.
    1-day DEL: 8.4 mg/kg
    14-day DEL: 0.6 mg/kg/day
    30-day DEL: 0.3 mg/kg/day

Dermal
    Insignificant.

Example: *methanol*

Inhalation
    TLV: 200 ppm = 262.1 mg/m^3
    It is not appropriate to use a TWA for methanol, because in this case accumulation of injury will be a function of the frequency of exposure above the threshold. Any exposure above the threshold will be cumulative. Therefore, to protect deployed forces from such scenarios a ceiling must be established.
    1-day DEL: 262.1 mg/m^3
    14-day DEL: 262.1 mg/m^3
    30-day DEL: 262.1 mg/m^3

Intermediate toxicodynamic half-lives

Recovery from injury caused by compounds having a toxicodynamic half-life of 3.6 h or longer, but shorter than years, will be incomplete after 1 day. In the best-case scenario of 3.6 h, recovery will be 99% complete. However, even for such compounds, $c \times t = k$ would be running at about 1% residual damage. This might be of little consequence if exposure is intermittent, but in some instances it might represent a hazard. A better illustration of this point can be made by using nitrosamines as examples. Nitrosamines are *strong* alkylating agents with short toxicokinetic half-lives (Druckrey 1967). However, the repair half-life of the DNA adducts is about 20 to 40 days. Consequently, the steady state of DNA damage will not be reached until about 200 days (on average). Thereafter, damage will accumulate according to $c \times t = k$. Just like a single dose of a chemical having very long toxicokinetic half-lives can cause cancer (Rozman 1999), single doses of dialkylnitrosamines can also cause cancer (Druckrey et al. 1964). If one mole (approximate LD_{50}) of dimethylnitrosamine is administered to rats, and assuming that 0.0001% of it will end up binding to DNA, this will still yield 6×10^{17} adducts. With a 30-day toxicodynamic half-life this will leave a 900-day old rat still with about 6×10^8 adducts. It is very likely that the traditional distinction between initiators and promoters in carcinogenesis is due to the respective compounds having toxicokinetic or toxicodynamic processes as rate-determining steps in their mechanism of action.

Example: *dimethyl-or diethylnitrosamine*
  TLV: This is a compound listed in the TLV booklet without a value.
  Dimethylnitrosamine's carcinogenicity was studied by Druckrey et al. (1963) under isoeffective conditions (100% carcinomas). Different daily dose rates of diethylnitrosamine yielded a $c \times t = k$ equal to 73,248 ± 5,234 (SE) mg/kg/day. Druckrey et al. (1967), like everybody else, viewed the daily dose rate as dose. Therefore, they plotted the daily dose rate versus time to derive a slope, which yielded the equation $c \times t^{2.3} = k$. This erroneous view led to the introduction of the notion about the reinforcing action (200-fold) of low doses. This mistake was due to the fact that their studies were not conducted under isotemporal conditions. Therefore, some rats received on the average 68 dose rates, whereas others received up to 840 dose rates. In fact, the difference in terms of cumulative dose was only 15-fold between the highest and lowest dose, which is comparable to the difference in induction time (12-fold). Suffice to say that Druckrey et al.'s (1963) data are in fact very consistent with $c \times t = k$, when viewing the dose as the sum of all dose rates.

  Derivation of DELs from the $c \times t$ data:
  $c \times t = 73,248 \pm 15,700$ (SD)
  Rat: $c \times t_{lifespan} = 73,248$ mg/kg/day
  Lifespan of rat: 900 days
  $c = 73,248/900 = 81.4$ mg/kg

This is the minimum dose required to cause cancer in rats after lifetime exposure. If it was chosen to protect rats from the carcinogenic effects of diethylnitrosamine to the extent of 99.94% (3 SD), then this dose would be:
  $c \times t = 73,248 \pm 15,700$ (SD)
  $73,248 - 47,100 = 26,148/ 900 = 29.1$ mg/kg

However, humans do not live 900 days, so let us assume 75 years (27,375 days). Under assumption of equal sensitivity this would yield a minimum carcinogenic dose in humans of $26,148/ 27,375 \cong 1$ mg/kg If human in vivo repair of DNA adducts were known, this number could be adjusted quite accurately, and species differences could be dealt with in a scientific rather than arbitrary fashion.

  A small safety factor might be applied by risk managers to move from a LOAEL to a NOAEL. The number should be small, because individual sensitivity was corrected for based on normal distribution rather than on arbitrary assumptions.

Inhalation
  0.5 mg/kg × 70 kg = 35 mg/kg
  35 mg/20 m^3 = 1.75 mg/20 m^3 (air inhaled/ 24 h)

1-day DEL: 1.75 mg/m^3
14-day DEL: 0.13 mg/m^3
30-day DEL: 0.06 mg/m^3

Oral
1-day DEL: 0.5 mg/kg
14-day DEL: 0.04 mg/kg/day
30-day DEL: 0.016 mg/kg/day

Dermal

Because it is a small amphophilic molecule, it will be readily absorbed through the skin. If needed, the oral data apply.

Very short toxicodynamic half-lives

The distinction between toxicokinetic and toxicodynamic half lives becomes fuzzy for compounds of very short recovery half-lives (<3.6 h), because for both of them another time scale (frequency of exposure) becomes the dominant time function. A very short recovery half-life implies rapid reversibility, or repair, or adaptation. Infrequent exposure to such compounds will have the least toxicological consequences, although in the case of air this could become rapidly fatal.

The efficient repair of oxygen-induced DNA repair appears to be a good example for rapid reversibility (Ames, 1989; Fraga et al. 1990). It takes continuous exposure to air over a lifetime to result in accumulation of oxidative damage in the form of aging.

Acknowledgement

Even though I am sole author of this paper for technical reasons, Dr. John Doull's intellectual contribution to the conceptualization of time along with dose as variables of toxicity must be recognized. Although I did much of the thinking and all of the writing, his daily probing of the ideas and his profound knowledge of toxicology were invaluable in the development of the concepts presented.

REFERENCES

Aas, P., S.H. Sterri, H.P. Hjermstad, and F. Fonnum. 1985. A method for generating toxic vapors of soman: toxicity of soman by inhalation in rats. Toxicol. Appl. Pharmacol. 80:437-445.

Ames, B.N. 1989. Mutagenesis and carcinogenesis: endogenous and exogenous factors. Environ. Mol. Mutagen. 14 (Suppl. 16):66-77.

Anzueto, A., G.G. Berdine, G.T. Moore, C. Gleiser, D. Johnson, C.D. White, and W.G. Johanson, Jr. 1986. Pathophysiology of soman intoxication in primates. Toxicol. Appl. Pharmacol. 86:56-68.

Anzueto, A., R.A. deLemos, J. Seidenfeld, G. Moore, H. Hamil, D. Johnson, and S.G. Jenkinson. 1990. Acute inhalation toxicity of soman and sarin in baboons. Fundam. Appl. Toxicol. 14:676-687.

ATSDR (Agency for Toxic Substances and Disease Registry). 1997. Pp. 153-173. In: Toxicological Profile for Benzene. ATSDR. Atlanta, GA.

Aungst, B. and D.D. Shen. 1986. Gastrointestinal absorption of toxic agents. Pp. 29-56. In: Gastrointestinal Toxicology, K. Rozman and O. Hänninen, eds. Amsterdam/New York/Oxford: Elsevier.

Benschop, H.P. and L.P. De Jong. 1991. Toxicokinetics of soman: species variation and stereospecificity in elimination pathways. Neurosci. Biobehav. Rev. 15:73-77.

Bliss, C.I. 1940. The relation between exposure time, concentration and toxicity in experiments on insecticides. Ann. Entomol. Soc. Am. 33:721-766.

Brugnone, R., L. Perbellini, G. Maranelli, G. Gugleilmi, and F. Lombardini. 1992. Reference values for blood benzene in the occupationally unexposed general population. Int. Arch. Occup. Environ. Health 64:179-184.

Busvine, J.R. 1938. The toxicity of ethylene oxide to Calandra oryzae, C. granaria, Tribolium castaneum, and Cimex lectularius. Ann. Appl. Biol. 25(3):605-635.

Caratero, A., M. Courtade, L. Bonnet, H. Planel, and C. Caratero. 1998. Effect of continuing gamma irradiation at a very low dose on the life-span of mice. Gerontology 44:272-276.

Cometto-Muñiz, J.E. and W.S. Cain. 1984. Temporal integration of pungency. Chemical Senses 8(4):315-327.

Druckrey, H. and K. Küpfmüller. 1948. Quantitative Analyse der Krebsentstehung Zeitschr. f. Naturforschg. 36:254-266.

Druckrey, H., R. Preussmann, S. Ivankovic, and D. Schmähl 1967. Organotrope carcinogene Wirkungen bei 65 verschiedenen N-Nitroso-Verbindungen an BD-Ratten. Zeitsch. für Krebsforschg. 69:103-201.

Druckrey, H., D. Schmähl, R. Preussmann and S. Ivankovic. 1963. Quantiative Analyse der carcinogenen Wirkung von Diäthylnitrosamin. Arzneim.-Forschg. 13: 841-846.

Druckrey, H., D. Steinhoff, R. Preussmann, and S. Ivankovic. 1964. Erzeugung von Krebs durch eine einmalige Dosis von Methylnitroso-Harnstoff und verschiedenen Dialkylnitrosaminen an Ratten. Zeitsch. f. Krebsforschg. 66:1-10.

El-Masri, H.A., R.S. Thomas, G.R. Sabados, J.K. Phillips, A.A. Constan, S.A. Benjamin, M.E. Andersen, H.M. Mehendale, and R.S. Yang. 1996. Physiologically based pharmacokinetic/pharmacodynamic modeling of the toxicologic interaction between carbon tetrachloride and Kepone. Arch. Toxicol. 70:704-713.

Flury, F. and W. Wirth. 1934. Zur Toxikologie der Lösungsmittel. Archiv f. Gewerbepath. u. Gewerbehyg. 5:1-90.

Fraga, C.G., M.K. Shigenaga, J.W. Park, P. Degan and B.N. Ames. 1990. Oxidative damage to DNA during aging: 8-hydroxy-2'-deoxyguanosine in rat organ DNA and urine. Proc. Natl. Acad. Sci. U.S.A. 87(12): 4533-4537.

Gardner, D.E., D.L. Coffin, M.A. Pinigin, and G.I. Sidoronko. 1977. Role of time as a factor in the toxicity of chemical compounds in intermittent and continuous exposure. Part 1: Effects of continuous exposure. J. Toxicol. Environ. Health 3:811-820.

Gardner, D.E., F.J. Miller, E.J. Blommer and D.L. Coffin. 1979. Influence of exposure mode on the toxicity of NO_2. Environ. Health Perspect. 30:23-29.

Garrettson, L.K. 1983. Lead. Pp. 1017-1023. In: Clinical Management of Poisoning and Drug Overdose, 2nd Ed., L.M. Haddad and J.F. Winchester, eds. Philadelphia: W.B. Saunders.

Gibaldi, M. and D. Perrier. 1975. Renal impairment. Pp. 253-266. In: Pharmacokinetics, M. Gibaldi and D. Perrier, eds. New York/ Basel: Marcel Dekker.

Goldenfeld, N. and L.P. Kadanoff. 1999. Simple lessons form complexity. Science 284:87-89.

Goyer, R.A. 1996. Toxic effects of metals. Pp.691-736. In: Casarett and Doull's Toxicology, 5th Ed., C.D. Klaassen, ed. New York.: McGraw Hill.

Gregus, Z. and C.D. Klaassen. 1986. Enterohepatic circulation of toxicants. Pp. 57-118. In: Gastrointestinal Toxicology, K. Rozman and O. Hänninen, eds. Amsterdam /New York/ Oxford: Elsevier.

Hartung, R. 1987. Dose response relationships. Pp. 29-46. In: Toxic Substances and Human Risk, R.G. Tardiff and J.V. Rodricks, eds. New York :Plenum Press.

Hodgson, E., I.S. Silver, L.E. Butler, M.P. Lawton, and P.E. Levi. 1991. Metabolism. Pp. 107-167. In Handbook of Pesticide Toxicology, Vol. I., W.J. Hayes, Jr. and E. R. Laws, Jr. eds. San Diego: Academic Press.

Hoel, D.G. and P. Li. 1998. Threshold models in radiation carcinogenesis. Health Phys. 75:241-250.

Kim, Y.C. and G.P. Carlson. 1986. The effect of unusual workshift on chemical toxicity. II. Studies on the exposure of rats to aniline. Fundam. Appl. Toxicol. 7:144-152.

Kleiber, M. 1975. Body size and metabolic rate. Pp. 179-222. In: The Fire of Life: An Introduction to Animal Energetics, revised Ed., M. Kleiber, ed. Huntington/New York: Robert E. Kreiger.

Kleiber, M. 1975. Energy. Pp. 104-130. In: The Fire of Life: An Introduction to Animal Energetics, revised Ed., M. Kleiber, ed. Huntington/New York: Robert E. Kreiger.

Koch, C. and G. Laurent. 1999. Complexity and the nervous system. Science 284: 96-98.

Lauffenberger, D.A. and J.J. Linderman. 1993. Cell surface receptor/ligand binding fundamentals. Pp. 9-72. In: Receptors, D.A. Lauffenburger and J.J. Linderman, eds. New York/ Oxford: Oxford University Press.

Lintern, C.M., J.R. Wetherell, and M.E. Smith. 1998. Differential recovery of acetylchlorinesterase in guinea pig muscle and brain regions after soman treatment. Human Exp. Toxicol. 17(3):157-162.

Littlefield, N.A., J.H. Farmer, D.W. Gaylor, and W.G. Sheldon. 1980. Effects of dose and time in a long-term, low-dose carcinogenic study. J. Environ. Pathol. Toxicol. 3:17-34.

Mehendele, H.M. 1995. Toxicodynamics of low-level toxicant interactions of biological significance: inhibition of tissue repair. Toxicology 105:251-266.

Ostwald and Dernoscheck. 1910. Ober die Beziehung zwischen Adsorption und Giftigkeit. Kolloid-Zeitschr. 6(6):297-307.

Parkinson, A. 1996. Biotransformation of xenobiotics. Pp. 113-186. In: Casarett and Doull's Toxicology, 5th Ed., C.D. Klaassen, ed. New York: McGraw-Hill.

Peters, G. and W. Ganter. 1935. Zur Frage der Abtötung des Kornkäfers mit Blausäure. Zetschr. f. Angew. Entomol. 21(4):547-559.

Peto, R., R. Gray, P. Brantom, and P. Grasso. 1991. Effects on 4080 rats of chronic ingestion of N-nitrosodiethylamine or N-nitrosodimethylamine: a detailed dose-response study. Cancer Res. 51(23 Pt 2):6415-51.

Pitot, H.C. III and Y.P. Dragan. 1996. Chemical carcinogenesis. Pp: 221-225. In: Casarett and Doull's Toxicology, 5th Ed., C.D. Klaassen, ed. New York: McGraw-Hill.

Roth, W.L., S.W. Ernst, L.W. Weber, L. Kerecsen, and K.K. Rozman. 1994. A pharmacodynamically responsive model of 2,3,7,8-tetrachlorodibenzo-p-dioxin (TCDD) transfer between liver and fat after low and high doses. Toxicol. Appl. Pharmacol. 127:151-162.

Roth, W.L., L.W. Weber, and K.K. Rozman. 1995. Incorporation of first-order uptake rate constants from simple mammitary models into blood-flow limited physiological models via extraction efficiencies. Pharm. Res. 12:263-269.

Rozman, K.K. 1999. Delayed acute toxicity of 1,2,3,4,6,7,8-tetracholordibenzo-p-dioxin (HpCDD) after oral administration obeys Haber's rule of inhalation toxicology. Toxicol. Sci. 49:102-109.

Rozman, K.K. 1986. Fecal excretion of toxic substances. Pp. 119-145. In: Gastrointestinal Toxicology, K. Rozman and O. Hänninen, eds. Amsterdam/ New York: Elsevier.

Rozman, K.K. 1998. Quantitative definition of toxicity: a mathematical description of life and death with dose and time as variables. Med. Hypotheses 51:175-178.

Rozman, K.K. and J. Doull. 1998. General principles of toxicology. Pp. 1-11. In: Environmental Toxicology. Current Developments, J. Rose, ed. Amsterdam: Gordon and Breach. Sci. Publ.

Rozman, K.K. and C.D. Klaassen. 1996. Absorption, distribution and excretion of toxicants. Pp. 91-112. In: Casarett and Doull's Toxicology, 5th Ed, C.D. Klaassen, ed. New York: McGraw Hill.

Rozman, K.K., L. Kerecsen, M.K. Viluksela, D. Österle, E. Deml, M. Viluksela, B.U. Stahl, and J. Doull, J. 1996. A toxicologist's view of cancer risk assessment. Drug Metab. Rev. 28:29-52.

Rozman K, W.L. Roth, H. Greim, B.U. Stahl and J. Doull. 1993. Relative potency of chlorinated dibenzo-p-dioxins (CDDs) in acute, subchronic and chronic (carcinogenicity) toxicity studies: implications for risk assessment of chemical mixtures. Toxicology 77(1-2):39-50.

Scheufler, E. and K.K. Rozman. 1984. Effect of hexadecane on the pharmacokinetics of hexachlorobenzene. Toxicol. Appl. Pharmacol. 75:190-197.

Sidell, F.R. 1974. Soman and sarin: clinical manifestations and treatment of accidental poisoning by organophosphates. Clin. Toxicol. 7:1-17.

Sivam, P.S., B. Hoskins, and I.K. Ho. 1984. An assessment of comparative acute toxicity of diisopropyl-fluorophosphate, tabun, sarin and soman in relation to cholinergic and GABAergic enzyme activities in rats. Fundam. Appl. Toxicol. 4: 531-538.

Sterri, S.H., S. Lyngaas, and F. Fonnum. 1980. Toxicity of soman after repetitive injection of sublethal doses in rat. Acta Pharmacol. Toxicol. 46:1-7.

Storm, J.E. and K.K. Rozman. 1998. Derivation of an occupational exposure limit (OEL) for methylene chloride based on acute CNS effects and relative potency analysis. Regul. Toxicol. Pharmacol. 27:240-250.

Storm, J.E. and K.K. Rozman. 1997. Evaluation of alternative models for establishing safe levels of occupational exposure to vinyl halides. Regul. Toxicol. Pharmacol. 25:240-255.

Swenberg, J.A., F.C. Richardson, J.A. Boucheron, and M.C. Dyroff. 1985. Relationships between DNA adduct formation and carcinogenesis. Environ. Health Persp. 62:177-183.

Talbot, B.G., D.R. Anderson, L.W. Harris, L.W. Yarbrough, and W.J. Lennox. 1988. A comparison of in vivo and in vitro rates of aging of soman-inhibited erythrocyte acetylcholinesterase in different animal species. Drug Chem. Toxicol. 11(3):289-305.

Tripathi, H.L. and W.L. Dewey. 1989. Comparison of the effect of diisopropylfluorophosphate, sarin, soman and tabun on toxicity and brain acetyl cholinesterase activity in mice. J. Toxicol. Environ. Health 26:437-446.

Viluksela, M., B.U. Stahl, L.S. Birnbaum, K.W. Schramm, A. Kettrup, and K.K. Rozman. 1997. Subchronic/chronic toxicity of 1,2,3,4,6,7,8-heptachlorodibenzo-p-dioxin (HpCDD) in rats. Part 1. Design, general observations, hematology and liver concentrations. Toxicol. Appl. Pharmacol. 146:207-216.

Viluksela, M., B.U. Stahl, L.S. Birnbaum, K.W. Schramm, A. Kettrup, and K.K. Rozman. 1998. Subchronic/chronic toxicity of a mixture of four chlorinated dibenzo-p-dioxins in rats. I. Design, general observations, hematology and liver concentrations. Toxicol. Appl. Pharmacol. 151:57-69.

Warren, E. 1900. On the reaction of Daphnia magna to certain changes in its environment. Quart. J. Microsc. Sci. 43:199-224.

Weber, L.W., S.W. Ernst, B.U. Stahl, and K.K. Rozman. 1993. Tissue distribution and toxicokinetics of 2,3,7,8-tetrachlorodibenzo-p-dioxin in rats after intravenous injection. Fundam. Appl. Toxicol. 21:523-534.

Weng, G., U.S. Bhalla, and R. Iyengar. 1999. Complexity in biological signaling systems. Science 284:92-96.

Whitesides, G.M. and R.F. Ismagilov. 1999. Complexity in chemistry. Science 284: 89-92.

Winthrobe, M.M. and G.R. Lee. 1974. Hematologic alterations. Pp. 28. In Harrison's Principles of Internal Medicine, 7th Ed., M.M. Winthrobe, G.W. Thorn, R.D. Adams, E. Braunwald, K.J. Isselbacher and R-G. Pererdorf, eds. New York: McGraw-Hill.

Health Risks and Preventive Research Strategy for Deployed U.S. Forces from Toxicological Interactions Among Potentially Harmful Agents

by Raymond S. H. Yang[1]

ABSTRACT

The goal of this paper is to recommend to the Department of Defense (DOD) a preventive research strategy for deployed U.S. forces to prevent future illness from toxicological interactions from potentially harmful agents. By doing so, it is implicit that potential health risks exist in deployments because of possible exposures to multiple chemicals, drugs, and biologics under stressful environmental and occupational conditions similar to those in the Persian Gulf War. This conclusion was reached based on the author's knowledge of toxicological interactions among chemicals and other agents and his assessment of the available literature information to date. It should be emphasized that this is not an effort to provide an exhaustive review of the field of toxicological interactions of chemical mixtures and other stressors. In fact, some of the areas are so new that the knowledge base is embryonic at best. DOD, through the National Research Council (NRC), seeks expert advice because of the limited information in the area of adverse health effects resulting from multiple stressors, including exposure to chemical mixtures, drug mixtures, vaccine mixtures, and physical and biological agents under highly stressful and hazardous environmental and occupational conditions. Furthermore, psychological stress undoubtedly plays a role in the potential development of such adverse health effects. There is probably no one individual or any group of individuals who knows the answers to such complex situations. Therefore, the author's opinions are, in some cases, based on educated guesses.

Given the principal goal stated above, this paper:

1. Discusses the current thinking on toxicological interactions at low-exposure doses, principally to chemicals. However, known and potential toxicological interactions involving biological and physical agents, as well as stressful environmental conditions, are also discussed.

2. Provides an assessment based on experimental toxicological studies of the effects of agents known to be present in the Persian Gulf War. The concerns about the surprising toxicological interac-

---

[1]Center for Environmental Toxicology and Technology, Departments of Environmental Health, Colorado State University, Foothills Campus, Ft. Collins, CO, 80523-1680.

tions discovered after the Persian Gulf War are discussed. These new discoveries offer potential explanations for the Gulf War Syndrome.

3. Illustrates the importance of the mechanistic understanding of the disease process through research by summarizing some of the studies reported in the literature, which offers a possible explanation for the neurotoxicities of the Gulf War Syndrome.

4. Looks into the rediscovered area of hormesis, as well as the little-known area of multiple stressors. Their potential roles in the field of toxicological interactions are discussed.

5. Explains genetic polymorphism as a basis for sensitive populations. A specific example in experimental toxicology involving multiple stressors is given as an illustration.

6. Offers a preventive research strategy to DOD to avoid possible future Gulf War Illnesses in deployed forces. The rationale, significance, and how-to's for such a preventive research strategy are given in detail.

7. Discusses the ongoing and possible future development of predictive tools for toxicological interactions among chemicals, drugs, biologics, physical and biological agents, and other multiple stressors. Philosophical issues and future perspectives in the context of the present task are also discussed.

INTRODUCTION

A common definition of an "expert" is one who knows more and more about less and less. Implicitly, this suggests that an expert is very, very focused and is likely to be knowledgeable in a very narrow field. If this is true, what happens when an extremely broad and complex situation like Gulf War Syndrome arises? Do we find many experts in their own respectively focused fields and hope to put the pieces of the puzzle together to form the mosaic? Who is going to see the mosaic? The experts collectively? or a wise old man or woman who knows it all?

The National Research Council (NRC), under the sponsorship of the Department of Defense (DOD), initiated in January 1998 a project on Strategies to Protect the Health of Deployed U. S. Forces. The goal and central theme are succinctly expressed as follows:

> The project will advise DOD on a long-term strategy for protecting the health of our nation's military personnel when deployed to unfamiliar environments. Drawing on the lessons of the Persian Gulf War (PGW) and subsequent deployments, it will advise the DOD with regard to a strategy for managing the health and exposure issues faced during deployments to unfamiliar environments; these include infectious agents, vaccines, drug interactions, and stress. It also will include adverse reactions to chemical or biological warfare agents and other substances. In addition, the project will deal with the problem of limited and variable data in the PGW context; and in the development of a prospective strategy for improved handling of health and exposure issues in future deployments. The project will also assess the DOD's response to the recommendations of other expert reports, such as those of the Defense Science Board, the Presidential Advisory Committee on Gulf War Veterans Illnesses, the Institute of Medicine, etc. These tasks would be accomplished with a good understanding of DOD's need to make trade-offs or set acceptable levels of risk.

The broad charge was translated into the following four tasks:

Task 2.1: An analytical framework for assessing the risks to deployed forces from a variety of medical, environmental, and battle-related hazards, including chemical and biological agents (CBA);

Task 2.2: Improved technology and methods for detection and tracking of exposures to these risks;

Task 2.3: Improved technology and methods for physical protection and decontamination, particularly of CBA; and

Task 2.4: Improved medical protection, health consequences management and treatment, and medical record keeping.

I was approached by the NRC as an "expert" to write one of the six commissioned papers for Task 2.1. The word "expert" was placed in quotation marks because of the implication of narrowness discussed above. In the research work done in our laboratory on toxicological interactions of chemical mixtures, it is interdisciplinary team work in its broadest sense. As discussed later, this team is presently collaborating with petroleum-chemical engineers who have the vision of using a recently advanced computer-modeling technique, structure-oriented lumping (SOL), in biomedical research. From that perspective, I would have much preferred that the NRC approached me as a scientist with a vision, not an expert. If possible, I would like to strive for being the "wise old man" who can see the mosaic. It is with this perspective that I embarked upon the writing of this paper.

TOXICOLOGICAL INTERACTIONS AT LOW DOSES

What is a "toxicological interaction"? and what is a "low dose"? These two terms must be defined and clarified at the outset. The many definitions of toxicological interaction tend to cause confusion. For this paper, we will stick to a simple definition and an updated one. The simple definition of toxicological interaction is "any toxicological consequence deviating from additivity." The updated definition, which incorporates current thinking about multiple stressors into an earlier version (Lindenschmidt and Witschi 1990; Yang 1997), is: "Toxicological interaction is the combination of two or more chemicals, biological agents or disease vectors, physical agents, or stressful environmental conditions that results in a qualitatively or quantitatively altered biological response relative to that predicted from the action of a single chemical, agent, or stressor. The interaction of the chemicals, biological, physical agents, or stressful conditions might be simultaneous or sequential and the biological response might be increased or decreased."

Until very recently, "low dose" in toxicology has been an abstract entity. It usually implies anything from no observable effects to sublethal effects. In September 1998, a U.S. General Accounting Office (GAO) report to the Congress on *Chemical Weapons. DOD Does Not Have a Strategy to Address Low-Level Exposures* summarized the variety of definitions of low-level exposure provided by DOD officials (GAO 1998). Among these definitions is a quantitative one—$0.2\ LD_{50}$. Although one might argue that the toxicological manifestation of $0.2\ LD_{50}$ might range from no effects to frank toxicological effects depending on the steepness of the dose-response curve, it is indeed the first quantitative expression of low dose that I have ever seen. Because this paper is to provide insight into health risks and a preventive research strategy for future deployed U.S. forces from toxicological interactions among potentially harmful agents, low dose is defined here as $0.2\ LD_{50}$ or lower for any given chemical, drug, biological or physical agent. It should be noted that $0.2\ LD_{50}$ might occur from a near zero dose to very high doses or concentrations, such as moles per unit weight or volume, depending on the toxicity of the chemical.

How common are toxicological interactions?

Toxicological interactions, be they at high or low doses, are more prevalent than is realized. It is more of a problem of our ignorance and lack of attention to this area rather than the lack of existence of such interactions.

In a recent publication, Lazarou et al. (1998) estimated that there were over 2.2 million cases of serious adverse drug reactions (ADRs) in hospital patients in 1994 in the United States, and among these cases 106,000 were fatal. During their hospital stay, the patients in the survey statistics were given an average of eight drugs. Compared with other statistics of causes of death, these investigators indicated that ADRs became the fourth to sixth leading cause of death for that year in the United States.

The Lazarou et al. (1998) study is particularly significant to our task here in the following ways:

1. Although Lazarou et al. (1998) attributed ADRs as the cause of these deaths, and not specifically toxicological interactions, the fact that multiple drugs were given rendered toxicological interactions to be most likely the cause. This suggestion is strengthened by the fact that drug-to-drug interactions are so common that a separate volume of the Physicians Desk Reference is dedicated to drug interactions (PDR 1996). Further, in the relatively limited chemical world of central nervous system (CNS) depressant drugs, more than 200 ADRs were documented to have occurred as a result of the administration of two or more of these drugs more than 20 years ago (Zbinden 1976).

2. So many ADR deaths occurred that ADRs were ranked as the fourth to sixth leading cause of death in the United States. In addition, over 2 million cases of sublethal ADRs were identified in that year's hospital patient population. A logical question to follow is how many other cases of ADRs might have gone undetected, perhaps due to misdiagnosis, as the intrinsic problems of the patients?

3. These patients were in the hospitals where such things as the environmental conditions, nutrition, and medical care are presumably optimal. Therefore, multiple environmental and occupational stressors such as what deployed forces might face were not there. What would be the consequences if these hospital patients were also exposed to stressful environmental conditions?

4. These people are sick and weak and their homeostasis is dysfunctional at best. Therefore, they are a sensitive population to these ADRs.

5. Drugs, for therapeutic purposes, were not likely to be given at 0.2 LD_{50} levels. Most likely they were given at lower dosage levels. Thus, this indicates human lethality and other sublethal ADRs at very low-level exposures of multiple drugs.

For very low exposures resulting from environmental contamination, most practicing toxicologists would probably consider that toxicological interactions are unlikely. This is due to the common belief that these concentrations, usually at parts per billion (ppb) levels, are far below the saturation levels for most biological processes, particularly for the detoxifying enzyme systems. Are these common beliefs true? To answer this question, Yang (1994) went through some calculations for 1 ppb chloroform in drinking water due to the chlorination disinfection process. Yang indicated that this level of chloroform means there are still more than 5 quadrillion molecules in 1 liter of water. Using a series of illustrations and arguments, Yang concluded that (1) even at 1-ppb level, there are a huge number of molecules in our body; (2) these molecules are not present alone in the sense of chemical species, they are present along with other xenobiotics; (3) there is a very narrow range (probably less than 3 orders of magnitude) between "no effects" and "effects" in the various toxicity studies; (4) toxicological interactions seems possible, at least theoretically, at low-exposure concentrations; however, the sensitivity of detection might pose a problem. Yang's contention was, in part, supported by some experimental findings, particularly the clear dose-related in vivo cytogenetic toxicity in rats treated with an ultra low concentration (ppb levels) of a pesticide-fertilizer mixture (Kligerman et al. 1993), and marked carcinogenic activities in a mixture of very low doses (1/50 of TD_{50}) of 40 known carcinogens (Takayama et al. 1989).

Considering carcinogenicity as an endpoint in toxicological interactions, a number of studies were published in the literature on multiple chemical exposures. In one series of studies (Elashoff et al. 1987; Fears et al. 1988, 1989), binary mixtures of 12 known or suspected carcinogens were evaluated for tumorigenicity. These investigators observed synergism, antagonism, and lack of interactions. In a review by Arcos et al. (1988) on binary-combination effects of carcinogens, a total of 976 interactions involving almost 200 carcinogens in 10 chemical classes were uncovered. The predominant target organ was the skin, accounting for nearly 50% of all synergistic combinations. Similarly, Rao et al.

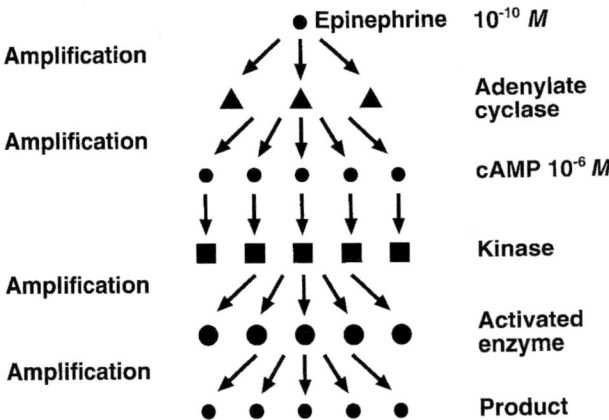

FIGURE 1 An example of cellular transduction and amplification. A single molecule of epinephrine resulted in the synthesis of thousands of cAMP molecules, which, through biological amplification, eventually raised the blood glucose level markedly. (Redrawn from Lodish et al. 1995.)

(1989) examined the literature on 600 tumor promoters or co-carcinogens and found 1,250 interactions involving chemicals from 21 classes.

If toxicological interactions are more prevalent than thought, why are there studies (Feron et al. 1995; Jonker et al. 1996; Cassee et al. 1998; Safe 1998) that support an additivity or less-than-additivity concept at the low-dose region? The answer to this question might be given from a number of different angles. First, some of these low-dose studies, including a number of papers from our laboratory (Pott et al. 1998; 1999; Benjamin et al. 1999; Dean et al. 1999), demonstrated antagonistic interactions, which are one form of toxicological interactions. Second, many of these studies that suggest that at low doses additivity or less than additivity prevails are based on acute or short-term toxic endpoints (Feron et al. 1995; Jonker et al. 1996). Third, because the real concern for environmental contamination is low-dose, long-term effects, acute and short-term toxicity studies cannot and should not be used to extrapolate to hazard identification for chronic toxicities. Finally, if environmental pollutants are active in any process that involves cascading amplification, such as hormonal effects or carcinogenic processes, they might cause toxicological interactions even at very low concentrations. For example, the concentration of epinephrine needed in the blood to stimulate glycogenolysis and release glucose from the liver and muscles can be as low as 10^{-10} M, a stimulus that generates a concentration of more than 10^{-6} M cAMP in the cell. Because three more catalytic steps precede the release of glucose, another 10^4 amplification can occur (Figure 1), so that blood glucose levels ultimately increase by as much as 50% (Lodish et al. 1995). If certain environmental pollutants can interfere with this process at the epinephrine level or similar processes with cascading and amplification effects, it is conceivable that disproportional toxicological interactions might happen.

Chemical-to-Chemical Interactions

In talking about chemical-to-chemical interactions, we are not specifically considering two or more chemicals reacting with one another to create one or more new chemicals before entering the body. Although this might be a case, we are referring to two or more chemicals causing toxicological consequences within the body deviating from additivity. The discussion in the last section indicates examples of toxicological interactions that may be classified as chemical-to-chemical interactions. Because this paper is not meant to be an exhaustive review of all known examples, more examples can be found in Goldstein et al. 1990; Calabrese 1991a,b; Pollak 1993; EHP 1994; FCT 1996; and Yang 1994, 1997. The additional examples given below are specifically centered around toxicological interactions following low-level exposures.

In the 1980s, the National Toxicology Program (NTP) initiated a large number of studies on the possible toxicological interactions on a number of target organs and systems by low-level exposures (ppm or ppb) to a 25-chemical mixture of groundwater contaminants from hazardous-waste sites, a pesticide-fertilizer mixture, or a herbicide-fertilizer mixture imitating groundwater contaminants in agricultural regions in California and Iowa. In one study, Germolec et al. (1989) reported that suppression of bone marrow stem-cell proliferation, as expressed by the number of colonies formed by the granulocyte-macrophage progenitor cells, as well as suppression of antigen-induced antibody-forming cells (sheep red blood cells) was observed in $B6C3F_1$ mice following 14-day and 90-day exposures to a drinking water cocktail of 25 groundwater contaminants. In another study, Kligerman et al. (1993) observed in vivo cytogenetic changes (increased sister-chromatid exchange) in Fischer 344 rats and $B6C3F_1$ mice following subchronic exposure to the California pesticide-fertilizer mixture. In this latter study, the six pesticides were at ppb levels, although ammonium nitrate, the only fertilizer given, was at ppm levels. In these studies, no systematic single chemical or submixture studies were conducted because of the complexity involved and limited resources. However, based on the experience and knowledge of the investigators, toxicological effects were deemed unlikely to happen with single-chemical exposure at the dose level tested.

It is interesting to draw parallels between the above two studies and certain findings in humans. For instance, studies conducted in Russia on children with compromised immune and endocrine systems living in different air-polluted, oil-waste regions revealed a dose-response effect of the anthropogenic pollution on T-suppressors as well as stimulation of immunoglobulin synthesis and reduction of phagocytic activity of the neutrophils (Etkina and Etkina 1995). In Greece, agricultural workers exposed to pesticides showed substantial clastogenic effects (chromosomal aberrations) in their lymphocytes without indication of increases in their basal frequency of sister chromatid exchange. Further, it was observed that individuals working exclusively in confined spaces, such as inside the greenhouse, showed higher chromosomal aberration levels than those working in open fields. No significant difference was found between smokers and nonsmokers (Kourakis et al. 1996).

Chemical-to-Physical Agent Interactions

Two examples are given below for chemical-to-physical agent interactions. In three NTP studies on the possible toxicological interactions between a 25-chemical mixture of groundwater contaminants and whole-body irradiation on hematopoiesis (Hong et al. 1991; 1992; 1993), exposure of the chemical mixture to $B6C3F_1$ mice enhanced the reduced bone marrow stem-cell proliferation resulting from radiation injury following repeated whole-body irradiation at 200 rads. Even 10 weeks after the cessation of chemical-mixture exposure, when all hematological parameters were normal, a residual effect of the chemical mixture might still be demonstrated as lower bone marrow stem-cell counts following irradiation (Hong et al., 1991). Another example of a chemical-to-physical agent interaction involved pesticides and ultraviolet (UV) light. It is commonly known that UV light will degrade hazardous chemicals such as pesticides. However, a study by McCabe and Nowak (1986) demonstrated that some pesticides act synergistically when combined with UV light.

Chemical-to-Biological Agent Interactions

In the broadest sense, chemical-to-biological interactions include pharmacodynamics of any toxicants because a chemical causes toxicity by interacting with a biological entity, be it an enzyme, nucleic acid, or a protein receptor. Thus, receptor-mediated toxicity such as TCDD-Ah receptor interactions, as well as multistage carcinogenesis from environmental chemicals, should be considered as part of chemical-to-biological interactions. However, for assessing risks to deployed forces, the concern is about the probability of chemical in conjunction with biological agents such as vaccines or disease vectors causing synergistic adverse health consequences. Examples given below are from some of the more recent publications, and they illustrate cases of chemical-to-biological agent interaction in the body leading to changes in pharmacokinetics and pharmacodynamics. Even though these examples mainly involve interactions between trace elements or heavy metals and bacterial or viral agents, a logical question to ask is how prevalent are these interactions among other chemicals and biological agents? These examples certainly suggest the likelihood of chemical-to-biological agent interactions leading to serious toxicities in humans.

Trace elements and heavy metals like copper, zinc, iron, and selenium have a significant influence on the function of the immune system. Srinivas et al. (1988) studied plasma levels of trace elements in 53 patients with acute bacterial and viral infections. They found that plasma concentrations of selenium, iron, and zinc were decreased in patients with bacterial infections (septicaemia, pneumonia, erysipelas, and meningitis). Patients with viral infections showed similar shifts of the trace elements but the changes were not as pronounced. In a series of studies from Sweden, Llback et al. (1992, 1993, 1994a,b, 1995) and Glynn et al. (1998) reported that:

1. An invading microorganism can increase the intestinal absorption and concomitantly alter the distribution of 109 Cd in Balb/c mice during viral infection (Coxsackie virus B3 [CB3]). Similar studies demonstrated the alteration of distribution of 63 Ni and 14C-cholesterol in CB3 infected mice.

2. Cadmium exposure for 10 weeks in female Balb/c mice with myocarditis (induced by CB3) resulted in a decreased maturation and mobilization of T and B lymphocytes, but increased humoral immune host responses.

3. A 10-week low-dose (0.002 M) administration of NiCl might contribute to the progression of target organ pathology in infection-induced diseases of an autoimmune or inflammatory character, such as diabetes and myocarditis.

4. The magnitude of inflammatory lesions in the hearts of CB3 infected mice can be affected by the potentially toxic heavy metals—cadmium, nickel, and methyl mercury. The infection is associated with a changed distribution, such as a cadmium accumulation in the spleen and kidneys. New target organs for nickel during the infection were the heart, pancreas, and lungs, in which the inflammatory lesions were present. The increased uptake was correlated with the disturbed function of the immune cells and an increased inflammatory reaction. Nickel and methyl mercury appeared to have a direct effect on immune cells that resulted in changed natural killer-cell activity and decreased mobilization of macrophages, and CD4+ and CD8+ cells into the inflammatory lesions.

Two other studies provide a glimpse of the diversified and intriguing domain of chemical-to-biological agent interactions. Novick et al. (1997) reported that free ionic zinc (Zn^{2+}) in saliva shortens duration and severity of common cold symptoms. They proposed that Zn^{2+} forms a complex with proteins of critical nerve endings and interrupts nerve impulses. Further, they suggested that Zn^{2+} binds with surface proteins of human rhinovirus (HRV) and blocks docking of HRV on intercellular adhesion molecule-1 on somatic cells, thereby interrupting HRV infection. In the world of plants, chemical-to-biological interactions might also be present. Ghoshroy et al. (1998) showed that exposure of tobacco plants to nontoxic concentrations of cadmium completely blocked viral disease caused by turnip vein-clearing virus. Cadmium-mediated viral protection was due to inhibition of the spread of the virus from the inoculated into uninoculated leaves.

On a much broader level involving ecological parameters, the study by Porter et al. (1984) summarized later, serves as an example of chemical-to-biological interaction.

Known Versus Unknown Interactions

The preceding sections have provided many examples of toxicological interactions; they also gave a glimpse of the known toxicological interactions at low doses. However, from the perspective of deployed forces, the possible toxicological interactions unknown to us are surprising and frightening. The examples of toxicological interactions given below, which were not known until the publications appeared several years after the PGW, serve as an illustration.

Two reports from Duke University on the synergistic neurotoxical effects in hens of pyridostigmine bromide (PB), *N,N*-diethyl-*m*-toluamide (DEET), and permethrin or chlorpyrifos in combination (Abou-Donia et al. 1996a,b) had provided some insights to the possible mechanistic basis for the neurotoxic symptoms observed in the veterans afflicted with Gulf War Syndrome. Of course, hens were used in these studies because they are a good animal model for organophosphate-induced delayed neurotoxicity (OPIDN). PB (prophylactic antinerve gas agent), DEET (insect repellant), permethrin (pyrethroid insecticide), and chlorpyrifos (organophosphorus insecticide) were used by the allied forces in the Persian Gulf War. Although each of these chemicals individually caused little or no toxicity at the doses tested, synergistic neurotoxical interactions were observed when they were given together as binary or trinary mixtures. The synergistic neurotoxical interactions were seen with multiple endpoints, including clinical signs, locomotor dysfunction, histopathological changes, plasma butyrylcholinesterase, brain acetylcholinesterase, and neurotoxicity-target esterase, body-weight changes, survival time, and mortality.

Another surprise involved pyridostigmine and the blood-brain barrier. To many scientists, pyridostigmine was generally considered to be safe and not likely to be involved in the neurotoxical aspects of Gulf War Syndrome because of the common belief that pyridostigmine does not penetrate through the blood-brain barrier. However, in 1996, Friedman et al. in Israel reported that, after mice were subjected to stress (forced swim), the blood-brain barrier literally opened up to pyridostigmine such that the value for a defined effect in 50% of exposed animals (ED_{50}) in vivo for brain acetylcholinesterase (AChE) lowered to 1% of that under nonstressed conditions. This finding was further backed up by increased brain levels of *c-fos* oncogene (which might be involved in the induction of AChE transcription) and AChE mRNAs in the stressed and pyridostigmine-treated mice. The results from the above study suggest that peripherally acting drugs such as pyridostigmine administered under stress might reach the brain with an amplification of their action by more than 100-fold and produce serious neurological damage (Friedman et al. 1996; Jamal 1998).

Such heretofore unknown toxicological interactions should raise the consciousness of the scientific community in at least two ways:

1. The findings provided a basis for hypothesizing about what might have happened to the Gulf War veterans with long-term neurotoxical consequences. As Friedman et al. (1996) suggested, the transcriptional responses (i.e., mRNA increases for *c-fos* and AChE) they observed in mice under stress plus pyridostigmine-treatment predict the induction of secondary and tertiary processes that, in turn, might have a number of neurotoxicological consequences. Specifically, Friedman et al. (1996) raised the

possibility that the observed pyridostigmine-induced enhancement of the capacity to produce AChE reflects a potential selective feedback mechanism that would diminish cholinergic overactivation.

2. Clinicians and scientists who hold the view that "what we don't know doesn't exist" should be humbled. Indeed, our knowledge in this area is at an embryonic stage.

A third interesting surprise involves the potentiation of PB toxicity in mice by, among others, caffeine. Chaney et al. (1997) reported that male ICR mice received ip injections of either a selected adrenergic drug or caffeine (5 mg/kg), followed 15 minutes later by an intraperitoneal (ip) injection of PB at 1, 2, or 3 mg/kg. Using isobolographic analyses, Chaney et al. (1997) concluded that synergism was demonstrated between PB and several commonly used classes of adrenergic agents and caffeine.

In line with the above discussion, it is also interesting to note the following reports:

1. Hanin (1996) summarized the work on stress and a leaky blood-brain barrier (BBB) and reported that "Acute immobilization stress in rats, cold or isolation exposure in mice and exposure of rats to conditions of acute as well as chronic summer heat, all resulted in increased penetration of the BBB by drugs, neurotransmitters and viruses that are normally excluded"

2. Hubert and Lison (1995) investigated potential muscular damage produced by short-term PB treatment in resting and exercising rats. They showed that, following physical exercise, PB significantly exacerbated the biochemical changes (increased creatine phosphokinase and urinary creatine excretion rate) reflecting a loss of integrity in skeletal muscles.

3. Casale et al. (1993) examined the potential of four carbamate and four organophosphate anti-cholinesterase (anti-ChE) insecticides to inhibit interleukin 2 (IL-2)-dependent proliferation of mouse T cells. Carbaryl and dichlorvos are the most potent agents and the mechanistic basis might be the inhibition of serine hydrolase-dependent immune functions including IL-2 signaling. Casale et al. (1993) proposed that these anti-ChE insecticides may be important immune dysregulators.

4. Rook and Zumla (1997) suggested the symptoms of Gulf War Syndrome might be compatible with the interaction between multiple Thorium (Th) 2-inducing vaccinations and stressful circumstances. They indicated that the mood changes and depression that commonly accompany Gulf War Syndrome can be accounted for by Th 2-mediated disorders.

5. Ben-Nathan et al. (1991) reported that the neurovirulent, noninvasive Sindbis virus strain (SVN), when injected intracerebrally into the mouse's brain, causes acute encephalitis and death but is unable to pass the blood-brain barrier to invade the brain when injected intraperitoneally. However, when mice were subjected to cold or isolation stress, the blood-brain barrier opened up to the SVN, leading to encephalitis and death.

Mechanistic Considerations

When dealing with toxicological interactions of chemical mixtures, as is the case with single chemicals, mechanistic information is critical, particularly in the development of predictive tools. A summary of mechanistic information is presented in a schematic form (Figure 2) taken from a number of studies related to the possible explanations of neurotoxicities in the PGW veterans (Abou-Donia et al. 1996a,b; Friedman et al. 1996; Haley and Kurt 1997; Jamal 1998).

The top half of the diagram deals with pharmacokinetics and the bottom half depicts pharmacodynamics, what happens inside of the blood-brain barrier. From the top left to right, Figure 2 illustrates three possible exposures and the related pharmacokinetic scenarios in those PGW veterans who might be both members of a sensitive population and who might have had higher levels of exposures to the

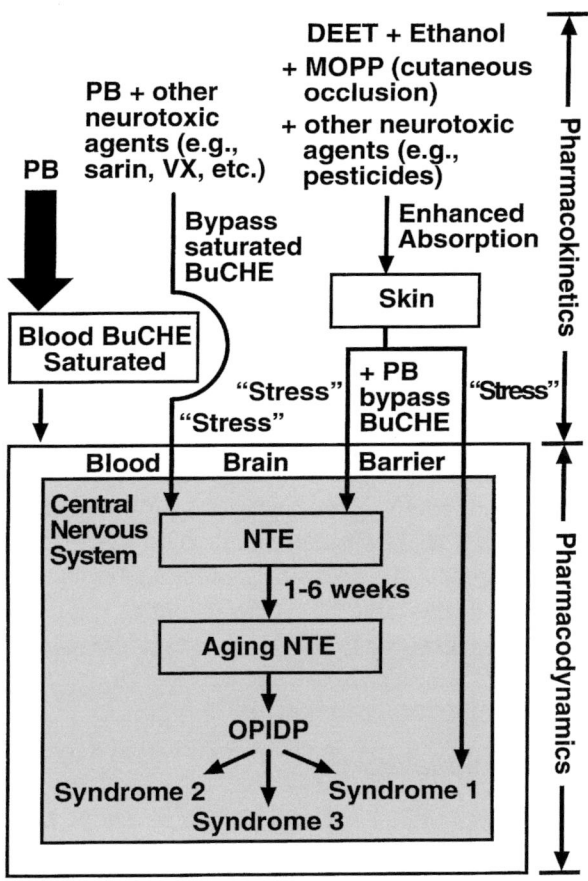

FIGURE 2 A schematic of proposed mechanisms responsible for the neurotoxicities observed in PGW veterans. The synthesis of this schematic was based on mechanistic information proposed in Abou-Donia et al. (1996a,b), Friedman et al. (1996), Haley and Kurt (1997), and Jamal (1998). BuChE = butyrylcholinesterase; DEET= N,N-diethyl-m-toluamide; MOPP = military operations protective posture; NTE = neuropathy target esterase; OPIDP = organophosphate-induced delayed polyneuropathy; PB = pyridostigmine bromide; VX = nerve gas.

chemicals and drugs implicated as the culprits. First, under normal circumstances, PB upon intake enters into the blood stream where butyrylcholinesterase (BuChE, also called pseudocholinesterase or plasma cholinesterase) binds with PB and renders it unavailable to other possible targets. Thus, BuChE is a body's natural protective mechanism. However, if this protective mechanism is overwhelmed (saturated) because there are also other neurotoxical agents such as sarin and VX in addition to PB then the possibility exists that some of these molecules might bypass BuChE's protective shield and enter the blood-brain barrier. In the third scenario, soldiers had to wear gear called a military operations protective posture (MOPP), which is the equivalent of a "walking Turkish bath" in desert weather conditions. Because the soldier perspires profusely, the MOPP becomes a most efficient occlusion for the body surface. Under such a condition, DEET, ethanol, and other neurotoxic agents such as pesticides might penetrate the skin at much higher rates than normal. Again, if there are PB molecules already bound to BuChE, these other neurotoxical agents might enter the blood-brain barrier without much resistance. Because of stress factors such as not eating or sleeping well, bad food and weather, and fear of death (paralleling the study by Friedman et al. [1996]) the penetration of neurotoxical agents might be further enhanced as indicated in Figure 2. Once these neurotoxical agents are in the CNS, they (mainly organophosphates [OP] and related compounds) react with neuropathy target esterase (NTE, formerly known as neurotoxic esterase). The OP-NTE complex undergoes molecular rearrangement over a 1- to 6-week period to form a byproduct that is axonotoxic and might lead to organophosphate-induced delayed polyneuropathy (OPIDP). The spectrum of clinical effects in OPIDP ranges from permanent impairment involving distal, wasting peripheral neuropathy and spinal cord spasticity to vague cognitive and behavioral changes (Haley and Kurt 1997). Haley and Kurt categorized the clinical manifestations into three syndromes. Syndrome 1 is impaired cognition, a milder form of neurotoxicity that resembles the chronic effects of pesticide exposure and poisoning. Syndrome 2 is confusion-ataxia, the most disabling form of neurotoxicity in PGW veterans. This syndrome might be the result of toxicological interactions from sublethal exposures to chemical nerve agents in soldiers whose protective pool of BuChE was already diminished by preexposure to PB or pesticides. Syndrome 3 is arthro-myo-neuropathy, which might result from heavy percutaneous absorption of DEET in soldiers whose BuChE pool was already saturated by PB, allowing more of the absorbed DEET to diffuse into the CNS.

It is important to make one point clear here. Whether this summary of mechanistic basis for possible explanation of neurotoxicities in the Gulf War Syndrome is 100% in line with the latest advances in neurotoxicology is not the main issue. The significance is that a group of independent scientists came up with an explanation of the neurotoxicity observed in veterans with Gulf War Syndrome. From my perspective, such a schematic summary of disease processes based on mechanistic information might serve as a conceptual model for the development of an integrated physiologically based pharmacokinetic/pharmacodynamic (PBPK/PD) model, as discussed later. With verification using available quantitative data, this model might possess predictive capability for computer simulations of possible future, similar scenarios in deployed U.S. forces. Further, with potential additional information provided by cutting-edge researchers in neurotoxicology or from advances in future studies, the PBPK/PD model might be refined and improved.

Hormesis and Potentially Beneficial Interactions

Hormesis, defined by Stebbing (1982) as the stimulatory effects caused by low levels of toxic agents, was originally developed under different terminologies over a century ago. Its origin, scientific development, historical perspectives, and modern implications have been ably reviewed by a number of contemporary scientists such as Stebbing 1982; Calabrese 1997; Calabrese and Baldwin 1997a,b; Stebbing 1997; Appleby 1998; Bailer and Oris 1998; Gaylor 1998; Johnson and Bruunsgaard 1998; Morré 1998; Morse 1998; Sielken and Stevenson 1998; Teeguarden et al. 1998. Dr. Edward J. Calabrese and his colleagues at University of Massachusetts should be credited for the most recent resurgence of scientific interest in hormesis.

The research group headed by Dr. Calabrese searched various computer databases and came up with over 8,000 studies potentially relevant to hormesis. Following a set of criteria related to experimental design, the types of responses and the magnitude and statistical significance of such responses, and the capacity of data replication, Calabrese (1997) and Calabrese and Baldwin (1997a) reported that 500 studies have shown evidence of hormesis to some degree. These investigators summarized their findings as follows.

1. Low-dose stimulatory responses are not restricted to any particular taxonomic group but are observed broadly across the microbial, plant, and animal kingdoms.

2. The types of agents shown to cause hormesis consist of all chemical classes and different types of physical stressors, including various kinds of radiation.

3. Hormesis involves a wide range of biological effects, including growth, longevity, reproduction, disease incidence, and behavioral changes.

To provide an actual example of the hormesis concept, Calabrese (1997) used the differential effects of antibiotics as an illustration. Antibiotics are supposed to kill or prevent bacteria from reproducing.

However, low doses of streptomycin would actually enhance reproduction of certain harmful bacteria even though it kills these bacteria at high doses. In fact, a higher killing capacity of the microbe to the host can be induced by the administration of low doses of streptomycin. This latter scenario is certainly an example of chemical-to-biological interaction in a very negative sense to the host.

Because hormesis is a stimulatory effect at low doses of a toxic agent, it generally has the connotation of being "good." In parallel with the concept of essential metal elements for our growth and homeostasis, hormesis might thus be considered as a form of beneficial effect from otherwise toxic substances at higher doses. Therefore, hormesis is an important consideration here because it occurs at low to very low doses and because, assuming that hormesis might occur with multiple chemicals, including chemical mixtures with interactions, it might provide a basis for the argument that not all interactions are bad.

MULTIPLE STRESSORS AND SENSITIVE POPULATIONS

This section will cover the emerging subject of toxicological interactions (thus possible adverse health effects) that extend beyond chemical challenges to other forms of stress. The subject of sensitive populations as determined by genetic polymorphism will also be considered.

Multiple stressors: What are they? How much do we know? What is the biochemical basis of stress and response?

Any chemical, physical, or biological insult to the body is a form of stress and can together form multiple stressors. However, in the context of the Gulf War Syndrome, multiple stressors might also include environmental hardship (extreme heat, poor resting conditions, poor food or waste intake, heavy and nonbreathable equipment and clothing, insect or other pests), occupational hazard (dangerous tasks, injuries from work, exposure to fuels, burning oil field, possible nerve gases, radioactive residues), and psychological stress (the threat of death and injuries, fear of exposure to chemical and biological warfare agents, away from home, poor living conditions). Indeed, in their publication, Haley and Kurt (1997) listed 18 suspected wartime causes of illnesses in veterans of the Persian Gulf War. These are chemical warfare agents; environmental pesticides; pesticides in uniforms; pesticides in flea collars; DEET-containing insect repellents; pyridostigmine bromide; ciprofloxacin; chloroquine; multiple immunizations; smoke from oil well fires; fumes from jet fuel in the environment; fumes from burning jet fuel in tents; petroleum in drinking water; depleted uranium in munitions; chemical agent-resistant coating (CARC) paint on vehicles; combat stress; smoking; and alcohol or cocaine use. The reality is probably even more complex than that. Although some of these individual stressors might have been studied and reported in the literature, little or no information is available on the possible combined actions of multiple stressors.

Stress is defined as a state of disharmony, or threatened homeostasis (Chrousos and Gold 1992). If the homeostasis is disrupted due to physical or psychological stress, intricate neural and biochemical events in the brain and in the endocrine and immune systems act jointly to counter the effects of stress and to reestablish homeostasis (Ember 1998). If homeostasis is not reset, debilitating illness results. Biochemically and physiologically, our hypothalamus-pituitary-adrenal gland axis is mobilized under stress and the glucocorticoid hormone cortisol is secreted. The sympathetic nervous system also is activated to release the catecholamines, epinephrine and norepinephrine. Cortisol and the catecholamines are the principal stress hormones.

The process of the body adapting to regain homeostasis is called allostasis. In humans, high allostatic loads (too much stress hormones) can suppress the immune system, decrease bone mineral density, weaken muscles, promote atherosclerosis (leading to heart disease), hike insulin resistance (leading to diabetes), and accelerate memory loss. Low allostatic load (too little stress hormones) can result in elevated autoimmune and inflammatory responses. Some PGW veterans suffer symptoms consistent with either too much or too little stress hormones (Ember 1998).

Environmental Stressors From Different Regions of the World

The world has extremely diverse weather and geographical conditions, with a wide range of temperature, humidity, and barometric conditions. Associated with these wide range of variables are the different plant, animal, and microbial forms. Any of these almost infinite number of combinations can be an environmental stressor. Because U.S. forces might be deployed anywhere in the world in the future, the studies of some extreme examples of such weather and geographical variables will be wise. This point is taken into consideration later in the proposed preventive research strategy.

Anthropogenic Stressors During Wars

During the Persian Gulf War, oil wells were set on fire, which created pollution in disastrous proportion. The employment of nerve gas was also suspected. In other war scenarios in urban and rural areas, anthropogenic stressors might include setting fires to buildings and equipment, contaminating water and food sources, destroying roads and bridges, decaying human and farm and pet animal corpses, and purposefully destroying chemical plants, releasing highly toxic chemicals. All these could magnify the already existing long list of stressors to the deployed U.S. forces.

Synergistic Interaction Stressors and Chemical, Biological, and Physical Agents

One landmark study that serves as an illustration of synergistic interaction stressors is that of Porter et al. (1984). These investigators evaluated the combined effects of food, water, an immunosuppressant and plant growth regulator (chlorocholine chloride), a virus (Venezuelan equine encephalitis virus), and an environmental contaminant (PCB) on the growth and reproduction of laboratory mice and deer mice. Using a fractional factorial experimental design, they demonstrated interactive effects among the variables tested. For instance, malnourished mice were more sensitive to virus exposure and environmental pollutants. An important interaction was also observed between chlorocholine chloride and water availability. In standard toxicological testing with water ad libitum, chlorocholine chloride enhanced growth of the young. In water stress conditions (80% of normal unlimited consumption), chlorocholine chloride suppressed growth. Porter et al. (1984) concluded that "Interactions of certain 'harmless' chemicals at low levels may prove deleterious than higher doses of 'dangerous' toxicants acting alone."

Specifically regarding to Gulf War Syndrome, other than the proposed mechanisms for neurotoxicity discussed earlier, Rook and Zumla (1997) also postulated the possibility of changes with the clinical manifestation of depression and mood as interactive effects from exposure to multiple Th 2-inducing vaccinations under stressful circumstances.

Human Variability: Genetic Polymorphism and Sensitive Population

The major advances made in the past decades in the area of genetic polymorphism have been in human responses to drugs. One of the greatest causes of interindividual variation of the effects of drugs, and hence of different clinical implications, is genetic variability in drug metabolism (Meyer and Zanger

1997; West et al. 1997). In that sense, genetic polymorphisms are the results of mutations in the genes for the enzymes critical in drug metabolism; the drug-metabolizing enzyme might have an increased or decreased level or be totally absent. Relatively high frequencies of such variant alleles exist in the human population (Meyer and Zanger 1997); for instance, glucose-6-phosphate dehydrogenase (G6PD) deficiency, the most common inherited enzyme-related idiosyncrasy, affects an estimated 400 million people (Eichelbaum and Evert 1996). Another interesting yet alarming feature of genetic polymorphism is the magnitude of the differences. Just as blue and brown eyes can occur in siblings, the interindividual variabilities in drug metabolism might vary by as much as 10-fold to greater than 1000-fold differences (Inaba et al. 1995). Such high magnitudes, if translated by direct-proportionality into acute drug toxicities, would rival any known toxicological interactions.

Based on the fact that genetic polymorphisms have been shown for most drug-metabolizing enzymes (Meyer and Zanger 1997; West et al. 1997), it is conceivable that genetic polymorphism might exist in a wide variety of biological processes. Indeed, a number of reports implicated the association of genetic polymorphism to environmental toxicology and diseases, including cancers (Hirvonen 1995; Ikawa et al. 1995; Rannug et al. 1995; Raunio et al. 1995; Weber 1995; Bartsch and Hietanen 1996; Feigelson et al. 1996; McFadden 1996; Aposhian 1997; Hong and Yang 1997). In one paper, McFadden (1996) speculated on a possible association of several degenerative neurological and immunological diseases with impaired sulfation of phenolic xenobiotics. Rannug et al. (1995), on the other hand, indicated that although CYP2D6 phenotype and genotype have mainly been related to the incidence of lung cancer, the results from 13 different studies showed an absence of any significant correlation between these parameters. This demonstrates that although genetic polymorphism is an exciting area of research with a great deal of vibrant activities, it is probably still in its infancy.

One specific example of genetic polymorphism that has direct bearing here is a study conducted and reported jointly by scientists from Israel, Denmark, and the United States (Loewenstein-Lichtenstein et al. 1995). In this study, the researchers reported that an Israeli soldier, who suffered severe symptoms following pyridostigmine prophylaxis during the Persian Gulf War, was determined to be homozygous for atypical BuChE. Homozygous carriers of atypical BuChE (under 0.04% in Europe but up to 0.6% in certain subpopulations) are known to suffer postanaesthesia apnea and hypersensitivity to the anti-ChE insecticide parathion. This soldier's serum BuChE and recombinant atypical BuChE had far less binding affinity or sensitivity toward PB and other anti-ChEs. These authors concluded that genetic differences among BuChE variants might explain at least partially some of the long-term adverse consequences associated with the collection of symptoms of the Gulf War Syndrome.

Normal Physiology Versus Abnormal Physiology

The abnormal physiology relevant here is the higher permeability of the blood-brain barrier to PB and other neurotoxical agents when an animal is under stress (Friedman et al. 1996; Hanin 1996); muscular damage produced by short-term PB treatment in exercising rats (Hubert and Lison 1995); important immune dysregulation caused by carbamate and OP anti-ChE insecticides (Casale et al. 1993); and sensitivity of individuals who possess genetic polymorphism with respect to xenobiotic metabolism and pharmacokinetics as discussed earlier.

Chronic Pain and Fatigue Syndromes

Chronic pain or fatigue, as clinical features of an amorphous illness, have been described for centuries in the medical literature. Although a variety of terms have been used to describe these symptoms, the currently preferred terms are Chronic Fatigue Syndrome and fibromyalgia (Clauw and Chrousos 1997). Systemic conditions characterized by chronic pain and fatigue include Chronic Fatigue Syndrome, fibromyalgia, somatoform disorders, and multiple chemical sensitivity (Clauw and Chrousos 1997). Gulf War Syndrome and Sick Building Syndrome share considerable homology with these illnesses.

In a comprehensive review, Clauw and Chrousos (1997) proposed an integrated model for potential pathogenic mechanisms for the symptoms in chronic pain and fatigue syndromes. The salient points are:

"there is a group of individuals who are genetically predisposed to develop the entire spectrum of illness. Susceptible individuals commonly experience a number of organ-specific illnesses before finally progressing to develop the more debilitating systemic conditions later in life. These illnesses may develop indolently or abruptly, and in the latter instances typically follow exposure to a stressor or series of stressors. Once an individual develops this illness, there is evidence of blunting of the human stress response, which may be manifest as: blunting of one or more hypothalamic-pituitary axes, globally increased peripheral and/or visceral nociception, or instability of the autonomic nervous system. These different axes of the stress response can either independently or concurrently function aberrantly, which may in part be responsible for the tremendous heterogeneity of symptoms. In this model, psychiatric illnesses can occur concurrently and significantly modulate disease activity and symptom expression, and vice versa. Finally, in this paradigm, changes in the immune system and in the peripheral tissues are de-emphasized because there are data suggesting that these anomalies occur because of these central alterations in the stress system."

It should be noted that the symptoms of Chronic Fatigue Syndrome have been described very frequently in patients with Chronic Neuropsychiatric Syndrome of OP compounds (see Jamal 1997).

Gulf War Illnesses: Are Gulf War illnesses real? Can they happen again? What can be done?

In answering the first question, one must try to put all the available pieces of the puzzle together to see what the mosaic tells us. The pieces of the puzzle available to us, in a broad and general sense, are: (1) the potential exists for synergistic toxicological interactions among PB, DEET, permethrin, and chlorpyrifos plus drugs and biologics; (2) under stress, our body might be more susceptible to other insults from chemical, physical, and biological agents; and (3) genetic polymorphism is prevalent in humans, and the magnitude of such manifestations might be very large in extremely sensitive populations. More specific pieces of the puzzle are presented earlier in the sections on Known versus Unknown Interactions and Mechanistic Considerations. My interpretation of the mosaic is that the Gulf War Syndrome is scientifically and biologically plausible. Therefore, I believe that it is real. As to the second question, given the potentially unlimited combinations among environmental and occupational conditions, prophylactic use of drugs, chemicals, and biologics, and the anthropogenic factors for future deployment of U.S. forces, problems similar to the Gulf War Syndrome can happen again.

What can we do about it? First, we must keep an open mind. Aldous Huxley stated, " Facts do not cease to exist because they are ignored." This paper has reviewed one surprise after another with respect to toxicological interactions from multiple stressors. A good scientist or clinician should never have the attitude that "what I don't know doesn't exist." Second, with the situation DOD is now in, a short-term, stop-gap preventive strategy must be in place to uncover the potential dangers, such that they can be dealt with before our soldiers must face them. Third, a long-term strategy in investing in basic research specifically toward multiple stressor interactions must be implemented. The details are given in the following section.

PREVENTIVE RESEARCH STRATEGY

Why preventive measures? The short answer is that we want to avoid any future Gulf War Illnesses in deployed forces. The importance, significance, and how-to's are given in the following sections.

DOD has been criticized for not having a strategy to address low-level exposures (GAO 1998). The very fact that DOD has commissioned NRC with the four tasks mentioned at the beginning is an indication of DOD's desire to map out an overall strategy for future deployed forces that goes beyond just low-level exposures. If the recent directive on *Deployment Health Surveillance and Readiness* (JCS 1998) from the Office of the Chairman, The Joint Chiefs of Staff, is any indication, DOD has only pushed forward in epidemiology study-related areas. Although epidemiological studies from past experiences provide useful information, they are generally after the fact, and they suffer from lack of sensitivity and the confounding problems of dealing with chemical mixtures or multiple stressors.

The potential target areas for the U.S. military forces to be deployed are throughout the world; thus, they cover many different geographical regions and their respective weather and environmental conditions. Adding to these conditions is the potential large number of exposure scenarios combining prophylactic drugs, biologics, chemicals, and anthropogenic factors. To avoid or minimize possible future serious health hazards to U.S. military personnel as a result of these combination exposures, preventive measures are critically needed. Because we cannot conduct toxicological experiments on humans, animal and cell-culture models are probably the next best available approach for preventive research.

In formulating plans for carrying out preventive research, it is important to utilize the recent advances in experimental biology and toxicology to assess the health effects of U.S. troops in potential scenarios of multiple exposures of drugs, biologics, and chemicals, as well as possible environmental stresses in different regions of the world. Because of the complexity of the multiple agents and factors involved, the resource-intensive nature of present-day experimental toxicology might only be a short-term solution in terms of preventive research. The long-term strategy should involve the development of predictive capability. In this regard, the integration of more innovative, efficient toxicological methodologies with computer modeling might be the only realistic way to deal with this dilemma, as discussed later.

An Integrated Experimental Toxicology Program
Assessing Multiple Stressors

The program suggested below covers both the short-term (from the present to about 5 years) and the long-term (5 years and beyond) objectives. As DOD does not seem to have a strategy for preventive research on potential health effects in future deployed forces, the short-term program should be implemented as soon as possible. The long-term program will take time because it has to mature in parallel to the advances in biomedical research in general. Thus, a relatively small but persistent support might be prudent for the long-term investment.

The short-term program is largely described in a report by the Committee to Study the Interactions of Drugs, Biologics, and Chemicals in U.S. Military Forces, of the Institute of Medicine (IOM 1996). In that report, the following recommendation was made:

"Ideally, for the most complete assessment of the potential interactions of drugs, biologics, and chemicals in the U.S. military forces, a process such as the following should be adopted. Different regions of the world should be characterized according to weather and geographical conditions; ecosystems; abundance of plant, animal, and microbial species; prevalence of diseases; possible anthropogenic pollutants;

and other environmental conditions. Within each region, a list of the potential dangers military personnel might face regarding possible exposures to warfare agents, chemicals, environmental and physical stresses, diseases, pests, prophylactic drugs and biologics, and so on should be compiled and analyzed. Then, under the climatic conditions of each of these regions, animal studies should be carried out to detect at least the four major toxicity categories (i.e., immunotoxicity, developmental and reproductive toxicity, neurotoxicity, and carcinogenicity).

However, to conserve resources and as a starting point, the committee suggests the following prototype experiments with the understanding that more specific scenarios may be incorporated into the experimental design of subsequent studies as needed. At the minimum, the following combination exposure scenarios should be studied for each of the toxicities mentioned above:

1. the complete combination: drugs, biologics, chemicals whose use is anticipated;
2. drugs whose use is anticipated;
3. biologics whose use is anticipated;
4. chemicals to which exposure is anticipated; and
5. controls

The doses of each entity to be used in the animal studies should be the anticipated level of exposure to the soldiers (on a milligram-per-kilogram, millimole-per-kilogram, or units-per-kilogram basis), which would be the baseline study dose, plus two other dose levels (10 times and 100 times this baseline dose). This recommendation may be considered as a first tier screening for possible adverse health hazards. Any toxicological interaction detected within any of the groups should be a warning flag to DOD, and a decision must be made with respect to the risks and benefits involved in using the agents. Beyond this first tier, any additional studies should be on a case-by-case basis guided by the recommendations of an expert panel of investigators.

Some of the conventional toxicity testing protocols may not be applicable in these studies because they are either too expensive and resource-intensive or not sensitive enough with respect to toxic responses, or both. Therefore, there is a need for continuing refinement and improvement of experimental toxicology methodologies by using the latest advances in molecular biology and genetics and in computer sciences. For example, to deal more effectively with interactions, investigators can use and integrate state-of-the-art advances in (1) computational technology; (2) physiologically based pharmacokinetic and pharmacodynamic modeling; (3) model-directed, unconventional, focused, mechanistically based, short-term toxicology studies; and (4) other mathematical and statistical modeling tools."

To consider further the above approach suggested by the IOM (1996), a number of refinements and modifications may be added:

1. The different regions of the world need not be so many as to add undue burden to the budget of the preventive research program. Depending on the most likely areas U.S. Forces might be deployed, one might simply have extremely hot or extremely cold regions. Within the former, one might consider combining extreme heat with extreme humidity or extreme dryness. These might easily be simulated in laboratory conditions. If elevation might present a potential factor, hyper- or hypobaric conditions can be reproduced in the laboratory as well. In this way, dealing with a large number of environmental factors can be avoided.

2. Even within the first tier there could be priority setting if research funding limitation becomes an issue. For instance, DOD might decide that, as a starter, only one complete set of experiments will be done under the weather conditions of Desert Storm and Desert Shield (for a region in the world where extreme heat, dry, and desert conditions prevail). Of course, in this case, a complete set of experiments should also be conducted under normal laboratory conditions as controls; these control data might be shared with other sets of future experiments in which other regions of the world would be considered.

3. In the IOM (1996) report, a minimum of five exposure scenarios, the complete combination, drugs, biologics, chemicals, and controls (one control group assuming a common vehicle for the groups) was proposed for toxicological interaction studies. However, additional exposure scenarios such as physical agents, disease vectors (as opposed to biologics, which could include only the vaccines applied to the soldiers), or stress factors such as those described by Friedman et al. (1996) might be added to the design as needed.

4. As our cell and molecular biology methodologies advance further, it is conceivable that cell culture systems might be used in the first tier and save the more resource-demanding animal experimentations for confirmatory studies.

5. Psychological stress was considered to be an important factor in the development of Gulf War Syndrome. Therefore, in neurotoxicity studies, a subset of experiments should be designed by neurobehavioral experimental toxicologists in conjunction with psychologists to assess psychological stress as a factor in the toxicological interactions among multiple stressors.

As part of the short-term program, research efforts to learn maximally from the Persian Gulf War should also be encouraged. For instance, Jamal (1998), in his review article on the potential causes and mechanisms of the Gulf War Syndrome, recommended that more multinational studies be done because such an approach could identify various subgroups with different exposure patterns to various risk factors. In particular, Jamal (1998) indicated that the absence of the Gulf War Syndrome in the French troops, who were not exposed to as many of the risk factors that the American and British soldiers experienced, remains crucial to the understanding of the Gulf War Syndrome.

The long-term program should be aimed at the development of predictive capability. The reason is quite obvious. With so many biologics, chemicals, drugs, physical and biological agents, and environmental and anthropogenic factors to consider, it is impossible to keep on doing experiments, particularly with the methods of present-day experimental toxicology. Because toxicology is really the integration of pharmacokinetics (the fate of chemicals or other agents in the body) and pharmacodynamics (the mechanistic interactions of chemicals or other agents in the body), a systematic research effort to investigate pharmacokinetics and pharmacodynamics in representatives of different classes of biologics, chemicals, and drugs, singly and in combination, will provide the database for PBPK/PD modeling or biologically based dose-response (BBDR) modeling. These studies might be conducted in mammals such as the most commonly used laboratory rats and mice for the generation of a database for PBPK/PD modeling. They might also be conducted in cell cultures for the generation of a database for BBDR modeling. In both cases, the latest advances of molecular biology and genetics should be utilized as much as possible. Only through such integration of more innovative, efficient toxicological methodologies, with modern computational technology and the application of engineering concepts to biomedical research, would we have a chance to develop a predictive approach to deal with this extremely complex area.

Data Analyses, Interpretation, and Utility for DOD

For statistical analyses of the experimental outcome from the above-proposed research, the IOM (1996) report has a section that translates the normal statistical jargon into easy-to-understand English. The following passages provide the fundamentals for statistical analyses of toxicological interactions of multiple agents:

"In the simplest case of two agents, each of which produces a single response, one can plot in two dimensions the set of doses (x, y), where x is the dose of Agent 1 and y is the dose of Agent 2 that produces identical responses. The line connecting this set of doses is an isobole, and its graph is an isobologram (see Figure 1 in Machado and Robinson 1994). Thus, an isobologram is analogous to a topographic map, in which identical responses correspond to identical elevations. In the simple two-agent case, the two-dimensional plot of isobolograms permits a simple, quantitative interpretation: a straight line is indicative of an additive effect of the two agents, that is, no interaction. A convex isobologram is evidence that the response from the combination of the two agents is less than the sum of their responses, which is an antagonistic interaction. A concave isobologram is evidence that the response from the combination of the two agents is greater than the sum of their responses, which is a synergistic interaction.

Combination of more than two agents must be studied in higher-dimensional space, where lines become surfaces and straight lines become planar surfaces. In 1981, Berenbaum quantified and generalized the isobologram to higher dimensions and used it to detect and characterize interactions of a combination of drugs or chemicals, showing that the contours of the constant response of the dose-response surface are planar if the components of the combination have an effect that is additive. In direct analogy to the two-agent case, if the observed response to the combination is statistically greater than that predicted under additivity, it is concluded that a synergistic interaction has taken place. For increasing dose-response relationships, if the observed response to the combination is statistically less than that predicted under additivity, it is concluded that an antagonistic interaction has taken place. If there is no statistical difference between the response predicted under additivity and the response observed upon exposure to the combination, it can be concluded that the components of the combination do not interact. The logic of the approach outlined above was used by Finney (1964), Berenbaum (1985), and Kelly and Rice (1990), among others, to detect and characterize interactions involving combinations of agents.

The real strength of this approach is that relatively few data are required to implement it. Under the assumption of additivity, in particular, the estimated dose-response surface can be calculated from the dose-response curves for the single agents; such data are likely to be available as a result of earlier product development research. One then needs only to collect additional data on the results of exposure to the combination of interest at the specified doses of the constituents.

The required single-agent dose-response data are likely to include multiple control groups, one for each agent under study, especially if these data were collected from several studies. Ideally, such control data can be used to estimate the background rate of response, although an important consideration is their proper inclusion in the analyses. If all of the single-agent control data are collected simultaneously, there should not be any problem combining them. However, when single-agent data are found in the literature or are collected at points in time that are remote to the time of collection of the combination data, then the problem is similar to the historical control problem discussed by Prentice et al. (1992). In extending earlier approaches, Gennings and Carter (1996) used a single parameter for the background (control) rate and developed a methodology that can be used to detect and characterize interactions by incorporating this parameter into the additivity model three different ways: as a fixed-effects parameterization, as a random-effects approach following Prentice et al. (1992), and as an approach involving the use of estimating equations (Liang and Zeger 1986)."

The approach for detecting interactions outlined above is directly applicable to the study of a particular complex mixture of biologics, chemicals, and drugs, as advocated earlier. Let B represent a given combination of biologics, let C represent a given combination of chemicals, and let D represent a given combination of drugs. The complex mixture is represented by $B+C+D$. One set of experiments designed to provide data to be analyzed by the methodology described above determines responses to the following sets of exposures:

Control, $B+C+D$, 10 $(B+C+D)$, 100 $(B+C+D)$;
    Control, B, 10 B, 100 B;
    Control, C, 10 C, 100 C; and
    Control, D, 10 D, 100 D.

The first set of exposure yields the combination agent data, and the next three sets yield the single-agent data for *B*, *C*, and *D*, respectively."

As for the interpretation and utility of the results, for the purposes of DOD, the most critical ones would be synergistic toxicological interaction. From such findings, one must seriously consider that similar synergistic toxicological interaction might happen in humans. Accordingly, preventive measures, such as modifying the vaccination protocols to fewer numbers, refraining from using prophylactic agents for nonlife threatening problems, and designing better protective masks and suits to minimize environmental harshness and possible chemical and biological warfare agents might be planned in advance.

Independent Scientific Board of Counselors

The establishment of an Independent Scientific Board of Counselors, if done properly, will be essential to the success of DOD's strategy in protecting future deployed forces. This board will review and approve preventive research activities; it will review the results from such research and determine the subsequent course of action. The composition for this board should include, at a minimum, scientific expertise in the areas of neurotoxicology, immunotoxicology, reproductive and developmental toxicology, carcinogenesis, statistics, computer modeling, toxicological interactions, and multiple stressors. Other types of expertise could be added as such needs arise. The members on this board must have an appreciation of the complexity of the problems related to dealing with deployed forces; therefore, they must also have unusually open minds to accommodate risky research and unconventional thinking.

The single most important function for such a board is to deal with science; the science of today and tomorrow, not yesterday. Therefore, it is absolutely essential that the board members should be those who are engaging actively in related research work. The appointment of a board member should never be based solely on political reasons or prestige of position or institution.

Existing Approaches for Assessing and Predicting Toxicological Interactions

Prediction of health effects usually involves some type of mathematical modeling, which ranges from the classical compartmental pharmacokinetic modeling to the currently advanced PBPK/PD modeling and quantitative structure-activity relationship (QSAR) modeling. Some successes, including those from our laboratory, of prediction of pharmacokinetics, pharmacodynamics, and toxicity (including lethality) following exposure to simple chemical mixtures are already evident in the literature (Andersen and Clewell 1983; Purcell et al. 1990; Sato et al. 1990; Thakore et al. 1991; Tardif et al. 1993; 1995; Barton et al. 1995; El-Masri et al. 1996a,b,c; Pelekis and Krishnan 1997; Tardif et al. 1997; Feng et al. 1998; Yang et al. 1999). The toxicological endpoints of prediction, for instance, include an interaction threshold (El-Masri et al. 1996a,b) and acute lethality due to hepatic injuries (El-Masri et al. 1996c; Feng et al. 1998; Yang et al. 1999).

For more complex mixtures, the integration of PBPK/PD, QSAR modeling, and lumping analysis (a modeling tool in the petroleum industry) might formulate a predictive tool for the health effect (Verhaar et al. 1997). The development of predictive capability of toxicities (including carcinogenicity) for chemical mixtures might borrow from the experience of petroleum-chemical engineers. In the 1960s, the application of lumping analysis rendered it possible to predict gasoline production, fairly adequately, based on a few "lumps" rather than the thousands of individual component chemicals of the petroleum (Kuo and Wei 1969; Wei and Kuo 1969). Thus, even though relatively little is known about the complex mixture of petroleum, a predictive tool was developed and applied from computer modeling. More recent advances and development in lumping analysis incorporated molecular structures and chemical reaction rules, and the end result–structure-oriented lumping (SOL)–is a powerful tool that can be used to simulate the chemical processes going on in a oil refinery (Quann and Jaff 1996; Quann 1998). Coupled with QSAR, SOL can make much more accurate predictions for boiling points, specific gravity, and absolute viscosity for homologous series. Thus, SOL can literally simulate a oil refinery, providing valuable information regarding product yield of fuel gas, gasoline, jet fuel, diesel and heating oil, lubricating oils, asphalt, and coke. The overall achievement of such a modeling approach, therefore, is not only tremendous economic gain but also much more efficient operation for oil refineries and companies.

A reasonable question to ask is, drawing the parallel that a cell is like a chemical plant, should we not be able to utilize a modeling approach, such as the SOL, to develop a predictive tool for health effects from chemical mixtures (Yang et al. 1998)?

New Tools: Computer Modeling and Molecular Biology

Having actively engaged in the research area of the toxicology of chemical mixtures for the last 16 years or so, I have long since become resigned to the fact that the conventional animal toxicological testing methods would not work for chemical mixtures (Yang 1996, 1997; Yang et al. 1998). By adding other multiple stressors such as biologics, physical and biological agents, and environmental stressful conditions, the situation is even more complex. To have a reasonable chance to deal with multiple stressors as a long-term strategy, there is probably no choice but to fully utilize and integrate (1) computational technology; (2) mathematical and statistical modeling; (3) mechanistically based, short-term toxicological studies; and (4) cellular and molecular biology methodologies. To conserve resources and to be able to handle complex experimental designs, an experimental approach for multiple stressors must at least meet the following critical requirements: (1) be relatively simple, short-term, and inexpensive; (2) apply the best science; (3) display an understanding of the mechanisms of toxicity; (4) have broad applicability; and (5) have predictive capability. Using carcinogenicity as an endpoint, a brief description of one possible approach integrating biomedical research with computer modeling follows.

On the biological front, cell-culture systems of human keratinocytes, will be the main thrust for the evaluation of carcinogenic potentials of the selected stressors. There are many phenotypical and genotypical changes accompanying transformation of human keratinocytes; some are early and others are late events. To cover these changes, primary human keratinocytes, which are commercially available, can be used to study the early events (Dlugosz et al. 1995). A number of immortal cell lines such as HaCat (Boukamp et al. 1988), RHEK-1 (Rhim et al. 1985), and NM-1 (Baden et al. 1987) can be used to study the later events. Selected pertinent biomarkers such as TGFa, TGFb, c-*myc*, c-*ras*, and p53 might be studied and time-course quantitative information obtained. Such quantitative information might be utilized to calibrate and verify BBDR models.

On the modeling front, the following conceptual BBDR model (Figure 3), which is a published modification (Portier et al. 1990) of the widely known two-stage Moolgavkar-Vinzon-Knodson (MVK) cancer model, can be used.

In this modified four-stage model, the investigators added damaged normal cells and damaged intermediate cells to provide for the two additional stages. Thus, the emphasis for additional cell types is on genetic aberration, such as formation of DNA adducts, single strand breaks, gene amplification, and chromosomal translocation. Similarly, additional stages might be added to the MVK model by

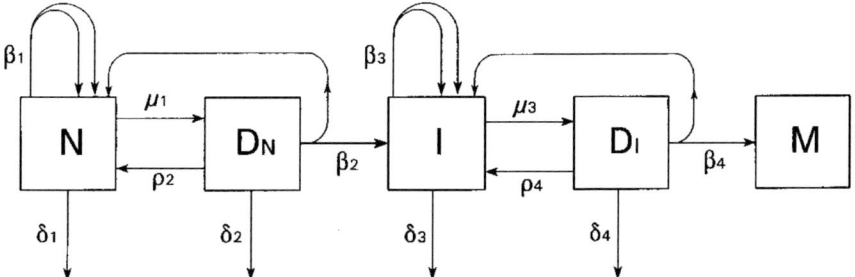

FIGURE 3 A four-stage model of carcinogenesis with clonal expansion and repair. N = normal cells; D_N = damaged normal cells; I = intermediate cells; D_I = damaged intermediate cells; M = malignant cells; β_i = birth rate; δ_i = death or differentiation rate; μ_i = genetic aberration rate; ρ_i = repair rate. (Reproduced from Portier et al. 1990, with permission.)

inserting cell types with a variety of early or late phenotypical or genotypical changes as long as these changes can be measured quantitatively. A model like this incorporates mechanistic information and, at each cellular stage, the birth, death, and mutation rates are either measurable or can be estimated. Therefore, this is a biologically based model. Because quantitative changes are expected to be related to doses, and the application of this model will certainly involve dose-response simulation and assessment, it is also a dose-response model. When considered in its totality, such a model is a BBDR model.

PBPK/PD models have, up to this point, been associated with whole, multicellular organisms such as mammals, fish, and plants. They describe the interrelationship of physiology, pharmacokinetics, and pharmacodynamics among different organs or lumps of organs or tissues. Although cells have their own physiology and organelles, PBPK/PD modeling has not often been considered with cellular systems. It is possible that a PBPK/PD model can be developed for the cell-culture system when the cell culture vessel is considered as the boundary of the system. Further, as technological advances are made, pharmacokinetics and pharmacodynamics at the subcellular organelle levels might be quantitatively determined. Under those circumstances, the mass balance and transfer, as well as receptor interactions at the subcellular organelle levels, might be described mathematically, and the resulting model, a PBPK/PD model for the cell-culture system, becomes verifiable.

Once the integration of computer modeling and the latest advances of molecular and cell biology becomes a reality, specific toxic responses (e.g., carcinogenic potential, neurotoxicity, developmental toxicity, immunotoxicity) might be assessed at much higher sensitivity levels and be much less expensive. Further development of computer modeling with the incorporation of other technologies, such as SOL, QSAR, and Monte Carlo simulation will enable us to formulate predictive capabilities. As these predictive capabilities are refined and improved through continued research, evaluation of toxicological interactions from multiple stressors might become more and more a matter of computer simulation. Such a developmental strategy will enable us to handle extremely complex situations involving multiple stressors.

Difficulties in Assessing and Predicting Agent Interactions

Presently, there is some success in predicting toxicological interactions of simple chemical mixtures using the integrated approach of computer modeling and mechanistic toxicology (Andersen and

Clewell 1983; Purcell et al. 1990; Sato et al. 1990; Thakore et al. 1991; Tardif et al. 1993; 1995; Barton et al. 1995; El-Masri et al. 1996a,b,c; Pelekis and Krishnan 1997; Tardif et al. 1997; Feng et al. 1998; Yang et al. 1999). However, there are two major limitations with the results of integrated approaching. One is that the results are relevant only with respect to the specific cases, with little or no extrapolative capability. The other is that all cases dealing with simple chemical mixtures of no more than three chemicals. To overcome these limitations, the next breakthrough must be based on the thorough understanding of the fundamental biology involved in the disruption of homeostasis and the development of a computer model able to handle very complex situations.

Opportunities on the Horizon

Thinking positively and considering that the complexity of issues related to chemical mixtures and multiple stressors are challenges for our intellectual capability, there are many opportunities to be explored and utilized. Nowhere are such opportunities more abundant than in the interdisciplinary research effort that goes beyond the traditional boundaries of fields of studies. For example, can toxicologists look to engineers for help in dealing with the issues of toxicological interactions of chemical mixtures? This author's preliminary experience is that toxicologists can indeed team up with engineers to produce synergistic creativity. The example given below on the potential utilization of SOL is but one such opportunity.

The basic concept of SOL is that any petroleum molecule can be described and represented by a set of 22 structural features or groups called "increments" (Quann and Jaff 1996; Quann 1998); one might consider these increments as the molecular puzzle pieces that form the mosaics of different hydrocarbon molecules. Each of the up to 6,000 hydrocarbon molecules in SOL modeling forms a "vector," a horizontal line to account for the presence or absence of the "increments," which are the 22 columns for the "vectors." This formulates a kind of molecular fingerprint for each of the 6,000 chemicals. The computer can search this matrix of $22 \times 6,000$ and locate each molecule easily. In addition to this accounting of hydrocarbon molecules, the possible chemical reactions for each of these 6,000 molecules (approximately an order of magnitude greater in numbers; or 60,000 reactions) are also incorporated into the model, according to chemical reaction rules that determine and account for the structural changes (i.e., changes of increments and vectors) of molecules involved in such reactions. Computer programs generate the entire network of chemicals and chemical reactions using sorting procedures to automatically construct the differential rate and energy balance equations for reaction modeling. Expanding further, SOL becomes a molecular-based model for the entire oil refinery by integrating individual-process models.

The idea is that we do not need to know everything, but we have enough information about the overall mosaic to be able to see it. The end result of SOL in petroleum engineering is a much more accurate and powerful predictive capability for both the unknown components and the endpoints of interest such as boiling point, specific gravity, and absolute viscosity of homologous series of petroleum chemicals (Quann and Jaff 1996; Quann 1998).

For the purpose of dealing with the toxicology of chemical mixtures (or to a higher level, the toxicology of multiple stressors), the specific significance of SOL might best be explained in the following way. If SOL can be applied successfully in petroleum engineering to deal with mixtures containing hundreds of thousands of chemical components plus an order of magnitude higher numbers for the chemical processes involved, why can it not be applied to chemicals or chemical mixtures in biological systems? After all, biochemical, cellular, and physiological processes are a collection of chemical and physical processes. There is certainly a tremendous gold mine of knowledge in the literature on physiological and biochemical processes in the cells. Even if our knowledge is incomplete about some of these processes (like our incomplete knowledge about all the components in petroleum catalytic-cracking processes), computer modeling might be utilized to estimate and predict some of the knowledge for which we do not have enough resources to obtain data empirically. Ultimately, with continuing advances in computer technology and cell biology, it should be possible to model a cell and its related chemical and physical processes for endogenous substances as well as xenobiotics. Such a development might start out with the modeling of as many of the molecular and biochemical pathways as possible for one type of disease process (e.g., cancer). The linkage of these pathways forms a network, and the connection of different networks for different disease processes would eventually provide the mosaic of a homeostatic or disrupted cell that we are looking for. Once this is achieved, molecular-based whole organ, biological system, or even whole body modeling for a human being will not be far behind. Only through this level of modeling the fundamentals of molecular, biochemical, and physiological processes at homeostatic state versus its disruption by chemicals or other stressors is there a real chance of predicting toxicological interactions of various chemical mixtures.

Philosophical Issues

The discussion of a number of issues might help DOD's effort to formulate strategies to protect the health of deployed U.S. forces.

The first issue is related to the balance between long-term investment versus urgency for answers. The health problems related to the Gulf War Syndrome and the potential adverse health effects under possible conditions for future deployment of U.S. forces cannot be resolved or predicted by quick fixes. The principal reason is that the true answers to those problems are dependent on scientific research and discovery. Because of the complexity and difficulty of the problems, the answers would most likely be uncovered based on painstakingly slow accumulation of knowledge. This is why a long-term strategy in research is necessary. From a different perspective, U.S. forces might need to be deployed anytime, and there must be some information to make health-related decisions. This is where the short-term preventive strategy comes in. As pointed out by the Senate Committee on Veterans' Affairs in the *Report of the Special Investigation Unit on Gulf War Illnesses* in 1998, "The men and women who have served in our nation's military deserve better than what ill Gulf War veterans have experienced."

The second issue relates to the fragmentation and polarization of the scientific community toward certain studies, particularly when they are in the limelight of the news media. Although scientific debates and challenges are healthy and necessary, if they have gone overboard, particularly when scientific opinions are colored by special agendas or emotionalism, the scientific community as a whole becomes the loser. Clinical and epidemiological research on the Gulf War Syndrome yielded results that ranged from no correlation, to some correlation, all the way to strong correlation with Gulf-War-related activities (Gouge et al. 1994; Jamal et al. 1996; Amato et al. 1997; Haley 1997; Haley and Kurt 1997; Haley et al. 1997a,b; Landrigan 1997). Some of these studies led to "war" across the Atlantic Ocean. I have witnessed firsthand part of the controversies surrounding the Abou-Donia et al. (1996a,b) studies and the Haley and Kurt (1997) study. These studies were all published in peer-reviewed journals; thus, at least part of the scientific community approved of these studies. As a scientist without any involvement in any of these studies, I would like to discuss the Abou-Donia et al. (1996a,b) studies objectively to illustrate a point. These two studies will be referred to as the Abou-Donia studies from hereon.

Even though the findings of the Abou-Donia studies were exciting and they might provide some pieces of the puzzle for the mysterious Gulf War Syndrome, a part of the scientific community did not embrace these results. There are probably two principal reasons for such reluctance.

1. Do animal models, particularly the chicken, reflect what's happening in humans?

The short answer is yes! From the days of the use of canaries by miners as a preventive measure from occupational hazard, the application of modern experimental biology and toxicology in assessing human health hazard has come a long way. Modern medicine has been built upon the foundation of biomedical research using animal studies. Besides, it is morally and ethically wrong to conduct human toxicological experiments even if there are means to do it. The NRC, in its recent publication on *Science and Judgment in Risk Assessment* (NRC 1994a), indicated the following advantages of animal studies:

- Animals can be used to collect toxicity information on chemicals before marketing, whereas epidemiological data can be collected only after human exposure.
- Animal studies can be controlled, so establishing causation is not in general difficult.
- The quantitative relationship between exposure (or dose) and extent of toxic response can be established.
- The animals and animal tissues can be thoroughly examined by toxicologists and pathologists, so the full range of toxic effects produced by a chemical can be identified.
- The exposure duration and routes can be designed to match those experienced by the human population of concern.

The utility of animal studies in human health hazard assessment might also be underscored by one of the conclusions reached by the Committee to Review the Health Consequences of Service During the Persian Gulf War (IOM 1995) which recommended for immediate action that "appropriate laboratory animal studies of interactions between DEET, PB [pyridostigmine bromide], and permethrin should be conducted."

However, NRC (1994a) also pointed out that laboratory animals are not human beings. Thus, although animal studies are useful in assessing adverse human health problems, their potential limitations must be recognized. In this context, it should also be pointed out that great variabilities in pharmacological and toxicological responses exist in human populations as well (see discussion of human variability above).

2. Because the Abou-Donia studies did not establish dose-response relationships, are they applicable to interpreting the Gulf War Syndrome in Gulf War veterans? Are the doses used in these studies relevant?

For obvious reasons of complexity of design and limitation of resources, both Abou-Donia studies were conducted at single dose levels; thus, a dose-response relationship was not established. This is certainly a weakness of the studies; however, it does not negate the interesting findings with respect to the unanticipated toxicological interactions in the binary and trinary chemical mixtures. These studies certainly suggest the possibility of such toxicological interactions in mammals, including humans. In that sense, scientists and clinicians, in their evaluation of the Gulf War Syndrome in PGW veterans should be well advised to take the above findings into consideration. This was indeed done by some (Haley and Kurt 1997; Jamal 1998).

In their first interaction study (Abou-Donia et al. 1996a), the dose regimen for 5 days/week for 2 months included concentrations of PB in water at 5 mg/kg/day by gavage; DEET neat at 500 mg/kg/day, subcutaneously (sc); and in permethrin in corn oil at kg/day, sc. In their second interaction study (Abou-Donia et al. 1996b), the dose regimen for 5 days/week for 2 months included concentrations of PB in water at 5 kg/day by gavage; DEET neat at 500 mg/kg/day, sc; and chlorpyrifos in corn oil at 10 mg/kg/day, sc. The same doses were given in single-chemical or mixture groups. The researchers have provided very thorough background information on these chemicals and the readers are referred to the original papers for detailed information. The rationale given for the selection of these dose levels and provide my commentary follow.

PB was issued to the military personnel as 30-mg tablet and the recommended dose regimen was one tablet three times daily. That would mean a daily combined dose of 90 mg/person. Assuming an average human body weight of 70 kg, this translates to 1.3 mg/kg/day. In setting their dose, the investigation obviously also considered the human PB therapeutic dose for myasthenia gravis at 200 to 1,400 mg a day (thus equivalent to 2.9 to 20 mg/kg/day), as well as the known acute toxicity in rats (oral LD_{50} for PB, 61.6 mg/kg/day). However, comparing the two scenarios strictly on a mg/kg/day basis, the PB dose employed in the studies is about 4 times higher than the intake by the Gulf War veterans. Using 0.2 LD_{50} as a definition of low dose as discussed at the beginning of this paper, the PB dose employed by the investigators is about 10 times lower than the 0.2 LD_{50} of the rats, estimated at about 12 mg/kg/day. To put it in a different way, assuming that absorption, distribution, metabolism, and elimination are the same between the hen and human, the area under the plasma concentration and time curve (AUC) in the hen would have been 4 times larger than that of the human on a per kilogram body-weight basis. In addition, the human dose was divided into three equal portions daily, whereas the hen dose was given by gavage in one bolus. Therefore, pharmacokinetically, the hen would have had much higher plasma concentration, perhaps 10 times higher, than that of the human. Depending on the window of opportunity for toxicological interactions, this difference can be significant.

DEET is used as an insect repellent against mosquitoes, biting flies, ticks, and other insects. Because there are no reliable estimates of DEET usage among service personnel during the Persian Gulf War, the Abou-Donia studies used a 1986 National Institute for Occupational Safety and Health study of the employees in the Everglades National Park to estimate a reasonably close dosage. In that study (McConnell et al. 1986), the mean weekly estimated dermal application of DEET was 14.6 g, which was equivalent to 42 mg/kg/day for a 70-kg person. It is noteworthy that the top 5% heavy users among the workers in the McConnell et al. (1986) study applied 66.3 g and the top 1% heavy users applied as high as 392.6 g for that weekly period, which was equivalent to applying 189 or 1,122 mg/kg/day, respectively. Given the above information, the selection of neat DEET at a concentration of 500 mg/kg/day, sc, by the Abou-Donia researcher appeared to have been high, even though it is within the upper limit. Considering further that the rat oral LD_{50} for DEET is 3,000 mg/kg, using the earlier low-dose definition of 0.2 LD_{50}, it could argued that the 500 mg/kg/day selected for the Abou-Donia studies is still within the low-dose range. Nevertheless, a question that might be on every concerned scientist's mind is "would the Abou-Donia researcher have observed the same toxicological interactions if the DEET dose was set at the estimated mean dose for an Everglades worker at 42 mg/kg/day in their experiments?" An additional point that might have bothered people is the sc injection mode of application in the Abou-Donia studies. Although it is understandable that the feathers are an obstruction for a topical application to chickens, an sc injection certainly bypasses the skin-penetration kinetics and the corn oil solvent would further complicate the absorption kinetics, if applied topically.

For permethrin or chlorpyrifos, both insecticides, the rationale for dose selection was not clear in the Abou-Donia studies. Once again, if using the earlier low-dose definition of 0.2 LD_{50}, and given the fact that the chicken oral LD_{50} for permethrin and chlorpyrifos are 9,000 mg/kg and 50 mg/kg, respectively, the 500 mg/kg/day for permethrin and 10 mg/kg/day for chlorpyrifos selected for the Abou-Donia studies are both within the low-dose range. Here, the same concerns on sc injection and corn oil as described above would also apply. There is one exposure assessment in the literature (NRC 1994b), however, in which the investigators concluded that, "The average lifetime dermal dose for military personnel from wearing permethrin-impregnated BDUs [body dress uniforms] (permethrin impregnation at a concentration of 0.125 mg/cm^2) was calculated to be

6.8×10^{-5} mg/kg per day." If we take this estimate without questioning and compare it with the dose of permethrin Abou-Donia et al. (1996a) applied in this study, there is more than a 7 million-fold difference. Therefore, on the surface, the investigators have seemingly used a totally unrealistically high dose of permethrin in this study. However, upon closer examination, the NRC (1994b) figure of 6.8×10^{-5} mg/kg per day might be unrealistically low. The logic used to reach this suggestion is as follows: The impregnation of BDUs with permethrin is presumably intended to kill insects upon contact. The idea here is that enough selective toxicity favoring humans exists such that a brief contact to the insects will kill them whereas prolonged dermal exposure to human is safe. The soldiers wear BDUs all day long; thus, their exposure to permethrin must be more than the exposure levels for the insects that land and crawl on the BDUs for a brief time. Even assuming the insects, in their brief landing and crawling, get the equivalent exposure (6.8×10^{-5} mg/g per day) as the soldiers in their BDUs (being sweaty) all day long, I have never known any insecticide that has the lethal effectiveness at 0.000068 mg/g per day. Therefore, something is very wrong in the NRC (1994b) estimate.

Taking the Abou-Donia studies in their totality, and despite their potential weaknesses, my opinion is that they are useful studies, particularly in the context of the Gulf War Syndrome. Given our initial total ignorance of the Gulf War Syndrome and thinking about the tasks ahead of us, I would rather have the knowledge Abou-Donia et al. (1996a,b) contributed in hand in assessing the overall situation. This is particularly true when some of the experimental design weaknesses in the Abou-Donia studies might easily be rectified by follow-up studies in which more resources might be invested to support more thorough dose-response experimental designs.

FUTURE PERSPECTIVES

The task before DOD is a formidable, but not an impossible, one. It will not be easy; it will require resources; and it will take a long-term, visionary commitment. Any war is a formidable task and DOD has repeatedly demonstrated its ability to live up to the expectation of the nation. Likewise, DOD, with its resources and the available help from the scientific community, should be able to map out a preventive research strategy for the protection of future deployed U.S. forces.

LIST OF ABBREVIATIONS

BBRD	biologically based dose response
BDU	battle dress uniform
BuCHE	butyrylcholinesterase
DEET	*N,N*-diethyl-*m*-toluamide
DOD	Department of Defense
MOPP	military operations protective posture
MVK	Moolgavkar-Venzon-Knudson
NTE	neuropathy target esterase
NTP	National Toxicology Program
OPIDN	organophosphate-induced delayed neurotoxicity
OPIDP	organophosphate-induced delayed polyneuropathy
PBPK/PD	physiologically based pharmacokinetics/pharmacodynamics
PB	pyridostigmine bromide
PCNA	proliferating cell nuclear antigen

QSAR   quantitative structure-activity relationship
SOL   structure-oriented lumping

ACKNOWLEDGEMENT

The concept development and related research work on chemical mixture toxicology and multiple stressors were supported in part by a Superfund Basic Research Program Project Grant (P42 ES05949) and a research grant (RO1 ES-09655) from the National Institute of Environmental Health Sciences (NIEHS) and a cooperative agreement (#U61/ATU881475) from Agency for Toxic Substances and Disease Registry (ATSDR). Without such generous support for biomedical research, this work could never have been possible.

REFERENCES

Abou-Donia, M.B., K.R. Wilmarth, A.A. Abdel-Rahman, K.F. Jensen, F.W. Oehme, and T.L. Kurt. 1996b. Increased neurotoxicity following concurrent exposure to pyridostigmine bromide, DEET, and chlorpyrifos. Fundam. Appl. Toxicol. 34:201-222.

Abou-Donia, M.B., K.R. Wilmarth, K.F. Jensen, F.W. Oehme, and T.L. Kurt. 1996a. Neurotoxicity resulting from coexposure to pyridostigmine bromide, DEET, and permethrin: Implications of Gulf War chemical exposures. J. Toxicol. Environ. Health 48:35-56.

Amato, A.A., A. McVey, C. Cha, E.C. Matthews, C.E. Jackson, R. Kleingunther, L. Worley, E. Cornman, and K. Kagan-Hallet. 1997. Evaluation of neuromuscular symptoms in veterans of the Persian Gulf War. Neurology 48:4-12.

Andersen, M.E. and H.J. Clewell. 1983. Pharmacokinetic interaction of mixtures. Pp. 226-238. in: Proceedings of the Fourteenth Annual Conference on Environmental Toxicology, AFAMRL-TR-83-099, Dayton, OH.

Aposhian, H.V. 1997. Enzymatic methylation of arsenic species and other new approaches to arsenic toxicity. Ann. Rev. Pharmacol. Toxicol. 37:397-419.

Appleby, A.P. 1998. The practical implications of hormetic effects of herbicides on plants. BELLE Newsletter. 6(3):23-24.

Arcos, J.C., Y.T. Woo, and Y.D. Lai. 1988. Database on binary combination effects of chemical carcinogens. J. Environ Sci. Health Part C Environ. Carcinog. Rev. 6(1):1-150.

Baden, H.P., J. Kubilus, J.C. Kvedar, M.L. Steinberg, and S.R. Wolman. 1987. Isolation and characterization of a spontaneously arising long-lived line of human keratinocytes (NM-1). In Vitro Cell. Develop. Biol. 23:205-213.

Bailer, A.J., and J.T. Oris. 1998. Incorporating hormesis in the routine testing of hazards. BELLE Newsletter. 6(3):2-5.

Barton, H.A., J.R. Creech, G.S. Godin, G.M. Randall, and C.S. Seckel. 1995. Chloroethylene mixtures: Pharmacokinetic modeling and in vitro metabolism of vinyl chloride, trichloroethylene, and trans-1,2-dichloroethylene in rat. Toxicol. Appl. Pharmacol. 130:237-247.

Bartsch, J. and E. Hietanen. 1996. The role of individual susceptibility in cancer burden related to environmental exposure. Environ. Health Perspect. 104(Suppl. 3):569-577.

Ben-Nathan, D., S. Lusting, and H.D. Danenberg. 1991. Stress-induced neuroinvasiveness of a neurovirulent non invasive sindvis virus in cold or isolation subjected mice. Life Sci. 48:1493-1500.

Benjamin S.A., R.S.H. Yang, J.D. Tessari, L.W. Chubb, M.D. Brown, and C.E. Dean. 1999. Lack of preneoplastic foci in rats exposed to a hazardous waste groundwater mixture in a medium-term hepatic initiation/promotion assay. Toxicology Submitted for publication.

Berenbaum, M.C. 1981. Criteria for analyzing interactions between biologically active agents. Adv. Cancer Res. 35:269-335.

Berenbaum, M.C. 1985. The expected effect of a combination of agents: The general solution. J. Theo. Biol. 114:413-431.

Boukamp, P., R.T. Petrussevska, D. Breitkreutz, J. Hornung, A. Markham, and N.E. Fusenig. 1988. Normal keratinization in a spontaneously immortalized aneuploid human keratinocyte cell line. J. Cell Biol. 106:761-771.

Calabrese, E.J. 1991a. Multiple Chemical Interactions. Chelsea, MI: Lewis. 704 pp.

Calabrese, E.J. 1991b. Alcohol Interactions with Drugs and Chemicals. Chelsea, MI: Lewis. 82 pp.

Calabrese, E.J. 1997. Hormesis revisited: New insights concerning the biological effects of low-dose exposures to toxins. Environ. Law Reporter 27:10526-19532.

Calabrese, E.J. and L.A. Baldwin. 1997a. The dose determines the stimulation (and poison): Development of a chemical hormesis database. Int. J. Toxicol. 16:545-559.

Calabrese, E.J. and L.A. Baldwin. 1997b. A quantitatively-based methodology for the evaluation of chemical hormesis. Human Ecolog. Risk Assess. 3:545-554.

Casale, G.P., J.L. Vennerstrom, S. Bavari, and T. Wang. 1993. Inhibition of interleukin 2 driven proliferation of mouse CTLL cells, by selected carbamate and organophosphate insecticides and congeners of carbaryl. Immunopharmacol. Immunotoxicol. 15:199-215.

Cassee, F.R., J.P. Groten, P.J. van Bladeren, and V.J. Feron. 1998. Toxicological evaluation and risk assessment of chemical mixtures. Crit. Rev. Toxicol. 28:73-101.

Chaney, L.A., R.W. Rockhold, J.R. Mozingo, A.S. Hume, and J.I. Moss. 1997. Potentiation of pyridostigmine bromide toxicity in mice by selected adrenergic agents and caffieine. Vet. Human Toxicol. 39:214-219.

Chrousos, G.P. and P.W. Gold. 1992. The concepts of stress and stress system disorders. Overview of physical and behavioral homeostasis. JAMA 267:1244-1252.

Clauw, D.J., and G.P. Chrousos. 1997. Chronic pain and fatigue syndromes: Overlapping clinical and neuroendocrine features and potential pathogenic mechanisms. Neuroimmunomodulation 4:134-153.

Dean, C.E., Jr., S.A. Benjamin, L.S. Chubb, J.D. Tessari, and R.S.H. Yang. 1999. Interaction of co-planar and non-planar PCBs in promotion of altered hepatic foci. [Abstract]. The Toxicologist. 48:235.

Dlugosz, A.A., A.B. Glick, T. Tennenbaum, W.C. Weinberg, and S.H. Yuspa. 1995. Isolation and utilization of epidermal kertinocytes for oncogene research. Meth. Enzymol. 254:3-21.

EHP. 1994. Envrionmental Health Perspectives Supplements, Toxicological Evaluation of Chemical Interactions, National Institute of Environmental Health Sciences, Volume 109, Supplement 9, November. 167 pp.

Eichelbaum, M. and B. Evert. 1996. Influence of pharmacogenetics on drug disposition and response. Clin. Exp. Pharmacol. Physiol. 23:983-985.

Elashoff, R.M., T.R. Fears, and M.A. Schneiderman. 1987. Statistical analysis of a carcinogen mixture experiment. I. Liver carcinogens. J. Nat. Cancer Inst. 79:509-526.

El-Masri, H.A., A.A. Constan, H.S. Ramsdel, and R.S.H. Yang. 1996b. Physiologically based pharmacodynamic modeling of an interaction threshold between trichloroethylene and 1,1-dichloroethylene in Fischer 344 Rats. Toxicol. Appl. Pharmacol. 141:124-132.

El-Masri, H.A., J.D. Tessariand R.S.H. Yang. 1996a. Exploration of an interaction threshold for the joint toxicity of trichloroethylene and 1,1-dichloroethylene: utilization of a PBPK model. Arch. Toxicol. 70:527-539.

El-Masri, H.A., R.S. Thomas, G.R. Sabados, J.K. Phillips, A.A. Constan, S.A. Benjamin, M.E. Andersen, H.M. Mehendale, and R.S.H. Yang. 1996c. Physiologically based pharmacokinetic/pharmacodynamic modeling of the toxicologic interaction between carbon tetrachloride and kepone. Arch. Toxicol. 70:704-713.

Ember, L.R. 1998. Surviving stress. C&EN 76(21):12-24.

Etkina, E.L. and I.A. Etkina. 1995. Chemical mixtures exposure and children's health. Chemosphere 31:2463-2474.

FCT (Food and Chemical Toxicology). 1996. Volume 34, Number 11/12, pp. 1025-1199.

Fears, T.R., R.M. Elashoff, and M.A. Schneiderman. 1988. The statistical analysis of a carcinogen mixture experiment. II. Carcinogens with different target organs, N-methyl-N-nitro-N-nitrosoguanidine, N-butyl-N-(4-hydroxybutyl)nitrosamine, dipentynitrosamine, and nitrilotriacetic acid. Toxicol. Ind. Health 4:221-255.

Fears, T.R., R.M. Elashoff, and M.A. Schneiderman. 1989. The statistical analysis of a carcinogen mixture experiment. III. Carcinogens with different target systems, aflatoxin B1, N-butyl-N-(4-hydroxybutyl)nitrosamine, lead acetate, and thiouracil. Toxicol. Ind. Health 5:1-23.

Feigelson, H.S., R.K. Ross, M.C. Yu, G.A. Coetzee, J.K. Reichardt, and B.E. Henderson. 1996. Genetic susceptibility to cancer from exogenous and endogenous exposures. J. Cell. Biochem. (Suppl.) 25:15-22.

Feng, L., R.S. Thomas, D. Ewert, S.A. Saghir, S.A. Benjamin, and R.S.H. Yang. 1998. PBPK/PD model for the toxicologic interactions of three chemicals: Kepone, carbon tetrachloride, and 1,1,2,2-tetrachloroethane. [Abstract]. The Toxicologist 42:342.

Feron, V.J., J.P. Groton, J.A. van Zorge, F.R. Cassee, D. Jonker, and P.J. van Bladeren. 1995. Toxicity studies in rats of simple mixtures of chemicals with the same or different target organs. Toxicol. Lett. 82/83:505-512.

Finney, D.J. 1964. Statistical Methods in Biological Assays, 2nd Ed. London: Charles Griffin.

Friedman, A., D. Kaufer, J. Shemer, I. Hendler, H. Soreq, and I. Tur-Kaspa. 1996. Pyridostigmine brain penetration under stress enhances neuronal excitability and induces early immediate transcriptional response. Nature Med. 2:1382-1385.

GAO (United States General Accounting Office). 1998. Chemical Weapons. DOD Does Not Have a Strategy to Address Low-Level Exposures. United States General Accounting Office Report to Congressional Requesters, GAO/NSIAD-98-228. Washington D.C.: United States General Accounting Office. (September 1998). 39 pp.

Gaylor, D. 1998. Safety assessment with hormetic effects. BELLE Newsletter. 6:6-8.

Gennings, C. and W.H. Carter, Jr., 1996. Utilizing concentration-response data from individual components to detect statistically significant departures from additivity in chemical mixtures. Biometrics 51:1264-1277.

Germolec, D.R., R.S.H. Yang, M.P. Ackermann, J.G. Rosenthal, G.A. Boorman, M. Thompson, P. Blair, and M.I. Luster. 1989. Toxicology studies of a chemical mixture of 25 groundwater contaminants: (II) Immunosuppression in B6C3F1 mice. Fundam. Appl. Toxicol. 13:377-387.

Ghoshroy, S., K. Freedman, R. Lartey, and V. Citovsky. 1998. Inhibition of plant viral systemic infection by non-toxic concentrations of cadmium. Plant J. 13:591-602.

Glynn, A.W., Y. Lind, E. Funseth, and N.G. Ilback. 1998. The intestinal absorption of cadmium increases during a common viral infection (coxsackie virus B3) in mice. Chem. Biol. Interact. 113:79-89.

Goldstein, R.S., W.R. Hewitt, and J.B. Hook. 1990. Toxic Interactions. San Diego: Academic Press. 488 pp.

Gouge, S.F., D.J. Daniels, and C.E. Smith. 1994. Exacerbation of asthma after pyridostigmine during Operation Desert Storm. Mil. Med. 159:108-111.

Haley, R.W. 1997. Is Gulf War Syndrome due to stress? The evidence reexamined. Am. J. Epidemiol. 146:695-703.

Haley, R.W., and R. Kurt. 1997. Self-reported exposure to neurotoxic chemical combinations in the Gulf War. A cross-sectional epidemiologic study. JAMA 227:231-237.

Haley, R.W., R. Kurt, and J. Hom. 1997a. Is there a Gulf War Syndrome? Searching for syndromes by factor analysis of symptoms. JAMA 227:215-222.

Haley, R.W., J. Hom, P.S. Roland, W.W. Bryan, P.C. van Ness, F.J. Bonte, M.D. Devous, Sr., D. Mathews, J.L. Fleckenstein, F.H. Wians, Jr., G.I. Wolfe, and T.L. Kurt. 1997b. Evaluation of neurologic function in Gulf War Veterans. A blinded case-control study. JAMA 227:223-230.

Hanin, I. 1996. The Gulf War, stress and a leaky blood-brain barrier. Nature Med. 2:1307-1308.

Hirvonen, A. 1995. Genetic factors in individual responses to envrionmental exposures. J. Occup. Environ. Med. 37:37-43.

Hong, J.Y. and C.S. Yang. 1997. Genetic polymorphism of cytochrome P450 as a biomarker of susceptibility to environmental toxicity. Environ. Health Perspect. 105(Suppl. 4):759-762.

Hong, H.L., R.S.H. Yang, and G.A. Boorman. 1991. Residual damage to hematopoietic system in mice exposed to a mixture of groundwater contaminants. Toxicol. Lett. 57:101-111.

Hong, H.L., R.S.H. Yang, and G.A. Boorman. 1992. Alterations in hematopoietic responses in mice caused by drinking a mixture of 25 groundwater contaminants. J. Environ. Pathol. Toxicol. Oncol. 11:1-10.

Hong, H.L., R.S.H. Yang, and G.A. Boorman. 1993. Enhancement of myelotoxicity induced by repeated irradiation in mice exposed to a mixture of groundwater contaminants. Arch. Toxicol. 7:358-364.

Hubert, M. and D. Lison. 1995. Study of muscular effects of short-term pyridostigmine treatment in resting and exercising rats. Human Exp. Toxicol. 14:49-54.

Ikawa, S., F. Uematsu, K. Watanabe, T. Kimpara, M. Osada, A. Hossain, I. Sagami, H. Kikuchi, and M. Watanabe. 1995. Assessment of cancer susceptibility in humans by use of genetic polymorphisms in carcinogen metabolism. Pharmacogenetics 5 (Spec No):S154-160.

Inaba, T., D.W. Nebert, B. Burchell, P.B. Watkins, J.A. Goldstein, L. Bertilsson, and G.T. Tucker. 1995. Pharmacogenetics in clinical pharmacology and toxicology. Can. J. Physiol. Pharmacol. 73:331-338.

IOM (Institutue of Medicine). 1995. Health Consequences of Service During the Persian Gulf War: Initial Findings and Recommendations for Immediate Action. Washington, D.C.: National Academy Press.

IOM (Institute of Medicine). 1996. Interactions of Drugs, Biologics, and Chemicals in U. S. Military Forces. Washington, D.C.: National Academy Press.

Jamal, G.A. 1997. Neurological syndromes of organophosphorus compounds. Adverse Drug React. Toxicol. Rev. 16:133-170.

Jamal, G.A. 1998. Gulf War Syndrome — a model for the complexity of biological and environmental interaction with human health. Adverse Drug React. Toxicol. Rev. 17:1-17.

Jamal, G.A., S. Hansen, F. Apartopoulos and A. Peden. 1996. The 'Gulf War Syndrome.' Is there evidence of dysfunction in the nervous system? J. Neurol. Neurosurg. Psychiat. 60:449-451.

JCS (Joint Chiefs of Staff). 1998. Memorandum : Deployment Health Surveillance and Readiness. MCM-251-98. Office of the Chairman, Washington, D.C. Dated 04 December 1998.

Johnson, T.E., and H. Bruunsgaard. 1998. Implications of hormesis for biomedical aging research. BELLE Newsletter. 6(3):17-19.

Jonker, D., R.A. Woutersen, and V.J. Feron. 1996. Toxicity of mixtures of nephrotoxicants with similar or dissimilar mode of action. Food Chem. Toxicol. 34:1075-1082.

Kelly, C. and J. Rice. 1990. Monotone smoothing with application to dose-response curves and the assessment of synergism. Biometrics 46:1071-1085.

Kligerman, A.D., R.E. Chapin, G.L. Erexson, D.R. Germolec, P. Kwanyuen, and R.S.H. Yang. 1993. Analyses of cytogenetic damage in rodents following exposure to simulated groundwater contaminated with pesticides and a fertilizer. Mutat. Res. 300:125-134.

Kourakis, A., M. Mouratidou, A. Barbouti, and M. Dimikiotou. 1996. Cytogenetic effects of occupational exposure in the peripheral blood lymphocytes of pesticide sprayers. Carcinogenesis 17:99-101.

Kuo, J.C.W., and J. Wei. 1969. A lumping analysis in monomolecular reaction systems: analysis of approximately lumpable system. Ind. Eng. Chem. Fundam. 8:124-133.

Landrigan, P.J. 1997. Illness in Gulf War Veterans. Causes and consequences. JAMA 227:259-261.

Lazarou, J., B.H. Pomeranz, and P.N. Corey. 1998. Incidence of adverse drug reactions in hospitalized patients. A meta-analysis of prospective studies. JAMA 279:1200-1205.

Liang, K.Y., and S.L. Zeger. 1986. Longitudinal data analysis for discrete and continuous outcomes. Biometrics 42:121-130.

Lindenschmidt, R.C., and H.P. Witschi. 1990. Toxicological interactions and other taarget organ toxicities. Pp. 409-442. In: Toxic Interactions, R.S. Goldstein, W.R. Hewitt, and J.B. Hook, eds. San Diego: Academic Press.

Llback, N.G., J. Fohlman, and G. Friman. 1993. Altered distribution of heavy metals and lipids in coxsackievirus B3 infected mice. Scand. J. Infect. Dis. (Suppl.) 88:93-98.

Llback, N.G., J. Fohlman, and G. Friman. 1994a. Changed distribution and immune effects of nickel augmented viral-induced inflammatory heart lesions in mice. Toxicology 91:203-219.

Llback, N.G., J. Fohlman, G. Friman, and A. Ehrnst. 1994b. Immune responses and resistance to viral-induced myocarditis in mice exposed to cadmium. Chemosphere 29:1145-1154.

Llback, N.G., J. Fohlman, G. Friman, and A.W. Glynn. 1992. Altered distribution of 109 cadmium in mice during viral infection. Toxicology 71:193-202.

Llback, N.G., U. Lindh, J. Fohlman, and G. Friman. 1995. New aspects of murine coxsackie B3 myocarditis — focus on heavy metals. Eur. Heart J. 16 (Suppl 0):20-24.

Lodish, H., D. Baltimore, A. Berk, S.L. Zipursky, P. Matsudaira, and J. Darnell. 1995. Pp. 885. In: Molecular Cell Biology. Third Ed. New York: W. H. Freeman & Company.

Loewenstein-Lichtenstein, Y., M. Schwarz, D. Glick, B. Nørgaard-Pedersen, H. Zakut, and H. Soreq. 1995. Genetic predisposition to adverse consequences of anti-cholinesterases in 'atypical' BCHE carriers. Nature Med. 1:1082-1085.

Machado, S.G., and G.A. Robinson. 1994. A direct, general approach based on isobolograms for assessing the joint action of drugs in pre-clinical experiments. Stat. Med. 13:2289-2309.

McCabe, M., and M. Nowak. 1986. Synergistic modulation of lymphocyte mitogenesis by carcinogenic xenobiotics. Bull. Environ. Contam. Toxicol. 37:187-191.

McConnell, R., A.T. Fidler, and D. Chrislip. 1986. Health Hazard Evaluation Determination. Report No. 83-085, NIOSH, U. S. Department of Health and Human Services. Washington, D.C.

McFadden, S.A. 1996. Phenotypic variation in xenobiotic mechanism and adverse environmental response: focus on sulfur-dependent detoxification pathways. Toxicology 111:43-65.

Meyer, U.A., and U.M. Zanger. 1997. Molecular mechanisms of genetic polymorphisms of drug metabolism. Annu. Rev. Pharmacol. Toxicol. 37:269-296.

Morré, D.J. 1998. A protein disulfide-thiol interchange protein with NADH: Protein disulfide reductase (NADH oxidase) activity as a molecular target for low levels of exposure to organic solvents in plant growth. BELLE Newsletter 6(3):25-33.

Morse, J.G. 1998. Agricultural implications of pesticide-induced hormesis of insects and mites. BELLE Newsletter. 6:20-23.

Novick, S.G., J.C. Godfrey, R.L. Pollack, and H.R. Wilder. 1997. Zinc-induced suppression of inflammation in the respiratory tract, caused by infection with human rhinovirus and other irritants. Med. Hypotheses 49:347-357.

NRC (National Research Council). 1994a. Pp. 58, 104, 92-105. In: Science and Judgment in Risk Assessment. Washington, D.C.: National Academy Press.

NRC (National Research Council). 1994b. Health Effects of Permethrin-Impregnated Army Battle-Dress Uniforms. Washington, D.C.: National Academy Press. 227 pp.

PDR. 1996. PDR Guide to Drug Interactions and Side Effects Indications. Montvale, NJ: Medical Economics Co. 1553 pp.

Pelekis, M., and K. Krishnan. 1997. Assessing the relevance of rodent data on chemical interactions for health risk assessment purposes: A case study with dichloromethane-toluene mixture. Regul. Toxicol. Pharmacol. 25:79-86.

Pollak, J.K. 1993. The Toxicity of Chemical Mixtures. The Centre for Human Aspects of Science and Technology. Sidney, Australia: The University of Sidney. 77 pp.

Porter, W.P., R.D. Hinsdill, A. Fairbrother, L.J. Olson, J. Jaeger, T. Yuill, S. Bisgaard, W.G. Hunter, and K. Nolan. 1984. Toxicant-disease-environment interactions associated with suppression of immune system, growth, and reproduction. Science 224:1014-1017.

Portier, C.J., D.G. Hoel, N.L. Kaplan, and A. Kopp. 1990. Biologically based models for risk assessment. Pp. 20-26. In: Complex Mixtures and Cancer Risk, H. Vainio, M. Sorsa, and A.J. McMichael, eds. Lyon, France: IARC.

Pott, W.A., S.A. Benjamin, and R.S.H. Yang. 1998. Antagonistic interactions of arsenic-containing mixtures in a multiple organ carcinogenicity bioassay. Cancer Lett. 133:185-190.

Pott, W. A., S.A. Benjamin, and R.S.H. Yang. 1999. Antagonism of hepatic preneoplastic foci by an arsenic-containing mixture: Role of apoptosis. [Abstract]. The Toxicologist 48:346.

Prentice, R.L., R.T. Smythe, D. Krewski, and M. Mason. 1992. On the use of historical control data to estimate dose response trends in quantal bioassay. Biometrics 48:459-478.

Purcell, K.J., G.H. Cason, M.L. Gargas, M.E. Andersen, and C.C. Travis. 1990. In vivo metabolic interactions of benzene and toluene. Toxicol. Lett. 52:141-152.

Quann, R.J. 1998. Modeling the chemistry of complex petroleum mixtures. Environ. Health Perspect. 106:1441-1450.

Quann, R.J., and S.B. Jaff. 1996. Building useful models of complex reaction systems in petroleum refining. Plenary Paper. Chem. Eng. Sci. 51: 1615-1635.

Rao, V.R., Y.T. Woo, D.Y. Lai, and J.C. Arcos. 1989. Database on promotors of chemical carcinogenesis. Environ. Carcinogenesis Rev. C7:145-386.

Rannug, A., A.K. Alexandrie, I. Persson, and M. Ingelman-Sundberg. 1995. Genetic polymorphism of cytochromes P450 1A1, 2D6 and 2E1: regulation and toxicological significance. J. Occup. Environ. Med. 37:25-36.

Raunio, H., K. Husgafvel-Pursiainen, S. Anttila, E. Hietanen, A. Hirvonen, and O. Pelkonen. 1995. Diagnosis of polymorphisms in carcinogen-activating and inactivating enzymes and cancer susceptibility — a review. Gene 159:113-121.

Rhim, J.S., G. Jay, P. Arnstein, F.M. Price, K.K. Sanford, and S.A. Aaronson. 1985. Neoplastic transformation of human epidermal keratinocytes by Ad12/SV40 and Kirsten sarcoma viruses. Science 227:1250-1252.

Rook, G.A.W., and A. Zumla. 1997. Gulf War Syndrome: is it due to a systemic shift in cytokine balance towards a Th2 profile? Lancet 349:1831-1833.

Safe, S.H. 1998. Hazard and risk assessment of chemical mixtures using the toxic equivalency factor approach. Environ. Health Perspect. 106 (Suppl. 4):1051-1058.

Sato, A., K. Endoh, T. Kaneko and G. Johansson. 1990. Effects of consumption of ethanol on the biological monitoring of exposure to organic solvent vapors: A simulation study with trichloroethylene. Brit. J. Ind. Med. 48:548-556.

Sielken, R.L., and D.E. Stevenson. 1998. Some implications for quantitative risk assessment if hormesis exists. BELLE Newsletter 6(3):13-17.

Srinivas, U., J.H. Braconier, B. Jeppsson, M. Abdulla, B. Akesson, and P.A. Ockerman. 1988. Trace element alterations in infectious diseases. Scand. J. Clin. Lab. Invest. 48:495-500.

Stebbing, A.R.D. 1982. Hormesis—the stimulation of growth by low levels of inhibitors. Sci. Total Environ. 22:213-234.

Stebbing, A.R.D. 1997. A theory for growth hormesis. BELLE Newsletter 6:1-11.

Takayama S, H. Hasegawa, and H. Ohgaki. 1989. Combination effects of fort carcinogens administered at low doses to male rats. Jpn. J. Cancer Res. 80(8):732-6.

Tardif, R., S. Lapare, G. Charest-Tardif, J. Brodeur, and K. Krishnan. 1993. Physiologically-based modeling of the toxicokinetic interaction between toluene and m-xylene in the rat. Toxicol. Appl. Pharmacol. 120:266-273.

Tardif, R., S. Lapare, G. Charest-Tardif, J. Brodeur, and K. Krishnan. 1995. Physiologically-based modeling of a mixture of toluene and xylene. Risk Anal. 15:335-342.

Tardif, R., G. Charest-Tardif, J. Brodeur, and K. Krishnan. 1997. Physiologically-based pharmacokinetic modeling of a ternary mixture of alkyl benzenes in rats and humans. Toxicol. Appl. Pharmacol. 144:120-134.

Teeguarden, J.G., Y. Dragan, and H.C. Pitot. 1998. Implications of hormesis on the bioassay and hazard assessment of chemical carcinogens. BELLE Newsletter 6:8-13.

Thakore, K.N., M.L. Gargas, M.E. Andersen, and H.M. Mehendale. 1991. PBPK derived metabolic constants, hepatotoxicity, and lethality of bromodichloromethane in rats pretreated with chlordecone, phenobarbital or Mirex. Toxicol. Appl. Pharmacol. 109:514-528.

Verhaar, H.J.M., J.S. Morroni, K.F. Reardon, S.M. Hays, D.P. Gaver, R.L. Carpenter, and R.S.H. Yang. 1997. A proposed approach to study the toxicology of complex mixtures of petroleum products: The integrated use of QSAR, lumping analysis, and PBPK/PD modeling. Environ. Health Perspect. 105 (Suppl. 1): 179-195.

Weber, W.W. 1995. Influence of heredity on human sensitivity to environmental chemicals. Environ. Mol. Mutagen. 25(Suppl. 26):102-114.

Wei, J., and J.C.W. Kuo. 1969. A lumping analysis in monomolecular reaction systems: analysis of the exactly lumpable system. Ind. Eng. Chem. Fundam. 8:114-123.

West, W.L., E.M. Knight, S. Pradhan, and T.S. Hinds. 1997. Interpatient variability: genetic predisposition and other genetic factors. J. Clin. Pharmacol. 37:635-648.

Yang, R.S.H. 1994. Toxicology of Chemical Mixtures: Case Studies, Mechanisms, and Novel Approaches. San Diego, CA: Academic Press. 720 pp.

Yang, R.S.H. 1996. Some current approaches for studying combination toxicology in chemical mixtures. Food Chem. Toxicol. 34:1037-1044.

Yang, R.S.H. 1997. Toxicologic interactions of chemical mixtures. Pp.189-203. In: Comprehensive Toxicology. Vol. 1, General Principles, Toxicokinetics, and Mechanisms of Toxicity, J. Bond, ed. Oxford, England: Elsevier Science Ltd.

Yang, R.S.H., R.S. Thomas, D.L. Gustafson, J.A. Campain, S.A. Benjamin, H.J.M. Verhaar, and M.M. Mumtaz. 1998. Approaches to developing alternative and predictive toxicology based on PBPK/PD and QSAR modeling. Environ. Health Perspect. 106 (Suppl. 6):1385-1393.

Yang, R.S.H., L. Feng, and S.A. Benjamin. 1999. Further refinement of a physiologically based pharmacokinetic/pharmacodynamic model for the toxicologic interaction between Kepone and carbon tetrachloride. [Abstract]. The Toxicologist 48:281.

Zbinden, G. 1976. Progress in Toxicology: Special Topics, Vol. 2. Berlin: Springer.

Appendix

Biographical Information on Commissioned Authors

Morton Lippmann is the director of the Human Exposure and Health Effects Program and the EPA Center for Particulate Matter Health Effects Research at the New York University School of Medicine. He received an S.M. in industrial hygiene from Harvard University and a Ph.D. in environmental health science from New York University. Before receiving his Ph.D. and joining the faculty at New York University, Dr. Lippmann worked as an industrial hygienist for the U.S. Atomic Energy Commission and the U.S. Public Health Service. He has served on several NRC committees, most recently as chair of the Committee on Toxicology's Subcommittee on Manufactured Vitreous Fibers.

Edward Martin is the president of Edward Martin and Associates, Inc., a consulting firm to the health-care industry and to major health-care information management and technology companies. He is the former acting assistant secretary of defense (health affairs) and the former principal deputy assistant secretary of defense (health affairs). Dr. Martin served 23 years in the U.S. Public Health Service (PHS), retiring at the rank of rear admiral. During his tenure with PHS, he served in a number of leadership capacities, including chief of staff for Surgeon General C. Everett Koop. Dr. Martin received his M.D. from the University of Kansas Medical School.

Joseph V. Rodricks is a principal at Life Sciences Consultancy as well as an adjunct professor at The Johns Hopkins University School of Public Health. He received his M.S. in organic chemistry and his Ph.D. in biochemistry from the University of Maryland. His work focuses on risk analysis and toxicology. Dr. Rodricks is the author of *Calculated Risks*, a widely used introduction to toxicology and risk analysis. He has served on several committees of the NRC, most recently on the Committee on Remediation of PCB-Contaminated Sediments.

Joan B. Rose is a professor in the marine science department at the University of South Florida. She received an M.S. in microbiology from the University of Wyoming and a Ph.D. in microbiology from the University of Arizona. Her research interests include methods for detection of pathogens in wastewater and the environment; water treatment for removal of pathogens; wastewater reuse; and occurrence of viruses and parasites in wastewater sludge. Dr. Rose serves on the NRC's Water Science and

Technology Board and on several NRC committees, including the Committee on Climate, Ecosystems, Infectious Diseases, and Health.

Karl Rozman is a professor in the Department of Pharmacology, Toxicology and Therapeutics at the University of Kansas Medical Center. He received a Ph.D. in organic and pharmaceutical chemistry from Leopold Franzen's University in Innsbruck, Austria. He is a board-certified toxicologist and advisor of governmental risk assessment groups at the national and international level. His research is primarily directed toward understanding the toxicokinetics and mechanisms of action underlying the toxicity of chlorinated aromatic hydrocarbons, particularly dioxins.

Raymond S. H. Yang is the director of the Center for Environmental Toxicology and Technology at Colorado State University and holds an appointment at the university as professor of toxicology. Since 1992, he has been the program director and principal investigator for the Project on Integrated Research on Hazardous Waste Chemical Mixtures, which is part of the National Institute of Environmental Heath Sciences (NIEHS) Superfund Basic Research Program. He is also program director for an NIEHS toxicology training grant on quantitative toxicology. Dr. Yang received an M.S. in toxicology and entomology and a Ph.D. in toxicology from North Carolina State University. His research interests include the toxicology of mixtures, pharmacokinetic and pharmcodynamic modeling, and risk assessment.